D0950237

**Pocket
Companion for

Medical-
Surgical
Nursing**

Pocket Companion for

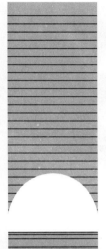

Medical-Surgical Nursing

DONNA D. IGNATAVICIUS, MS, RNC
ROXANNE AUBOL BATTERDEN, MS, RN, CCRN
KATHY A. HAUSMAN, MS, RN, CNRN

W.B. SAUNDERS COMPANY

Harcourt Brace Jovanovich, Inc.
Philadelphia, London, Toronto, Montreal, Sydney, Tokyo

W. B. SAUNDERS COMPANY
Harcourt Brace Jovanovich, Inc.

The Curtis Center
Independence Square West
Philadelphia, PA 19106

Library of Congress Cataloging-in-Publication Data

Ignatavicius, Donna D.
    Pocket companion for Medical-surgical nursing / Donna D. Ignatavicius,
    Roxanne Aubol Batterden, Kathy A. Hausman.
        p. cm.
    Companion v. to: Medical-surgical nursing / Donna D. Ignatavicius,
    Marilyn Varner Bayne. 1991.
        Includes index.
        ISBN 0-7216-3507-5
    1. Nursing—Handbooks, manuals, etc. 2. Surgical nursing—Handbooks,
manuals, etc. I. Ignatavicius, Donna D. Medical-surgical nursing.
II. Batterden, Roxanne Aubol. III. Hausman, Kathy A. IV. Title.
    [DNLM: 1. Nursing Process—handbooks. 2. Surgical Nursing—
handbooks. WY 39 I24p]
RT41.I36 1992, Suppl.
610.73—dc20
DNLM/DLC   91-31745

Editor: Michael Brown
Developmental Editor: Lee Henderson

Pocket Companion for
Medical-Surgical Nursing   ISBN 0-7216-4595-x

Last digit is the print
number: 9   8   7   6   5   4   3   2

ACKNOWLEDGMENTS

Thanks to Editor-in-Chief Michael J. Brown and Senior Developmental Editor Lee Henderson for their guidance in the development of *Pocket Companion for Medical-Surgical Nursing.* Special thanks to EDP Team Manager Lorraine B. Kilmer and Production Manager Frank Polizzano at W. B. Saunders Company, and to Geraldine McGowan at Editorial Services of New England, for making the impossible happen.

PREFACE

The *Pocket Companion for Medical-Surgical Nursing* covers 326 common diseases, disorders, and other subjects that you are likely to encounter in clinical practice. It was written to help meet the needs of the busy nursing student and the practicing nurse. It was designed for use as both an independent pocket reference tool and as an adjunct to *Medical-Surgical Nursing: A Nursing Process Approach.*

Knowing the fast pace of nursing practice, we made the *Pocket Companion* as easy to use as possible by

- Listing all diseases, disorders, and other topics alphabetically, by their most common names
- Providing alphabetic page tabs
- Formatting diseases and disorders consistently throughout
- Providing a comprehensive, practical index
- Including only the essential, need-to-know information and presenting it in a succinct, concise format

Like Ignatavicius and Bayne's *Medical-Surgical Nursing: A Nursing Process Approach*, the *Pocket Companion* incorporates the nursing process for the most common health problems. Assessment, high-priority Nursing Diagnoses, and step-by-step Interventions are included for each of these diseases and disorders. Discharge Planning sections outline the essential components to include when preparing a client for discharge from the hospital.

At the end of the coverage of each disease, disorder, or other topic, you will find space to tailor your *Pocket Companion* to your clinical practice by jotting down additional information pertinent to your clinical setting.

For those times when you need in-depth coverage of a particular topic, each entry concludes with a cross reference to detailed coverage in *Medical-Surgical Nursing: A Nursing Process Approach.*

All nursing diagnoses included in the *Pocket Companion* are those approved by the North American Nursing Diagnosis Association (NANDA) as of 1990.

As a further aid, a complete, alphabetized list of NANDA diagnoses is printed on the inside covers of the book.

The *Pocket Companion* concludes with four appendices: Nursing Interventions for Physiologic Changes Related to Aging; Guidelines for Common Client Problems; Isolation Precautions; and Quick Reference to High-Flow Oxygen Delivery Systems.

We hope that the *Pocket Companion for Medical-Surgical Nursing* will become a valued, trusted, practical aid to your clinical practice.

DONNA D. IGNATAVICIUS, MS, RNC
ROXANNE AUBOL BATTERDEN, MS, RN, CCRN
KATHY A. HAUSMAN, MS, RN, CNRN

CONTENTS

Abdominal Trauma

OVERVIEW

- Abdominal injuries account for 25% of deaths due to trauma.
- Two broad categories are
  1. Blunt trauma, 50% resulting from automobile accidents and the balance caused by assaults and falls, commonly affecting multiple abdominal organs
  2. Penetrating trauma, most often caused by gunshot wounds and stab wounds; the liver and small bowel are most commonly involved in stab wounds, and the small bowel in gunshot wounds.
- The major cause of death is hemorrhage.

COLLABORATIVE MANAGEMENT

- Immediate exploratory laparotomy and repair of abdominal injuries are performed if the client has signs of peritoneal irritation, such as rebound tenderness, or active bleeding.
- Superficial wounds are explored and cleaned under local anesthesia.
- The nurse assesses for abdominal trauma by
  1. Asking the client about the presence, location, and quality of pain
  2. Inspecting the abdomen for contusions, abrasions, lacerations, ecchymosis, penetrating injuries, and symmetry
  3. Auscultating the abdomen for absent or diminished bowel sounds and bruits
  4. Percussing for abnormal sounds such as resonance over the liver or dullness over the stomach or intestines
  5. Lightly palpating the abdomen to identify areas of tenderness, guarding, rigidity, and spasm
- Prior to surgery, the nurse
  1. Places large-bore intravenous catheters, as ordered
  2. Infuses intravenous fluids at a rapid rate, as ordered
  3. Obtains blood samples for analysis
  4. Inserts an indwelling Foley catheter
  5. Inserts a nasogastric tube to prevent vomiting
- The client who does not have overt signs of bleeding is admitted to the hospital for observation.

- The nurse assesses for and immediately reports
    1. Abdominal or referred pain
    2. Nausea
    3. Mental status changes
    4. Vital signs
    5. Vomiting
    6. Abdominal guarding
    7. Abdominal rigidity
    8. Rebound tenderness
    9. Skin temperature changes
    10. Absent bowel sounds
    11. Decreased urinary output
- Prior to discharge, the nurse teaches the client
    1. The signs and symptoms of bleeding
    2. To watch for and report to the physician
        a. Abdominal pain
        b. Nausea and vomiting
        c. Bloody or black stools
        d. Fever
        e. Weakness or dizziness
    3. Wound care, following surgery

For more information on abdominal trauma, see
*Medical-Surgical Nursing: A Nursing Process
Approach*, **pp. 1400–1401.**

Achalasia

OVERVIEW

- Achalasia is a progressively worsening dysphagia evidenced by chronic and vague complaints of difficult swallowing and of food sticking in the throat.
- The exact cause is unknown, but the accepted theory is a lack of peristalsis related to neuromuscular factors

and inadequate relaxation of the lower esophageal sphincter (LES).

COLLABORATIVE MANAGEMENT

Assessment
- The nurse records the client's
  1. Symptoms, including dysphagia, pain, or regurgitation
  2. Factors that aggravate the symptoms, such as position or diet
  3. Home treatments that relieve the symptoms, including over-the-counter drugs
  4. History of previous esophageal trauma or surgery
  5. Nutritional history, including diet habits, food intolerance, nutritional status, and weight loss

Planning and Implementation
NDx: POTENTIAL FOR ALTERED NUTRITION: LESS THAN BODY REQUIREMENTS

Nonsurgical Management
- The nurse
  1. Administers anticholinergic drugs, nitrates, gastrointestinal hormones, and calcium channel blockers to lower the esophageal pressure and relax the lower esophageal sphincter
  2. Teaches the client to avoid foods or habits that aggravate symptoms
  3. Encourages the client to experiment with diet changes, including semisoft foods and warm foods and liquids that may be better tolerated
  4. Teaches the client to eat several small meals per day instead of three large meals
  5. Instructs the client to sleep with the head of the bed elevated on blocks 6 to 10 inches or by reclining in a semisitting position

Surgical Management
- Surgery may be necessary and is aimed at facilitating food passage by dilating the unrelaxed esophageal sphincter or enlarging the sphincter by myotomy.
- For long-term refractory achalasia, *excision* of the affected portion of the esophagus may be attempted with or without replacement by a segment of colon or jejunum.
- *Sphincter dilation* for achalasia is performed under local anesthesia with a pneumatized dilator (a pressurized bag filled with water).
- A *myotomy* is performed to enlarge the sphincter

and requires a thoracotomy approach to expose the esophagus; muscle fibers are cut to open the esophagus to provide less obstruction for food passage.

• Nursing care for the client undergoing myotomy is similar to that described in Lung Cancer.

• The nurse informs the client undergoing dilation that he or she will be awake during the procedure but that a local anesthetic, such as benzocaine (Cetacaine), is sprayed on the oropharynx.

• Following dilation, the nurse
   1. Assesses for hemoptysis
   2. Teaches the client to expectorate rather than swallow secretions that accumulate in the oral cavity
   3. Evaluates secretions for bleeding
   4. Observes the client for symptoms of esophageal perforation
      a. Elevated temperature
      b. Chest or shoulder pain
      c. Subcutaneous emphysema in the chest and neck
      d. Changes in level of discomfort

Discharge Planning

• The nurse instructs the client about medications, diet, and proper positioning.

• Postmyotomy or postdilation instructions include notifying the physician for clinical manifestations of infection, hemorrhage, esophageal perforation, or respiratory complications due to reflux or aspiration.

For more information on achalasia, see *Medical-Surgical Nursing: A Nursing Process Approach*, **pp. 1285–1288.**

Acquired Immunodeficiency Syndrome

OVERVIEW

• Acquired immunodeficiency syndrome (AIDS) is an infection with the human immunodeficiency virus (HIV).

• HIV is transmitted via sexual contact, blood or blood products, use of contaminated needles, and from mother to newborn child.

• The Centers for Disease Control classification of HIV contains four categories:
  1. Acute infection
  2. Asymptomatic infection
  3. Persistent generalized lymphadenopathy, thrombocytopenia
  4. Other disease
     a. Constitutional symptoms such as persistent weight loss, fever, night sweats, diarrhea, fatigue, and the presence of some immune abnormalities by laboratory test
     b. Neurologic disease
     c. Secondary infectious diseases
     d. Secondary cancers
     e. Other conditions

COLLABORATIVE MANAGEMENT

Assessment

• The nurse records the client's
  1. History of when symptoms started, severity of symptoms, associated problems, and interventions to date
  2. Past medical history
  3. Sexual practices and history of sexually transmitted diseases
  4. Level of knowledge regarding the diagnosis, symptom management, diagnostic tests, treatment, community resources, and modes of transmission of the virus
  5. Familiarity with and use of safe sexual practices
  6. Knowledge of the risks associated with reproduction

- The nurse assesses for
  1. Shortness of breath, cough
  2. Fever
  3. Night sweats
  4. Fatigue
  5. Weight loss
  6. Lymphadenopathy
  7. Diarrhea
  8. Visual changes
  9. Headache
  10. Memory loss
  11. Confusion
  12. Seizures
  13. Personality changes
  14. Dry skin
  15. Rashes
  16. Skin lesions such as Kaposi's sarcoma (KS), herpes
  17. Pain and discomfort
  18. Changes in ability to perform activities of daily living (ADL)
  19. Availability of a support system, such as family and significant others
  20. Current employment status and occupation
  21. Social activities and hobbies
  22. Self-esteem and body image changes
  23. Suicidal ideation, depression
  24. Involvement with community resources or support groups

Planning and Implementation

NDx: INEFFECTIVE BREATHING PATTERN

- The nurse
  1. Assesses respiratory status frequently
  2. Monitors arterial blood gases, as ordered
  3. Provides oxygen and room humidification, as ordered
  4. Performs chest physiotherapy
  5. Encourages fluids as tolerated
  6. Elevates the head of the bed to facilitate breathing
  7. Helps the client pace activities to minimize shortness of breath
  8. Administers antipyretics to reduce fever
  9. Assists with ADL as needed

NDx: ALTERED NUTRITION: LESS THAN BODY REQUIREMENTS

- The nurse
  1. Monitors intake and output
  2. Obtains a calorie count
  3. Weighs the client daily

4. Provides meals or snacks with high caloric and nutritional value; offers high-calorie supplements (in consultation with a dietitian)
5. Helps the client select foods that are appealing and available
6. Gives enteral or parenteral feedings, as ordered, if needed
7. Provides a soft or bland diet
8. Provides meticulous mouth care
9. Administers supplemental vitamins, as ordered
10. Administers metronidazole (Flagyl), as ordered, for clients with giardiasis
11. Administers phenoxylate hydrochloride (Lomotil) to control diarrhea and a diet that includes less roughage and less fatty, spicy, or sweet food and no alcohol and caffeine

NDx: ALTERED THOUGHT PROCESSES

- The nurse
  1. Establishes baseline neurologic and mental status
  2. Observes for and reports changes in behavior that may be related to the loss and psychological stress experienced by the client
  3. Assists with ADL, as needed
  4. Reorients the client to the environment; uses calendars, clocks, and radios; puts the bed near the window if possible
  5. Paces the client's activities; gives simple directions and uses short and uncomplicated sentences
  6. Teaches the family and significant other techniques to use to help orient the client
  7. Administers anticonvulsants as ordered, for seizures

NDx: IMPAIRED SKIN INTEGRITY

- The nurse
  1. Monitors for progression of lesions
  2. Avoids pressure (uses egg crate, air, or water mattress)
  3. Uses careful hygienic measures
  4. Provides meticulous skin care
  5. Gives analgesics, as ordered, if needed
- KS is the most common skin lesion.
- Rapidly progressive KS is treated with chemotherapy.
- Radiation therapy is transiently effective.
- Interferon-alpha is quite effective, especially in clients with better immune function.
- Changes in appearance can be minimized by the use of make-up, long-sleeved shirts, and hats.

- Herpes simplex virus abscess is also a commonly seen skin lesion in clients with HIV
- The nurse
  1. Cleans the abscess with a diluted solution of povidone-iodine and leaves it open to the air or uses a heat lamp to help it dry
  2. Applies Domeboro soaks as ordered, which may promote healing
  3. Administers drug therapy with acyclovir (Zovirax), as ordered, which is potentially toxic to the kidney; thus, the client must maintain adequate hydration
  4. Implements wound and skin precautions

NDx: POTENTIAL FOR IINFECTION

- Clients with HIV are at high risk for *opportunistic* infections.
- Drug therapy includes azidothymidine or zidovudine (Retrovir). Side effects include macrocytic anemia, mild headache, nausea, and changes in white blood cell count or liver function tests.
- Opportunistic infections include
  1. Protozoal infection of the lungs
     a. *Pneumocystis carinii* pneumonia is manifested by tightness in the chest, shortness of breath, crackles (rales) in the lungs, persistent dry cough, low-grade or high-grade fever.
     b. *P. carinii* pneumonia is treated with trimethoprim-sulfamethoxazole (Bactrim) or pentamidine isothionate.
  2. Protozoal infections of the nervous system
     a. Protozoal neurologic infections are manifested by fever, headache, blurred vision, nausea and vomiting, stiff neck, mild confusion, mental status changes, seizures, personality and behavioral changes, and focal neurologic deficits
     b. *Toxoplasma gondii* encephalitis is treated with pyrimethamine (Daraprim) with sulfadiazine (Microsulfon).
  3. Protozoal infections of the gastrointestinal tract, including *Cryptosporidium*, a parasite that causes gastroenteritis with diarrhea and abdominal discomfort that can lead to wasting and electrolyte imbalance
  4. Fungal infections
     a. *Candida stomatitis* is manifested by food tasting "funny," mouth pain, difficulty swallowing, cottage-cheese-like exudate, and

inflammation on the mouth and back of the throat.

b. *C. esophagitis* is manifested by difficulty swallowing; clients are given ketaconazole (Nizorail) orally or amphotericin B intravenously.

c. *C. neoformans* or *Cryptococcus* meningitis is treated with amphotericin B and sometimes with flucytosine.

5. Bacterial infections, which are atypical

a. *Myobacterium avium-intracellulare* is treated experimentally with ansamysin, clofazimine, and amikacin.

b. *M. tuberculosis* is treated with isoniazid, rifampin, and ethambutol.

6. Viral infections, which play a significant role in the morbidity and mortality associated with AIDS

a. Herpes simplex is treated with acyclovir.

b. Cytomegalovirus is treated with ganciclovir.

7. Wasting syndrome (no clear-cut infectious etiology or obvious mechanical problems), which is manifested by weight loss, dry, itchy, irritated skin and diffuse rashes, eczema or psoriasis; petechiae, blood in urine or stool, or bleeding gums

NDx: SELF ESTEEM DISTURBANCE

• Self-esteem is affected by changes in appearance, in relationships with others, in day-to-day activity and in job performance and possibly by guilt about life-style.

• The nurse

1. Provides a climate of acceptance
2. Allows for privacy
3. Offers a safe environment
4. Encourages self-care, independence, control, and decision making
5. Helps formulate short-term goals that are attainable
6. Is honest with his or her feelings

NDx: ANTICIPATORY GRIEVING

• The nurse

1. Encourages the client and significant others to talk openly and honestly about their feelings
2. Refers to appropriate community and social resources for help with future planning (will, disability, hospice care, durable power of attorney)

- The nurse
  1. Explains the rationale for universal precautions to the client and visitors
  2. Visits the client frequently and provides for diversional activities
  3. Encourages the client to verbalize feelings about self, coping skills, and sense of ability to control the situation

Discharge Planning

- The nurse
  1. Identifies the actual and potential need for care, such as a visiting nurse, Meals on Wheels, a home health aide, and 24-hour supervision
  2. Identifies and corrects any hazards in the home prior to discharge
  3. Refers the client to support group(s)
- The nurse teaches the client/family
  1. The mode of transmission of HIV infection
  2. The need to notify sexual contacts
  3. Signs and symptoms of infections
  4. The importance of follow-up visits with the physician(s)

For more information on acquired immunodeficiency syndrome, see *Medical-Surgical Nursing: A Nursing Process Approach,* **pp. 632–645.**

Adrenal Hypofunction

OVERVIEW

- A decreased production of adrenocortical steroids (adrenal hypofunction) may occur secondary to inadequate secretion of adrenocorticotropic hormone (ACTH), dysfunction of the hypothalamic-pituitary control mechanism, or complete or partial destruction of the adrenal glands.

- Primary hypofunction, also referred to as *Addison's disease*, is due to chronic destructive disease, resulting in the loss of the major adrenal hormones cortisol and aldosterone.

- Secondary hypofunction is the result of failure in the hypothalamic or pituitary portion of the adrenal axis, which causes decreased cortisol and adrenal androgen production.

COLLABORATIVE MANAGEMENT

Assessment

- The nurse records the client's
  1. Description of symptoms
  2. Activity level
  3. Salt intake (salt craving)
  4. Past medical history
     a. Radiation to the head or abdomen
     b. Tuberculosis
     c. Intracranial surgery
     d. Medications such as steroids, anticoagulants, or cytotoxic drugs
- The nurse assesses for
  1. Gastrointestinal problems
     a. Anorexia
     b. Nausea, vomiting, diarrhea
     c. Abdominal pain
     d. Weight loss
  2. Increased or decreased skin pigmentation
  3. Hyperpigmentation of the mucous membranes, surgical scars, areolae, skin folds, and area over knuckles on the hand (not seen in secondary disease)
  4. Decreased body hair
  5. Hypoglycemia (cortisol hypersecretion)
     a. Sweating
     b. Headache
     c. Tachycardia
     d. Tremors
  6. Volume depletion (cortisol and aldosterone deficiencies)
     a. Postural hypotension
     b. Dehydration
  7. Emotional lability, forgetfulness

Planning and Implementation .

NDx: Fluid Volume Deficit

- The nurse
    1. Carefully measures intake and output
    2. Records the client's weight every day
    3. Takes vital signs frequently to detect postural hypotension and dysrhythmias
    4. Administers cortisone and hydrocortisone, as ordered to correct glucocorticoid deficiency
    5. Administers supplemental mineralocorticoids, such as fludrocortisone (Florinef), as ordered, to maintain electrolyte balance

NDx: Altered Tissue Perfusion

- The nurse
    1. Monitors vital signs frequently to detect hypotension and tachycardia
    2. Monitors and reports signs of adrenal crisis that may be caused by physical and emotional stress (manifested by hypotension, cold, pale skin, and decreased urinary output)

Discharge Planning

- The nurse teaches the client that
    1. Medications should be taken with meals or snacks
    2. Weight must be taken daily
    3. The physician is consulted regarding increasing dosage during increased stress
    4. A Medic Alert bracelet or necklace must be worn at all times
- Clients on a supplementary mineralocorticoid need a dietary consultation to help them select foods that are acceptable within sodium restrictions. The nurse and the dietitian stress the importance of constant sodium intake.

For more information on adrenal hypofunction, see *Medical-Surgical Nursing: A Nursing Process Approach,* **pp. 1544–1549.**

Adult Respiratory Distress Syndrome

- Adult respiratory distress syndrome (ARDS) is a form of acute respiratory failure characterized by dyspnea, hypoxemia, decreased pulmonary compliance, and the presence of pulmonary infiltrates.
- ARDS is caused by a diffuse lung injury, leading to extravascular lung fluid.
- The major site of injury is the alveolar capillary membrane.
- Multiple types of injury affect alveoli, which can no longer participate in gas exchange.
- Interstitial edema causes compression and obliteration of terminal airways, thereby reducing lung volume and lung compliance.
- Etiologies include serious nervous system injury, trauma, shock, cerebrovascular accident, tumors, sudden increases in cerebrospinal fluid pressure, sepsis, near drowning, burns, disseminated intravascular coagulation, multiple blood transfusions, hemolytic disorders, drug ingestion, and direct injury to the lung, such as by aspiration of gastric contents, radiation, near drowning, infections, and inhalation of toxic gases.
- Clients have a rapidly deteriorating respiratory status with increased work of breathing and deteriorating blood gas levels; hypoxemia persists despite high concentrations of oxygen.
- ARDS usually requires endotracheal intubation and mechanical ventilation with positive end-expiratory pressure (PEEP).

For more information on adult respiratory distress syndrome (ARDS), see *Medical-Surgical Nursing: A Nursing Process Approach*, **pp. 2057–2058.**

Allergy, Atopic

OVERVIEW

• Atopic allergic manifestations occur in persons who are genetically predisposed respond to a variety of environmental allergens by forming immunoglobulin E.

• Atopic allergy includes allergic asthma, allergic rhinitis (hay fever, seasonal allergies, perennial allergic rhinitis [e.g., to dust or molds]), urticaria, and eczematous dermatitis.

COLLABORATIVE MANAGEMENT

Assessment

• The nurse records the client's
   1. Symptoms
      a. Relationship to the environment (for example, only at work or only in a particular room of the house)
      b. Situational or seasonal variations
      c. Aggravating and relieving factors
      d. When they occur
      e. When and under what situation they first occurred
   2. History of hyposensitization therapy
   3. Known allergies
   4. Results of any prior skin testing
   5. Current medications
• The nurse assesses for
   1. Sneezing
   2. Rhinorrhea
   3. Nasal puritis
   4. Congestion
   5. Red, edematous, and pruritic eyes
   6. Increased lacrimation
   7. Sore throat
   8. Frontal headaches
   9. Increased fatigue
   10. Anorexia
   11. Depression
   12. Coughing
   13. Dyspnea
   14. Increased sputum production
   15. Urticaria

e nurse administers one or more of the following
s, as ordered

1. Chlorpheniramine maleate (Chlor-trimeton), 4 to
   8 mg, every 4 to 6 hours
2. Diphenhydramine hydrochloride (Benedryl), 25
   to 50 mg, every 4 to 6 hours
3. Terfenadine (Seldane), 60 mg every 12 hours
4. Phenylpropanolamine (Propagest), phenylephrine
   (Neo-Synephrine), or pseudoephedrine (Sudafed)

nasal decongestants are not recommended
use there is often a rebound effect

• Hyposensitiza... not relieved by antihistamines,
...adron) nasal spray is often used.
or immunotherapy, may be ... ferred to as desensitization
essary.

• The nurse
1. Administers gradually increasing subcutaneous
   doses of the allergen, which may lead to tolerance
2. Observes the client for 30 minutes after each
   injection for a possible systemic reaction
3. Is prepared for an anaphylactic reaction (has
   epinephrine and emergency equipment on hand)

Discharge Planning
• The nurse teaches the client/family about the need
for environmental control (especially for the client with
perennial allergic rhinitis)

1. Use nonallergenic materials for bedding
   (mattresses, pillows, blankets).
2. Enclose the mattress and box spring in airtight
   plastic covers.
3. Replace carpets with washable throw rugs and
   draperies with light, washable curtains.
4. Use pull shades rather than venetian blinds.
5. Launder bed linen frequently.
6. Have a heating and cooling system that both
   humidifies and filters the air.
7. Avoid smoking and smoke-filled areas.
8. Keep windows at home, in the car, and at the
   office closed; use an air-conditioner if possible.
9. Minimize early-morning activity (emission of
   pollen is greatest from 5 to 10 A.M.).
10. Stay indoors on windy days and days when
    humidity and pollen count are very high.
11. Take vacations in pollen-free places.

12. Do not mow the lawn, rake leaves, or wo the garden.
13. Do not keep many indoor plants if sensiti molds.
- The nurse
  1. Provides drug information as needed
  2. Teaches stress and anxiety-reduction technique to minimize symptoms
  3. Emphasizes the importance of follow-up visits with the physician(s)

For more information on atopic allergy, see *Medical-Surgical Nursing: A Nursing Process Approach,* **pp. 658–663.**

Alzheimer's Disease

OVERVIEW

- Alzheimer's disease is a chronic, progressive, degenerating disease that accounts for almost half of the dementias occurring in persons older than 65 years of age.

COLLABORATIVE MANAGEMENT

Assessment

- The nurse records the client's
  1. Age
  2. Current employment status and work history
  3. Ability to fulfill household responsibilities: grocery shopping, laundry, and meal planning
  4. Driving ability
  5. Ability to handle routine financial transactions
  6. Communication skills

7. Behavior
8. Family history of Alzheimer's disease
9. Past medical history, with particular attention to head trauma, viral illness, or exposure to metal or toxic waste

- The nurse assesses for
  1. Indicators of the stages of the disease
     a. Stage I: forgetfulness, mild memory loss, decreased interest in personal affairs, subtle changes in personality and behavior
     b. Stage II: confusion; obvious memory loss, especially short-term memory; hesitant speech; ritualistic, repetitive behavior
     c. Stage III: dementia; wandering, becomes lost; increasing motor deficits; incontinence; aphasia
     d. Stage IV: severe physical deterioration; total dependence for activities of daily living (ADL); does not recognize family or significant others
  2. Cognitive changes, such as deficits in attention, concentration, judgment, and perception
  3. Alterations in communication abilities, such as apraxia, dysarthria, and agnosia
  4. Indications of tremors, myoclonus, and seizure activity
  5. Reaction to changes in routine and environment
  6. Impaired social interaction, disinterest in hobbies, loss of interest in current events

Planning and Implementation
NDx: ALTERED THOUGHT PROCESSES

- The nurse
  1. Provides a structured, consistent environment
  2. Establishes a daily routine; explains changes in routine before they occur and again immediately before they take place
  3. Places familiar objects, clocks, and single-date calendars in easy view of the client
  4. Reorients the client to the environment frequently
  5. Assists the client to maintain independence in ADL as long as possible; places complete clothing outfits on a single hanger (if able to dress)
  6. Allows the client to participate in meal planning, grocery shopping, and other household routines as able
  7. Suggests adaptive devices for the home, such as grab bars in the bathroom

17

8. Develops an individualized bowel and bladder program
9. Attracts the client's attention before conversing
10. Keeps the environment free of distractions
11. Speaks slowly and distinctly in short, clear sentences
12. Allows sufficient time for the client to respond
13. Administers ergoloid mesylates (Hydergine, Niloric), as ordered; used in early stages to improve cognition; other agents have not proved effective
14. Administers amitriptyline (Elavil), doxepin (Sinequan), or imipramine (Tofranil) to treat depression, as ordered

NDx: POTENTIAL FOR INJURY

- The nurse
  1. Ensures that the client always wears an identification bracelet
  2. Ensures that alarms or other distractions for outside doors are working properly at all times
  3. Checks the client frequently
  4. Takes the client for walks several times per day and encourages the client to participate in activities to decrease his or her restlessness
  5. Restrains the client with a lap belt or chest restraint *only* if absolutely necessary
  6. Implements seizure precautions if there is a history of seizures
  7. Administers phenytoin (Dilantin) to treat seizures, as ordered
  8. Administers hypnotic or neuroleptic agents (Benadryl, Halcion, Haldol, Mellaril), as ordered, to treat agitation, assaultiveness, or hyperactivity
  9. Observes for side effects of neuroleptic agents, including increased confusion and extrapyramidal symptoms

NDx: INEFFECTIVE FAMILY COPING: COMPROMISED; ALTERED FAMILY PROCESS

- The nurse
  1. Advises the family to seek legal counsel regarding the client's competency and the need to obtain guardianship or durable power of attorney
  2. Refers the family to a local support group
  3. Encourages the family to maintain its own social network and to obtain respite care periodically
  4. Assists the family to identify and develop strategies to cope with the long-term consequences of the disease

NDx: SLEEP PATTERN DISTURBANCE

- The nurse
  1. Establishes prebedtime ritual
     a. Personal hygiene
     b. Quiet environment
     c. Back rub or small snack
  2. Keeps the client active during the day with a balance between active and passive activities; discourages the client from taking a nap, if possible
  3. Administers chloral hydrate, as ordered, for sleep

Discharge Planning

- The nurse
  1. Identifies and suggests corrections of hazards in the home prior to discharge
  2. Ensures that the client can correctly use all assistive-adaptive devices ordered for home use
  3. Ensures that assistive-adaptive devices are installed in the home before discharge
- The nurse teaches the client/family
  1. How to assist the client with ADL
  2. How to use assistive-adaptive equipment
  3. How to select and prepare food that the client is able to chew and swallow, with dietary consultation
  4. How to prevent wandering
  5. What to do in the event of seizure
  6. How to prevent the client from injury
  7. Drug information, if prescribed
  8. How to implement the prescribed exercise program
  9. The importance of follow-up visits with the physician and other therapists

For more information on Alzheimer's disease, see *Medical-Surgical Nursing: A Nursing Process Approach,* **pp. 915–921.**

Amenorrhea

OVERVIEW

- *Amenorrhea* is the absence of menstrual periods.
- *Primary amenorrhea*, menstruation that has failed to occur by age 16, is asssociated with anomalies of the reproductive tract; hypothalamic and pituitary disorders, such as delayed puberty; systemic diseases such as thyroid and adrenal dysfunction, diabetes, and malnutrition; ovarian disease; and malformations of the reproductive tract.
- *Secondary amenorrhea*, menstruation that has started but has stopped and has not recurred for 3 months, is associated with functional disorders such as pregnancy; menopause; lactation; cervical stenosis; Asherman's syndrome; polycystic ovary disease; pituitary tumor or insufficiency; psychogenic stress; excessive physical activities; medications such as antihypertensives, birth control pills, and phenothiazines; nutritional conditions such as obesity, anorexia nervosa, and sudden weight loss; and ovarian disease, failure, or destruction.

COLLABORATIVE MANAGEMENT

- Assessment includes
  1. Family history of menstruation
  2. Family history of genetic abnormalities
  3. Ambiguous genitalia at birth
  4. Development of secondary sex characteristics
  5. Nutritional habits
  6. Past surgery
  7. Emotional stress
  8. Physical characteristics of primary amenorrhea
     a. Anomalies of the genital tract, including external genitalia
     b. Short stature
     c. Lack of breast development
     d. Lack of pubic and axillary hair
  9. Factors involved in secondary amenorrhea
     a. Menstrual history
     b. Obstetric history
     c. History of sexual activity
     d. Symptoms of pregnancy
     e. Current and past eating habits and dieting
     f. Physical activity
     g. Hormonal deficiencies

    h. Drug history
    i. Galactorrhea
    j. Hirsutism
- Management is directed at correcting the underlying cause

1. Hormone replacement
2. Corrective surgery
3. Stimulation of ovulation
4. Periodic progesterone withdrawal
5. Counseling and emotional support

For more information on amenorrhea, see *Medical-Surgical Nursing: A Nursing Process Approach*, **pp. 1692–1693.**

Amputation

OVERVIEW

- Amputation is a removal of a part of the body.
- The psychological ramifications of the procedure are often more devastating than the physical impairment that results.
- *Traumatic* amputation occurs when a body part is severed unexpectedly, e.g., by a saw; attempts to replant it may be made.
- Methods of *surgical* amputation include
  1. *Open* or guillotine amputation, used for clients who have or are likely to develop an infection; the wound remains open, with drains to allow drainage to escape from the site until the infection clears
  2. *Closed* or flap amputation, whereby skin flaps are pulled over the bone end and are sutured in place as part of the amputation procedure

- Loss of all or any of the small toes presents minor disability.
- Loss of the great toe is significant because it affects balance, gait, and "push-off" ability during walking.
- Midfoot amputations and the Syme procedure (most of the foot is removed, but the ankle remains intact) are performed for peripheral vascular disease.
- Other lower extremity amputations are below-knee amputation (BKA), above-knee amputation (AKA), hip disarticulation (removal of the hip joint), and hemipelvectomy.
- *Upper extremity* amputations are generally more incapacitating because the arms and hands are needed for activities of daily living (ADL).

COLLABORATIVE MANAGEMENT
Assessment
- The nurse records the client's
  1. History of events that led to tissue destruction
  2. Age and sex
  3. Concurrent illnesses
  4. Smoking history
  5. Skin changes, e.g., color, temperature
- The nurse assesses for
  1. Skin color, temperature, sensation, and pulses in both the affected and unaffected extremities
  2. Capillary refill
  3. Concurrent medical problems
  4. The client's psychological preparation for an amputation
  5. Self-concept, self-esteem, and body image disturbance
  6. The family's reaction to the surgery

Planning and Implementation
NDx: IMPAIRED PHYSICAL MOBILITY
- The nurse
  1. Performs range-of-motion (ROM) and muscle-strengthening exercises
  2. Teaches the client to use assistive-adaptive devices (crutches, walker, etc.) before surgery, if appropriate
  3. Arranges for the client to see a prosthetist before surgery to begin planning for postoperative needs; some clients are fitted with a temporary prosthesis at the time of surgery

4. Initiates special measures for lower extremity amputations
   a. Ensures that the bed is equipped with a firm mattress and a trapeze and overhead frame
   b. Assists the client into a prone position every 3 to 4 hours for 20 to 30 minutes to prevent hip contractures
   c. Instructs the client to push the residual limb down toward the bed while supporting it on a pillow (for BKAs)
   d. Elevates the limb on a pillow for 24 hours after surgery (this is controversial; follow hospital policy)
   e. Inspects the limb daily to ensure that it lies flat on the bed surface
5. Takes measures to prevent complications of immobility, such as atelectasis, pneumonia, confusion, or thromboembolism

NDx: Body Image Disturbance

- Using the word *stump* when referring to the remaining portion of the limb is controversial.
- The nurse
  1. Assesses the client's verbal and nonverbal references to the affected area
  2. Asks the client to verbalize his or her feelings about changes in body image and self-esteem; the client may verbalize acceptance but refuse to look at the area during a dressing change
  3. Provides realistic information about potential changes in life-style, job, and recreational activities; however, many clients are able to return to previous activities due to advances in prosthetic devices
  4. Refers to a vocational counselor for evaluation as appropriate
  5. Helps the client set realistic goals and objectives
  6. Stresses the client's personal strengths
  7. Reassures the client and his or her sexual partner that an intimate relationship is possible; assists them to adjust to changes; refers them to a sexual counselor as needed

NDx: Anticipatory Grieving

- The nurse
  1. Prepares the client for care and sensations that will occur after surgery
  2. Reassures the client that feelings of loss and

grieving are normal and provides support as
needed

3. Refers the client to a local support group

NDx: PAIN

- The nurse provides relief measures for phantom limb
pain.
  1. The client complains of pain in the removed body
     part.
  2. The pain is described as burning, crushing, or
     cramping or as a numbness or tingling; the client
     feels that the missing part is in a distorted
     position.
  3. Pain is triggered by touching the stump.
  4. Pain is real to the client and is treated the same as
     stump pain with pain medication.

NDx: IMPAIRED SKIN INTEGRITY

- The nurse
  1. Recognizes that initial pressure dressings and
     drains are removed 48–72 hours after surgery
  2. Inspects the wound for signs of inflammation,
     e.g., redness and swelling
  3. Records the characteristics of drainage
  4. Follows hospital procedure for wrapping the
     stump; a stump shrinker or heavy stockinet may
     be used in place of an elastic bandage

NDx: ALTERED (PERIPHERAL) TISSUE PERFUSION

- The nurse
  1. Monitors the skin flap for adequate tissue
     perfusion
  2. Recognizes that the area should be warm, not hot
  3. Assesses for the presence of proximal pulses and
     compares to the other extremity

Discharge Planning

- The nurse
  1. Identifies and suggests corrections for hazards in
     the home prior to discharge (in collaboration with
     the physical and occupational therapy)
  2. Ensures that the client can correctly use all
     adaptive-assistive devices prior to discharge
  3. Provides a detailed plan of care at the time of
     discharge for clients to be transferred to a
     rehabilitation or long-term care facility
     (Rehabilitation may be lengthy. See
     Rehabilitation.)
- The nurse teaches care of the stump
  1. Rebandage every day with clean bandages.

2. Inspect for signs of inflammation or skin breakdown.
- The nurse teaches care of the prosthesis
  1. Refinish a wooden prosthesis once every 6 months.
  2. Clean it with mild soap and water, and dry it completely.
  3. Replace worn inserts and liners when heavily soiled.
  4. Check all mechanical parts periodically for unusual sound or movements.
  5. Grease mechanical parts as instructed by the prosthetist.
  6. Use garters to keep stockings or socks in place.
- The nurse emphasizes the importance of follow-up visits with the physician(s) and other therapists.

For more information on amputation, see *Medical-Surgical Nursing: A Nursing Process Approach,* **pp. 807–813.**

Amyotrophic Lateral Sclerosis

- Amyotrophic lateral sclerosis (ALS), also known as Lou Gehrig's disease, is a progressive degenerative disease involving the motor system.
- Mental status changes do not occur.
- The disease is characterized by fatigue, muscle atrophy, weakness, tongue atrophy, dysphagia, nasal quality to speech, and dysarthria.
- As the disease progresses, flaccid quadriplegia develops and respiratory muscles become involved, leading to pneumonia and death.

- There is no known cure.
- Treatment is symptomatic and directed toward the following: impaired physical mobility, total self-care deficit, altered nutritional status, ineffective breathing pattern and airway clearance, impaired gas exchange, and urinary and bowel incontinence.

For more information on amyotrophic lateral sclerosis, see *Medical-Surgical Nursing: A Nursing Process Approach,* **pp. 922–923.**

Anal Fissure

- An anal fissure is an elongated ulcerated laceration between the anal canal and the perianal skin.
- *Primary* fissures are idiopathic, with no known cause.
- *Secondary* fissures are associated with Crohn's disease, tuberculosis, leukemia, trauma from a foreign body, childbirth, or perirectal surgery.
- Constipated stool, diarrhea, or spasm of the anal sphincter are possible causes.
- An acute anal fissure is superficial and resolves spontaneously or with conservative treatment.
- Chronic fissures recur and require surgical treatment.
- Pain during and after defecation is the most common symptom, followed by bleeding outside the stool or on toilet tissue.
- Other symptoms associated with chronic fissures are pruritis, urinary frequency or retention, dysuria, and dyspareunia.
- Management of acute anal fissure is nonsurgical, with interventions aimed at local, symptomatic pain relief and stool softening to reduce trauma.

- Surgical excision of the fissure is performed if the area is nonresponsive to treatment.

For more information on anal fissure, see *Medical-Surgical Nursing: A Nursing Process Approach*, **p. 1405.**

Anal Fistula

- An anal fistula is an abnormal tractlike communication between the anal canal and the skin outside the anus.
- Most anal fistulas result from anorectal abscesses but can be associated with tuberculosis, Crohn's disease, and ulcerative colitis.
- Symptoms include pruritis or purulent discharge.
- Treatment depends on the cause and includes surgical excision, temporary colostomy, or treatment of the primary disorder.
- Symptomatic pain relief measures and stool softeners are used to reduce tissue trauma and discomfort.

For more information on anal fistula, see *Medical-Surgical Nursing: A Nursing Process Approach*, **pp. 1405–1406.**

Anaphylaxis

OVERVIEW

- Anaphylaxis is the rapid, systemic, simultaneous occurrence of a hypersensitive reaction in multiple organs.
- Anaphylaxis occurs within seconds to minutes of exposure to a causative allergen.

COLLABORATIVE MANAGEMENT
Assessment

- The nurse records the client's
  1. Symptoms
     a. Cause
     b. How quickly they appeared
     c. How rapidly they resolved
     d. Previous history of allergic reactions
- The nurse assesses for
  1. Apprehension
  2. Weakness
  3. Anxiety (the client may complain of a feeling of impending doom)
  4. Generalized pruritus and urticaria
  5. Erythema
  6. Angioedema of the eyes, lips, or tongue
  7. Cutaneous wheals or urticarial eruptions that are intensely pruritic and sometimes coalesce
  8. Bronchoconstriction and spasm, as well as mucosal edema and hypersecretion of mucus
  9. Respiratory assessment that reveals congestion, rhinorrhea, dyspnea, wheezing, rales, and diminished breath sounds
  10. Laryngeal edema
  11. Hypotension
  12. Rapid, weak, and possibly irregular pulse
  13. Diaphoresis
  14. Confusion
  15. Dysrhythmias
  16. Shock
  17. Cardiac arrest

Planning and Implementation
NDx: INEFFECTIVE AIRWAY CLEARANCE; INEFFECTIVE BREATHING PATTERN

- The nurse
  1. Establishes an airway IMMEDIATELY and has a tracheostomy set available

28

2. Administers supplemental oxygen via nasal cannula or face mask
3. Elevates the head of bed unless contraindicated secondary to hypotension
4. Administers epinephrine (1:1000), 0.2 to 0.5 mL, as ordered, as soon as the client displays symptoms of systemic anaphylaxis; may repeat every 15 to 20 minutes if needed
5. Administers diphenhydramine (Benedryl), as ordered, 25 to 100 mg, to treat angioedema and urticaria
6. Administers aminophylline, 6 mg/kg intravenously for severe bronchospasm, as ordered; then initiates maintenance therapy (0.3 to 0.5 mg/kg per hour)
7. Administers an inhaled beta-adrenergic agonist such as metaproterenol (Alupent) or albuterol (Proventil) every 2 to 4 hours, as ordered
8. Administers corticosteroids, as ordered, for persistent symptoms
9. Monitors arterial blood gases (ABGs)
10. Suctions the client as needed
11. Performs frequent respiratory assessments

NDx: ALTERED TISSUE PERFUSION
- The nurse
  1. Establishes an intravenous line with a large-gauge catheter
  2. Administers drug therapy as listed above
  3. Administers a rapid infusion of normal saline, as ordered; albumin or 5% plasma protein fraction may be given as a volume expander
  4. Administers vasoconstrictors such as norepinephrine or dopamine, as ordered (monitors central venous pressure and pulmonary arterial and capillary wedge pressures)
  5. Monitors cardiac rhythm (dysrhythmias can occur secondary to anaphylaxis or treatment)
  6. Records strict measurement of intake and output
  7. Monitors for mental status changes that could occur secondary to cerebral hypoxia

NDx: ANXIETY
- The nurse
  1. Stays with the client and provides reassurance
  2. Remains calm and speaks slowly
  3. Gives short, concise directions

Discharge Planning

- The nurse provides information regarding anaphylaxis
  1. Definition

2. How it occurs
3. Prevention
4. Medic Alert bracelet or necklace (stressing the importance of wearing it at all times)

• The nurse consults with the physician about the need for the client to carry an emergency anaphylaxis kit.

For more information on anaphylaxis, see *Medical-Surgical Nursing: A Nursing Process Approach,* **pp. 652–658.**

Aneurysm

OVERVIEW

• An aneurysm is an abnormal dilation of an artery as a result of localized weakness and stretching of the arterial wall.

• An aneurysm forms when the media, or the middle layer of the artery, is weakened, producing a stretching effect in the intima (the inner layer) and adventitia (the outer layer of the artery).

• The effect of blood pressure on the artery wall produces further weakness in the media and enlarges the aneurysm.

• The most common cause is arteriosclerosis; atheromatous plaque forms and weakens the intimal surface.

• The types of aneurysms include
  1. *Sacular,* an outpouching from a distinct portion of the artery wall
  2. *Fusiform,* the diffuse dilation involving the total circumference of the artery

3. *Dissecting*, a cavity formed when blood separates the layers of the artery wall
4. *False*, the complete rupture of an artery with subsequent aneurysm formation.

- The most common aneurysm site is the aorta.
- Abdominal aneurysms arise below the level of renal arteries but above the iliac bifurcation.
- Thoracic aneurysms develop between the origin of the left subclavian artery and the diaphragm.
- The thoracic aorta is the most common site for dissecting aneurysms.
- Femoral and popliteal aneurysms are relatively uncommon.
- Aneurysms can thrombose, embolize, or rupture.

COLLABORATIVE MANAGEMENT

Assessment

- The nurse records the client's
  1. Age
  2. Sex
  3. Race
  4. Cigarette use
  5. Hypercholesterolemia
  6. Hypertension
  7. Obesity
  8. Stress
  9. Familial predisposition
  10. Past medical history
  11. Medications, prescribed and over the counter
- The nurse assesses for
  1. Prominent pulsation in the upper abdomen
  2. Abdominal tenderness on palpation
  3. Abdominal or lower back pain
  4. Upper gastrointestinal bleeding
  5. Abdominal rigidity
  6. Chest pain with radiation to the neck, back, or shoulders
  7. Hoarseness or coughing
  8. Pulsating mass in the popliteal space
  9. Pulsating mass over the femoral artery
  10. Rupture of an aortic aneurysm
     a. Sudden onset of severe abdominal or back pain
     b. Shock
     c. Pulmonary edema symptoms
     d. Diminished heart sounds
     e. Aortic insufficiency murmur
     f. Blood pressure variations in arms

Planning and Implementation

NDx: POTENTIAL FOR ALTERED (PERIPHERAL, CEREBRAL, CARDIOPULMONARY, GASTROINTESTINAL, RENAL) TISSUE PERFUSION

Nonsurgical Management

• Hypercholesterolemia is treated by dietary restriction of fat and cholesterol.

• Alcohol intake is restricted.

• Antihypertensive drugs are prescribed to maintain normal blood pressure and decrease stress on the aneurysm.

• Cholesterol-lowering agents such as nicotinic acid (niacin) or lovastatin (Mevacor) are prescribed, if necessary.

Surgical Management

• Surgical removal of the aneurysm and replacement of the excised portion with graft placement may be performed as an elective or emergency procedure.

• The nurse provides preoperative care
  1. Administers large volumes of intravenous fluids to maintain tissue perfusion and blood pressure
  2. Assesses all peripheral pulses to serve as a baseline for comparison after surgery
  3. Provides routine preoperative care

• Postoperative care varies with the type of aneurysm repair.

• Care of the client with an abdominal aneurysm repair is similar to that provided for clients with other abdominal surgeries. The client is admitted to the critical care unit and is often maintained on a mechanical ventilator overnight.

• The nurse provides specific postoperative care, in addition to providing routine postoperative care. See Postoperative Care.
  1. Assesses vital signs every hour
  2. Assesses circulation by checking pulses distal to the graft site
  3. Reports signs of occlusion immediately to the physician, such as pulse changes, severe pain, cool to cold extremities below the graft, and white or blue extremities

• Aortic aneurysm repair requires assessment of renal function because the aorta is clamped during the repair, potentially compromising the blood flow to the kidneys.

• The nurse additionally
  1. Assesses hourly urinary output and urine color

2. Monitors daily blood urea nitrogen and creatinine levels

• Care of the client undergoing thoracic aneurysm repair is similar to other thoracic surgeries. (See Lung Cancer.)

• The nurse additionally
1. Assesses for signs of bleeding by monitoring chest tube drainage for excess drainage
2. Monitors for cardiac abnormalities

Discharge Planning

• The nurse instructs the client/family to control modifiable risk factors
1. Smoking
2. Hypertension with medication and diet
3. Hypercholesterolemia with diet and medication
4. Weight reduction
5. Stress

• The nurse
1. Teaches the client to restrict activities
   a. Avoid lifting heavy objects for 6 to 12 weeks postoperatively
   b. Use discretion in activities that involve pulling, pushing, or straining, such as vacuuming, changing bed linens, moving furniture, mopping or sweeping, raking leaves, mowing grass, and chopping wood
   c. Defer driving a car for several weeks
2. Provides written and oral wound care instructions, if needed
3. Provides pain management instructions, as ordered

For more information on aneurysms, see *Medical-Surgical Nursing: A Nursing Process Approach*, **pp. 2218–2224.**

Anorectal Abscess

- Anorectal abscesses result from obstruction of the ducts of glands in the anorectal region by feces, foreign bodies, or trauma.
- Stasis of the obstructing contents results in infection that spreads into adjacent tissue.
- Rectal pain is the first clinical manifestation.
- Local swelling, erythema, and tenderness on palpation appear a few days after the onset of pain.
- The diagnosis is made by physical exam and history.
- Simple perianal and ischiorectal abscesses can be excised under local anesthetic.
- More extensive abscesses require incision under regional or general anesthesia.

For more information on anorectal abscess, see *Medical-Surgical Nursing: A Nursing Process Approach*, **pp. 1404–1405.**

Anorexia Nervosa

OVERVIEW

- Anorexia nervosa is a serious eating disorder that takes the form of indirect self-destructive behavior and can become life threatening; it is the clinical syndrome of self-induced starvation.
- The anorectic refuses to eat because of an intense fear of losing control of eating and becoming fat.
- The disorder occurs primarily in females, and onset occurs during early adolescence.

- Medical sequelae occur from the effects of starvation and unhealthy behaviors, such as purging by vomiting or abuse of laxatives or diuretics.
- DSM-III-R diagnostic criteria include

    1. Refusal to maintain body weight over a minimal normal weight for age and height, e.g., weight loss leading to maintenance of body weight 15% below that expected or failure to make expected weight gain during a period of growth, leading to body weight 15% below that expected
    2. Intense fear of gaining weight or becoming fat although underweight
    3. Disturbance in the way in which one's body weight, size, or shape is experienced, e.g., the person claims to "feel fat" even when emaciated and believes that one area of the body is "too fat" even when obviously underweight
    4. In females, the absence of at least three consecutive menstrual cycles when otherwise expected to occur (primary or secondary amenorrhea)

COLLABORATIVE MANAGEMENT

Assessment

- The nurse records the client's

    1. Demographic data, including age, sex, socioeconomic status, education, and occupation
    2. History of medical problems, including gastrointestinal symptoms such as nausea, vomiting, esophagitis, irritable bowel syndrome, and constipation
    3. Concerns about physical functioning, such as weakness, fatigue, intolerance to cold, changes in sleep habits, swelling in body part, or seizures
    4. Weight history and data on current weight, height, and body build
    5. Sexual history, including onset of breast development; age, weight, and height at onset of menarche; menstrual history and details about amenorrhea, if present
    6. Attitudes and behaviors related to food and weight
    7. Reports of changes in appetite or denial of appetite, use of appetite-suppressant drugs, self-induced vomiting, and frequency of weighing self
    8. Typical pattern of eating
    9. Use of laxatives and diuretics and habits of hiding or throwing away food

10. History of psychiatric illness and treatment.
11. Family history of psychiatric illness and treatment

- The nurse assesses for
    1. Weight loss
    2. Amenorrhea
    3. Hypothermia (decreased core body temperature) to 95° F (35° C)
    4. Decreased blood pressure, heart rate, and respiratory rate
    5. Loss of muscle mass and subcutaneous fat
    6. Fine lanugo hair
    7. Hypokalemic metabolic acidosis from vomiting, laxatives, and diuretics
    8. Edema
    9. Discolored tooth enamel from exposure to gastric acid
    10. Psychosocial factors, including high academic achievement, motivation, and compliance; sense of ineffectiveness and low self-esteem; desire for parental approval and striving for perfection

Planning and Implementation

NDx: ALTERED NUTRITION: LESS THAN BODY REQUIREMENTS

- The nurse
    1. Provides a diet of 1200 to 1600 calories per day, with foods selected by the client
    2. Increases calories gradually to ensure steady weight gain of 2 to 4 lb/week and to avoid abdominal distention with gastric dilation
    3. Administers intravenous (IV) fluids or liquid feedings by nasogastric tube, as ordered, if the client persistently refuses food

NDx: PAIN (ABDOMINAL)

- Narcotic analgesics are **never** indicated because of potential decreased stomach and bowel motility.
- The nurse
    1. Administers acetaminophen (Tylenol), as ordered, for minor abdominal discomfort
    2. Administers antacids, as ordered, for the discomfort of indigestion.
    3. Provides a low-lactose, low-lipid diet; milk products and fats are slowly introduced during the second or third week of re-feeding and are withdrawn if cramping is severe

NDx: POTENTIAL FLUID VOLUME DEFICIT

- The nurse
  1. Provides hourly oral fluids, including water, juice, soda, coffee, and tea, but avoiding milk
  2. Administers isotonic IV fluids, as ordered, if oral fluids are refused or volume replacement is needed
  3. Maintains a strict record of intake and output

NDx: FLUID VOLUME EXCESS

- Diuretics are not recommended for refeeding edema; they are indicated in heart failure.
- Refeeding edema responds well to low-salt diets.
- Fluid restriction is limited to 1000 to 1500 mL/day.

NDx: CONSTIPATION

- The nurse
  1. Initiates a bowel regime, as ordered, including a bulk laxative such as psyllium (Metamucil) and a stool softener such as docusate (Colace)
  2. Administers a cathartic suppository such as bisacodyl (Dulcolax) or a sodium phosphate (Fleet) enema for persistent constipation

NDx: ANXIETY

- Extremely anxious clients may require an antianxiety agent prior to meals, e.g., a short-acting anxiolytic agent such as lorazepam (Ativan).
- The nurse
  1. Allows the client to control decisions and give input into nonfood-related issues
  2. Provides emotional support and encouragement during mealtimes and after meals and snacks
  3. Teaches relaxation techniques and guided imagery

NDx: BODY IMAGE DISTURBANCES

- The nurse
  1. Encourages the client to express feelings about body size and function and points out misconceptions to the client without arguing
  2. Provides positive feedback for accurate perception of body size and function and helps the client to accept changes

NDx: INEFFECTIVE COPING

- The nurse
  1. Administers antidepressants, as ordered, that are

indicated for depression; otherwise medication is not indicated
2. Arranges individual therapy with a psychiatrist, psychologist, or psychiatric liaison nurse as an inpatient and after discharge, as ordered
3. Teaches that support groups organized by recovering anorexics and/or families provide education and support during periods of stress for the client/family

NDx: POTENTIAL FOR NONCOMPLIANCE

- The nurse
  1. Monitors behavior and provides support combined with client motivation
  2. Instructs the client/family on specific information related to the illness and treatment plan, emphasizing the consequences of noncompliance

Discharge Planning

- Educational efforts are focused on teaching the client/family to recognize and understand the physical, behavioral, and emotional characteristics of the disease.

- The teaching plan is individualized to identify client specific problems.

- The nurse teaches the client/family
  1. Use of food patterns and exchanges (consult with a dietitian)
  2. Avoidance of family conflicts at mealtimes
  3. The importance of follow-up visits with the physician(s)

For more information on anorexia nervosa, see *Medical-Surgical Nursing: A Nursing Process Approach*, **pp. 1414–1434.**

Aortic Insufficiency/ Regurgitation

- In aortic insufficiency, the aortic valve leaflets do not close properly during diastole, causing the annulus to become dilated, loose, or deformed.

- Regurgitation of blood from the aorta into the left ventricle occurs during diastole; the left ventricle dilates to accommodate the greater blood flow and hypertrophies.

- Nonrheumatic causes include infective endocarditis, congenital anatomic aortic valvular abnormalities, and Marfan's syndrome, a generalized, systemic connective tissue disease.

- Signs and symptoms include
  1. Palpitations
  2. Dyspnea
  3. Orthopnea
  4. Paroxysmal nocturnal dyspnea
  5. Fatigue
  6. Angina
  7. Sinus tachycardia
  8. Blowing, decrescendo diastolic murmur

- Aortic valve surgery is the treatment of choice.

- The postoperative client requires lifetime anticoagulation therapy to prevent thrombus formation on the valve.

- For preoperative and postoperative care, see Coronary Artery Disease.

For more information on aortic insufficiency, see *Medical-Surgical Nursing: A Nursing Process Approach*, **pp. 2172–2178.**

Aortic Stenosis

- In aortic stenosis, the aortic valve orifice narrows, obstructing the left ventricular outflow during systole.
- Increased resistance to ejection or afterload results in left ventricular hypertrophy.
- As stenosis progresses, cardiac output decreases.
- The left atrium has incomplete emptying, and the pulmonary system becomes congested; right-sided failure may develop.
- Congenital valvular disease or malformation is the main cause.
- Signs and symptoms include
  1. Dyspnea on exertion
  2. Angina
  3. Syncope on exertion
  4. Fatigue
  5. Orthopnea
  6. Paroxysmal noctural dyspnea
  7. Harsh, systolic crescendo-decrescendo murmur
- Aortic valve replacement surgery is the treatment of choice.
- The postoperative client requires lifetime anticoagulation therapy to prevent thrombus formation on the valve.
- For preoperative and postoperative care, see Coronary Artery Disease.

For more information on aortic stenosis, see *Medical-Surgical Nursing: A Nursing Process Approach*, **pp. 2172–2178.**

Appendicitis

OVERVIEW

• Appendicitis is an inflammation of the vermiform appendix, the small, fingerlike pouch attached to the cecum of the colon.

• Appendicitis occurs when there is ulceration of the mucosa or when the lumen of the appendix is obstructed.

• Inflammation leads to infection as bacteria invade the wall of the appendix.

• Appendicitis is the most common cause of acute inflammation in the right lower abdominal quadrant.

COLLABORATIVE MANAGEMENT

Assessment

• The nurse records the client's
   1. Age and sex
   2. History of abdominal surgery (prior appendectomy)
   3. History of medical conditions
   4. Recent barium studies
   5. Dietary history, including fiber intake

• The nurse assesses for
   1. Sudden onset of abdominal pain originating in the epigastric or periumbilical area and shifting to the right lower quadrant
   2. Nausea and vomiting
   3. Anorexia
   4. Urge to defecate or pass flatus
   5. Abdominal tenderness, which may be absent in early stages or diffuse with localization to the right lower quadrant in later stages of inflammation (McBurney's point)
   6. Muscle rigidity and rebound tenderness

Planning and Implementation

NDx: Altered (Gastrointestinal) Tissue Perfusion

• The nurse keeps the client on nothing-by-mouth status and administers fluids intravenously, as ordered, prior to emergent surgical appendectomy (removal of the appendix).

• If abscess is present, surgical drains are inserted during surgery.

- If peritonitis is present, the client will have a nasogastric tube in place to prevent gastric distention.
- The nurse provides routine postoperative care.
- The nurse
  1. Assesses the abdominal drains for excess drainage
  2. Maintains the client's nasogastric tube if inserted intraoperatively for peritonitis
  3. Administers intravenous antibiotics, as ordered
  4. Assists the client out of bed on the evening of surgery, as ordered
  5. Administers narcotic analgesia, as ordered

Discharge Planning

- The nurse provides written postoperative instructions
  1. How to care for the incision
  2. How to take and monitor pain medication, as ordered
  3. How to increase fiber intake
  4. How to limit activity, including avoidance of heavy lifting
  5. How to inspect the incision for redness, tenderness, swelling, and drainage

For more information on appendicitis, see *Medical-Surgical Nursing: A Nursing Approach*, **pp. 1344–1347.**

Arteriosclerosis/ Atherosclerosis

OVERVIEW

- Arteriosclerosis describes a thickening or hardening of the arterial wall of the vascular system.
- *Atherosclerosis*, a type of arteriosclerosis, involves the formation of a plaque within the arterial wall.

- Atherosclerosis is the most common type of arterial obstruction; the process results in coronary artery disease (CAD), cerebrovascular disease (CVA), and peripheral vascular disease (PVD).

- The exact pathophysiologic mechanism of atherosclerosis is unknown.

- Atherosclerosis begins as a fatty streak on the intimal surface of an artery and develops into a fibrous plaque that partially or completely occludes the artery's blood flow.

- The final stage of atherosclerosis occurs when the fibrous lesion becomes calcified, hemorrhagic, ulcerated, or thrombosed.

COLLABORATIVE MANAGEMENT

Assessment

- The nurse records the client's
  1. Age
  2. Sex
  3. Race
  4. Weight and height
  5. Exercise habits
  6. Diet
  7. Family or client history of diabetes, hypertension, and hyperlipidemia
  8. Related vascular disorders such as CVA, myocardial infarction, or PVD
  9. Previous surgical procedures, such as coronary artery bypass, carotid endarterectomy, or lower extremity revascularization
  10. Angioplasty procedures
  11. Thrombolytic therapy
  12. Medications

- The nurse assesses for
  1. Pain related to decreased oxygen supply
  2. Change in function related to decreased oxygen supply
  3. Dry skin
  4. Atrophic changes, such as hair loss, muscle mass loss, and thickened or clubbed nails
  5. Pallor around the lips and nail beds
  6. Rubor of the skin
  7. Reddened areas
  8. Cellulitis
  9. Distended veins
  10. Varicosities
  11. Edema
  12. Ulcerations
  13. Discoloration of lower extremities

14. Arterial pulsation, including rate and intensity
15. Arterial bruits
16. Temperature differences in lower extremities
17. Prolonged capillary refill

Planning and Implementation

NDx: POTENTIAL FOR ALTERED PERIPHERAL TISSUE PERFUSION

- The nurse
    1. Encourages the client to stop smoking
    2. Teaches the client to limit dietary fat to 30% of total calories per day (with dietitian consult)
    3. Teaches the client to limit cholesterol intake, as prescribed
    4. Administers cholesterol-lowering agents such as nicotinic acid (niacin) or lovastatin (Mevacor), as ordered
    5. Reinforces the need for a routine exercise program

Discharge Planning

- The nurse teaches the client/family
    1. To follow a low-fat, low-cholesterol diet and an exercise program
    2. To report signs of occlusive atherosclerotic disease to the physician, such as discomfort in the chest, upper back, or jaw, which may or may not radiate down one or both arms; pain in the legs; episodes of weakness, dizziness, blurred vision, tingling, numbness, or loss of sensation in the face or extremities; or severe abdominal or back pain

For more information on arteriosclerosis/
atherosclerosis, see *Medical-Surgical Nursing: A
Nursing Process Approach*, **pp. 2187–2195.**

Asthma, Bronchial

OVERVIEW

• Bronchial asthma is a clinical disorder characterized by narrowing of the bronchial tree or airways, with two major types:
1. *Extrinsic*, which is precipitated by allergenic exposure (e.g., to pollens, molds, dust, or animal dander)
2. *Intrinsic*, which is precipitated by nonallergenic factors, such as viral infection, exercise, cold, cigarette smoke, changes in temperature or humidity, gasoline fumes, and paint fumes
• Emotional stress aggravates an asthma attack.

COLLABORATIVE MANAGEMENT

• Symptoms are typically variable in frequency and severity and acute or insidious in onset and include
1. Shortness of breath
2. Nonproductive cough
3. Feeling of tightness or pressure in the chest
4. Dyspnea
5. Tachypnea
6. Audible wheezes
7. Anxiety
8. Respirations that are increasingly rapid and shallow
9. Fatigue
10. Cyanosis
11. Confusion and lethargy
• Treatment includes
1. Control of exacerbating factors
2. Treatment of acute episodes
3. Maintenance drug therapy
4. Beta-adrenergic agents (epinephrine, isoproterenol, ephedrine), which relax bronchial smooth muscle and inhibit mediator release
5. Theophylline and derivatives, which act in a similar fashion
6. Oxygen to maintain a PO_2 level above 60 mmHg
7. Intake and output and electrolyte monitoring
8. Administration of intravenous fluids if necessary
9. Maintenance therapy with theophylline and bronchodilator

- Also see Chronic Obstructive Pulmonary Disease.

For more information on bronchial asthma, see *Medical-Surgical Nursing: A Nursing Process Approach*, **pp. 663–664.**

Autoimmune Thrombocytopenic Purpura

OVERVIEW

- Autoimmune thrombocytopenia purpura is also referred to as idiopathic thrombocytopenic purpura (ITP).
- The total number of circulating platelets is greatly diminished, although bone marrow platelet production is normal.
- An antibody (antiplatelet antibody) is made and coats the surface of the platelets, making the platelets more susceptible to attraction and destruction by phagocytic leukocytes.
- The spleen is the primary site of platelet destruction.
- When the rate of platelet destruction exceeds the rate of platelet production, the number of circulating platelets decreases, and blood clotting slows.

COLLABORATIVE MANAGEMENT
Assessment
- The nurse records the client's
    1. History of present illness
    2. Age and sex
    3. Medication use (aspirin and aspirin-containing products)

4. Family history of autoimmune disorders
5. History of overt and hidden bleeding
6. History of related symptoms
   a. Headaches
   b. Behavior changes
   c. Increased somnolence
   d. Decreased alertness
   e. Decreased attention span
   f. Lethargy
   g. Muscle weakness
   h. Diminished appetite
   i. Weight loss
   j. Increased fatigue

- The nurse assesses for
  1. Ecchymoses (bruises) on the arms, legs, upper chest, and back
  2. Petechial rash
  3. Mucosal bleeding

Planning and Implementation
NDx: POTENTIAL FOR INJURY

- The nurse
  1. Administers immunosuppressant drugs, such as corticosteroids and azathioprine (Imuran), as ordered, to inhibit immune system synthesis of autoantibodies directed against platelets
  2. Administers low-dose chemotherapy with agents such as vinca alkaloids and cyclophosphamide (Cytoxan), as ordered
  3. Administers platelet transfusions for acute, life-threatening bleeding
  4. Maintains a safe environment

- A splenectomy is performed for clients not responding to drug therapy.

Discharge Planning

- The disease is usually self-limiting in adults. It is chronic but controllable.
- The nurse
  1. Identifies signs and symptoms of decreased coagulation, bleeding, and infection
  2. Avoids aspirin and aspirin-containing products
  3. Reinforces prescribed medication treatment schedule
  4. Explains side effects of medications, including bone marrow suppression, which may lead to increased risk of infection

5. Emphasizes the importance of follow-up visits with the physician(s)

For more information on autoimmune thrombocytopenia purpura, see *Medical-Surgical Nursing: A Nursing Process Approach*, **pp. 2274–2276.**

Back Pain

OVERVIEW

- The areas of the back most commonly affected by back pain are the cervical and lumbar vertebrae.
- *Cervical back pain* is usually related to a ruptured disk between the fifth and sixth vertebrae or to nerve compression caused by osteophyte formation.
- *Low-back pain* (LBP) is typically caused by a herniated nucleus pulposus (usually between the fourth and fifth lumbar or fifth lumbar and first sacral vertebrae), ligament sprain, disk injury from hyperflexion, or muscle sprain or spasm.

COLLABORATIVE MANAGEMENT

Assessment

- The nurse records the client's
  1. Activity before the back pain occurred (pain may occur immediately or a few days later)
  2. Occupation
  3. History of arthritis or family history of arthritis
- The nurse assesses the client for
  1. Posture and gait
  2. Vertebral alignment and swelling
  3. Muscle spasm
  4. Pain radiating down the arm or leg
  5. Tenderness of the back and involved extremity

6. Sensory changes: paresthesia, numbness
7. Muscle tone and strength
8. Limitations in movement
9. Reaction to illness

Planning and Implementation

NDx: Pain

Nonsurgical Management

• Muscle relaxants such as cyclobenzapine hydrochloride (Flexeril) and nonsteroidal anti-inflammatory drugs such as aspirin or ibuprofen (Motrin) are often given.

• Epidural steroid injections may be administered in some cases.

• The purpose of traction is to separate the vertebrae and relieve pressure on the impinged nerve.

• Cervical traction includes
  1. Head halter
  2. Skeletal (halo traction)

• Low-back traction includes
  1. Pelvic
  2. Bilateral Buck's
  3. Hanging

• For care of the client in cervical traction see Spinal Cord Injury. For other types of traction see Fracture.

• Positioning includes a bed board and the Williams' position for LBP (semi-Fowler position, with knees flexed).

• Other approaches include a custom-fitted lumbosacral brace or corset for LBP, moist heat, deep-heat therapy such as ultrasound or diathermy, massage, transcutaneous electrical nerve syndrome (TENS), distraction, imagery, and music therapy.

• See Pain for additional information on acute and chronic pain management.

Surgical Management

• *Laminectomy* includes
  1. The removal of one or more vertebral laminae, plus osteophytes, and the herniated nucleus pulposus through a 3-in incision.
  2. A *spinal fusion* to stabilize the spine if repeated laminectomies are performed.
  3. A hospital stay of 2 to 5 days, depending on the procedure.

• *Chemonucleolysis* includes
  1. The injection of the affected disk with an enzymatic substance, chymopapain

(Chymodiactin), under local anesthesia and fluoroscopy.
2. A major complication is anaphylactic reaction (women are more likely to experience the reaction).
3. Testing for sensitivity with a fluoroallergosorbent test (FAST) prior to the procedure.
4. A special exercise program and precautions for 2 to 3 months before resuming full activity.
5. The possibility of exacerbation of symptoms for up to 6 weeks postprocedure.
- *Percutaneous lateral diskectomy* includes
   1. The insertion of a metal cannula adjacent to the affected disk under fluoroscopy and the threading of a special cutting tool through the cannula for removal of pieces of the disk that are compressing the nerve root.
   2. A major risk of infection and nerve root injury.
   3. A hospital stay of 2 to 3 days.
   4. Special exercises and precautions for 2 to 3 months before resuming full activity.
- *Microdiskectomy* includes
   1. Microscopic surgery through a 1-in incision.
   2. The possible complications of infection, dural tears, and missed disk fragments.
- The nurse provides preoperative care
   1. Provides routine preoperative care
   2. Warns the client that various sensations may be experienced in the affected leg or both legs because of manipulation of nerves and muscles during surgery
- The nurse provides postoperative care
   1. Takes vital signs and neurologic checks every 4 hours
   2. Assesses for fever and hypotension
   3. Checks the dressing for any drainage (clear drainage may indicate a cerebrospinal fluid leak)
   4. Measures intake and output (an inability to void may indicate damage to sacral spinal nerves)
   5. Recognizes that most clients may be out of bed with assistance the evening of surgery; clients with a spinal fusion may be on bed rest for 24 to 48 hours
   6. Logrolls the client every 2 hours
   7. Provides routine postoperative care

NDx: IMPAIRED PHYSICAL MOBILITY
- Exercises to strengthen the back are begun when acute pain subsides.

- The nurse
  1. Teaches the client to be careful when exposing the affected arm or leg to hot water
  2. Teaches the client to make sure when walking that the foot is placed firmly on the ground with each step (for clients with sensory compromise in the feet)

Discharge Planning

- The nurse teaches the client/family
  1. The prescribed exercise program (client mastery is ensured by observing correct performance on return demonstration, in collaboration with physical therapy)
  2. Restrictions on lifting and bending and on activities
  3. Principles of body mechanics
  4. The use of a firm mattress or bed board
  5. Drug information

For more information on back pain, see *Medical-Surgical Nursing: A Nursing Process Approach,* **pp. 813–819.**

Bartholin's Abscess

- A Bartholin's abscess is an infection of a Bartholin's cyst when bacteria (*Escherichia coli, Neisseria gonorrhoeae, Staphylococcus aureus, Streptococcus, Trichomonas vaginalis,* or *Mycoplasma hominis*) enter the duct.
- History reveals
  1. Complaints of perineal discomfort

2. Dyspareunia (painful intercourse)
3. Low-grade fever
4. Swelling of the labia
5. Purulent discharge
6. Difficulty sitting or walking
7. Tender mass on the side of the vaginal opening that is swollen and red

- The abscess usually ruptures spontaneously within 72 hours.
- Interventions include
    1. Bed rest
    2. Analgesics
    3. Application of moist heat
    4. Broad-spectrum antibiotics
    5. Incision and drainage of the abscess
    6. Total excision of the Bartholin's gland, if needed, in women over 40 years of age

For more information on Bartholin's abscess, see *Medical-Surgical Nursing: A Nursing Process Approach*, **p. 1715.**

Bartholin's Cysts

- Bartholin's cysts are one of the most common disorders of the vulva.
- The cysts result from obstruction of a duct; the secretory function of the gland continues, and the fluid fills the obstructed duct.
- The cause of the obstruction may be infection, congenital stenosis or atresia, thickened mucus near the ductal opening, or mechanical trauma.
- Cysts usually appear unilaterally, and size ranges from 1 to 10 cm.

- Assessment for small cysts includes
  1. No symptoms
  2. Client complains of dyspareunia, inadequate genital lubrication, or feeling a mass in the perineal area
- Assessment for large cysts includes
  1. Constant, localized pain
  2. Difficulty walking or sitting
  3. Swelling immediately beneath the skin in the posterior vulva
  4. Brown or sanguineous cyst
- For symptomatic cysts, surgical treatment with incision and drainage may provide temporary relief.
- Marsupialization (the formation of a pouch that serves as a new duct opening) may be performed to prevent recurrence.
- Local comfort measures and antibiotics may be given.

For more information on Bartholin's cyst, see *Medical-Surgical Nursing: A Nursing Process Approach*, **pp. 1714–1715.**

Basal Cell Carcinoma, Ocular

- Basal cell carcinoma of the eye most frequently occurs in the lower eyelid.
- Basal cell carcinoma does not metastasize, and multifacial lesions may be present.
- Vision is altered only when the lesion's size, weight, or location affects visual functioning.

- Treatment is surgical excision of the lesion and client education.

For more information on ocular basal cell carcinoma, see *Medical-Surgical Nursing: A Nursing Process Approach,* **p. 1069.**

Bell's Palsy

- Bell's palsy, or facial paralysis, is an acute paralysis of cranial nerve VII, with maximal paralysis reached within 2 to 5 days.
- Pain behind the face or ear may proceed paralysis by a few hours or days.
- The disorder is characterized by an inability to close the eye, wrinkle the forehead, smile, whistle, or grimace; the face appears masklike and sags.
- Treatment includes
  1. Prednisone (Deltasone)
  2. Analgesics for pain
  3. Protection of the eye from corneal abrasion or ulceration
  4. Application of warm, moist heat
  5. Dietary instruction if the client has difficulty chewing or swallowing

For more information on Bell's palsy, see *Medical-Surgical Nursing: A Nursing Process Approach,* **p. 987.**

Benign Prostatic Hyperplasia

OVERVIEW

- Glandular units in the prostate undergo tissue hyperplasia resulting in benign prostatic hypertrophy (BPH).
- The enlarged prostate extends upward into the bladder and inward, narrowing the prostatic urethral channel.
- The prostate obstructs urine flow by encroaching on the bladder opening, resulting in a hyperirritable bladder, producing urgency and frequency, bladder wall hypertrophy, and hydronephrosis and hydroureter.
- Urinary retention or incomplete bladder emptying results in urinary tract infections.

COLLABORATIVE MANAGEMENT

Assessment

- The nurse records the client's
  1. Age
  2. Urinary pattern and symptoms
     a. Frequency
     b. Nocturia
     c. Hesitancy
     d. Intermittency
     e. Diminished force and caliber of stream
     f. Sensation of incomplete bladder emptying
     g. Postvoid dribbling
     h. Hematuria
- The nurse assesses for
  1. Distended bladder
  2. Client readiness for digital prostatic examination
  3. Symptoms of renal insufficiency
     a. Nutritional deficiencies
     b. Edema
     c. Pruritis
     d. Pallor
     e. Ecchymosis

Planning and Implementation

NDx: POTENTIAL FOR INFECTION; POTENTIAL FOR INJURY

Nonsurgical Management
- Prostatic fluid may be released by prostatic massage, frequent intercourse, and masturbation.
- The nurse teaches the client to
  1. Avoid drinking large amounts of fluid in a short period
  2. Avoid alcohol and diuretics
  3. Void as soon as the urge is felt
  4. Avoid medications that increase urinary retention, such as anticholinergics, antihistamines, and decongestants

Surgical Management
- Surgery is performed in the client who develops acute urinary retention, chronic urinary tract infections secondary to residual urine in the bladder, hematuria; hydronephrosis, and bladder neck obstruction symptoms, such as urinary frequency and nocturia.
- The usual surgical interventions to treat BPH include
  1. *Transuretheral resection of the prostate (TURP)* involves the insertion of a resectoscope though the urethra and resection of the enlarged portion of the prostate.
  2. *Suprapubic*, or *transvesical, prostatectomy* involves an abdominal incision to expose the bladder. The prostate gland is enucleated through the bladder cavity, and repair to the bladder is done, if required.
  3. *Retropubic*, or *extravesical, prostatectomy* is accomplished by an abdominal incision above the symphysis pubis. A small incision is made into the prostate gland, and the gland is enucleated.
  4. *Perineal prostatectomy* is used primarily to remove prostate glands filled with calculi, to treat prostatic abscesses, to repair complications, or to treat poor surgical risks. The surgeon makes a U-shaped incision between the ischial tuberosities, the scrotum, and the rectum. The prostatic capsule is opened and enucleated.
- The nurse provides preoperative care
  1. Informs the client to expect an indwelling bladder catheter and possibly continuous bladder irrigation.
  2. Tells the client to expect hematuria and blood clots.
  3. Provides routine preoperative care.
- The nurse provides postoperative care
  1. Informs the client that he may feel the urge to void due to the large diameter of the Foley

catheter and the pressure of the balloon on the internal sphincter.
2. Instructs the client to try not to void around the catheter, which will cause the bladder to spasm.
3. Maintains continuous irrigation with normal saline solutions, as ordered by the physician.
4. Monitors the color of the output and adjusts the rate of the irrigation accordingly.
5. Hand irrigates the catheter, as ordered, to remove obstructive blood clots.
6. Monitors for frank bleeding.
7. Assesses the suprapubic catheter (in suprapubic prostatectomy), the catheter site, and the drainage system, if necessary.

Discharge Planning

- The nurse provides postoperative instructions
  1. Recognize that temporary loss of control of urination is normal and will improve
  2. Contract and relax the urinary sphincter frequently to reestablish urinary control
  3. Increase water intake to keep urine flowing freely
  4. Avoid strenuous activities to prevent injury
  5. Notify the physician for persistent hematuria
  6. Consume alcohol, soft drinks, and spicy foods in moderation to prevent irritation to remaining prostatic tissue

For more information on benign prostatic hyperplasia, see *Medical-Surgical Nursing: A Nursing Process Approach*, **pp. 1742–1750.**

Bladder Trauma

- Bladder trauma occurs because of blunt or penetrating injury to the lower abdomen.
- The most common cause is a fractured pelvis in which bone fragments puncture the bladder.

- Bladder trauma other than a simple contusion requires surgical intervention, including closure repair of the anterior or posterior bladder wall and peritoneal membrane.
- Anterior bladder wall injury requires a Penrose drain and Foley catheter.
- Posterior bladder wall injury requires a Penrose drain and Foley or suprapubic catheter.

For more information on bladder trauma, see *Medical-Surgical Nursing: A Nursing Process Approach*, **pp. 1880–1881.**

Blindness

OVERVIEW

- Blindness may be total or diminished in one or both eyes.
- Types of blindness include
    1. Color: unable to distinguish certain colors; primary colors seen as gray
    2. Legally blind: Best visual acuity with corrective lenses in the better eye is 20/200 or less or if the widest diameter of the visual field in that eye is no greater than 20 degrees
    3. Loss of peripheral vision
    4. Loss of central vision

COLLABORATIVE MANAGEMENT

- The nurse
    1. Orients the client to the immediate environment
        a. Describes the approximate size of the room
        b. Describes a focal point in the room to serve as a point of reference, such as a chair or the bed,

and then describes all other objects in relation to the focal point

   c. Accompanies the client to other important areas in the room (bathroom)

   d. Never leaves the client in the middle of an unfamiliar room

2. Assists the client in establishing the locations of personal objects, such as the call light, clock, and water pitcher

3. Never changes the location of objects without the client's consent

4. Sets up the meal tray and uses an imaginary clock placement to orient the client to food placement

5. Instructs the client to grasp her or his elbow while keeping the elbow close to the body and alerts the client to hazards such as steps or a narrow doorway when assisting with ambulation

6. Monitors the client's use of a cane (held in the client's dominant hand) to help detect obstacles

7. Knocks before entering the client's room; identifies self and the purpose of the visit

8. Provides for diversional activities

- Newly blind clients may experience a brief period of physical or psychological immobility, hopelessness, anger, or denial.

For more information on blindness, see *Medical-Surgical Nursing: A Nursing Process Approach,* **pp. 1010–1012.**

Bone Tumors, Benign

OVERVIEW

- Benign bone tumors are often asymptomatic and may be discovered on routine radiographic examination or as the cause of pathologic fractures.

- Types of benign tumors include
  1. Chondrogenic (from cartilage)
     a. Osteochondroma is the most common and generally involves the femur and tibia.
     b. Chondroma, or endochondroma, primarily affects the hands, feet, ribs, sternum, spine, and long bones and frequently causes pathologic fractures after trivial injury.
  2. Osteogenic (from bone)
     a. Osteoid osteoma most frequently involves the femur and tibia and causes unremitting bone pain.
     b. Osteoblastoma, often called the giant osteoid osteoma, affects the vertebrae and long bones.
     c. Giant cell tumors, unlike most other benign tumors, affect women older than 20 years of age.

COLLABORATIVE MANAGEMENT
Assessment
- The nurse records the client's
  1. Age and sex
  2. History of trivial trauma, fractures, or neoplasms
  3. Family history of neoplasms
- The nurse assesses for
  1. Severity, nature, and location of pain
  2. Local swelling around the involved area
  3. Muscle spasms or atrophy
  4. Anxiety and fear about diagnosis and surgery

Planning and Implementation
NDx: POTENTIAL FOR INJURY
- The nurse
  1. Maintains a hazard-free environment
  2. Increases dietary protein, vitamins C and D, calcium, and iron to promote healing

NDx: PAIN
- The nurse
  1. Administers analgesics and nonsteroidal anti-inflammatory drugs, such as ibuprofen (Motrin), as ordered
  2. Applies heat or cold
  3. Teaches imagery and relaxation techniques
- Curettage, a surgical procedure, is performed to excise the tumor tissue.

Discharge Planning

- The nurse stresses the importance of follow-up visits with the physician(s).

- Care and health teaching is the same as that for other general orthopedic surgery discussed in Fracture.

For more information on benign bone tumors, see *Medical-Surgical Nursing: A Nursing Process Approach,* **pp. 759–761.**

Bone Tumors, Malignant

OVERVIEW

- There are several types of *primary* tumors

  1. *Osteosarcoma*, or osteogenic sarcoma, is the most common and is most frequently found in the distal femur, proximal tibia, and humerus; the lesion typically metastasizes to the lungs within 2 years of treatment.
  2. *Ewing's sarcoma* is the most malignant and often extends into soft tissue and metastasizes to the lungs and other bones.
  3. *Chondrosarcoma* typically affects the pelvis and proximal femur near the diaphysis.
  4. *Fibrosarcoma* is an uncommon, slow-growing tumor that can metastasize to the lungs.

- *Secondary* tumors originate in other tissues, metastasize to bone, and are found most often in the older age group.

- The source of the original secondary tumor includes the prostate, the kidney, the thyroid, and the lungs.

- Secondary tumors primarily metastasize to the vertebrae, the pelvis, and the ribs.

COLLABORATIVE MANAGEMENT
Assessment
- The nurse records the client's
    1. History of previous radiation therapy for cancer
    2. General health status
    3. Family history of neoplasms
- The nurse assesses for
    1. Pain
    2. Local swelling
    3. Palpable mass
    4. Ability to perform activities of daily living (ADL)
    5. Low-grade fever, fatigue, and pallor (seen in Ewing's sarcoma)
    6. Level of support system to help the client cope with the diagnosis and treatment
    7. Anxiety and fear

Planning and Implementation
NDx: PAIN
Nonsurgical Management
- Analgesics and nondrug pain relief measures are used.

- Chemotherapeutic agents, given alone or in combination with radiation therapy and surgery, work best for small, metastatic lesions. The drugs selected are determined in part by the primary source of the tumor.

- Radiation therapy is as effective as surgery for Ewing's sarcoma in reducing the size of the tumor and thereby decreasing pain.

- Nursing care for clients receiving chemotherapy and/ or radiation therapy is discussed on pp. 91–103.

Surgical Management
- *Wide excision* is the removal of the lesion surrounded by an intact cuff of normal tissue and leads to cure of low-grade tumors only.

- *Radical resection* includes the removal of the lesion, the entire muscle, bone, and other tissues directly involved; bone deficits may be corrected with grafts.

- *Percutaneous cordotomy* may be done to treat intractable pain.

- The nurse provides preoperative care
    1. Provides routine preoperative care
    2. Provides psychological support; answers questions and explains routines and procedures
    3. Administers chemotherapy, as ordered
- The nurse provides postoperative care
    1. Assesses neurovascular status

2. Observes and records wound drainage
3. Maintains pressure dressing and suction as ordered
4. Begins muscle-strengthening and range-of-motion exercises as soon as permitted; a continuous passive motion (CPM) machine may be used
5. Assists with ADL as needed

NDx: ANTICIPATORY GRIEVING

- The nurse
  1. Allows the client/family to verbalize their feelings
  2. Refers questions outside the scope of nursing practice to the physician, spiritual counselor, or other appropriate professional
  3. Encourages the client/family to write down their questions and have them available when the physician visits

NDx: BODY IMAGE DISTURBANCE

- The nurse
  1. Recognizes and accepts the client's view about body image alteration
  2. Develops a trusting relationship with the client
  3. Allows the client to verbalize his or her feelings
  4. Emphasizes the client's strengths and remaining capabilities
  5. Assists the client to set realistic goals regarding life-style

NDx: POTENTIAL FOR INJURY

- The nurse
  1. Maintains a hazard-free environment to prevent falls and to minimize trauma
  2. Teaches strengthening exercises

NDx: ANXIETY

- The nurse
  1. Answers questions openly and honestly
  2. Explains all procedures and aspects of care, including the rationale and importance of each aspect

Discharge Planning

- The nurse
  1. Ensures that the client can correctly use all assistive-adaptive devices ordered for home use
  2. Teaches complications and side effects of radiation therapy, such as dry skin
  3. Teaches complications and side effects of chemotherapy, such as nausea and vomiting

4. Teaches wound care, as needed
5. Develops and reinforces a pain management program
   a. Drug information, including the importance of taking the correct dosage and at the right time
   b. Progressive relaxation techniques and music therapy
6. Reviews the prescribed exercise regimen
7. Emphasizes the importance of follow-up visits with the physician(s) and other members of the health care team
8. Refers the client to a local cancer support group

For more information on malignant bone tumors, see *Medical-Surgical Nursing: A Nursing Process Approach,* **pp. 761–768.**

Brain Abscess

- A brain abscess is a purulent infection of the brain in which pus forms in the extradural, subdural, or intracerebral area of the brain.
- The causative organisms are most often bacteria.
- A brain abscess is typically manifested by symptoms of a mass lesion and mild increased intracranial pressure, including
  1. Headache, nausea, and vomiting
  2. Mild lethargy and slight confusion
  3. Decreased peripheral vision
  4. Generalized weakness and possibly hemiparesis
  5. Ataxia, nystagmus, and dysconjugate gaze
- Drug therapy includes
  1. Antibiotics; metronidazole (Flagyl) if an anaerobic organism is the cause

2. Phenytoin (Dilantin) to prevent seizures
● Occasionally surgical drainage of an encapsulated abscess may be performed.

For more information on brain abscess, see *Medical-Surgical Nursing: A Nursing Process Approach,* **pp. 903–905.**

Brain Tumor

OVERVIEW

● Brain tumors arise anywhere within the brain structure and are named according to the cell or tissue from which they originate.

● Primary tumors originate within the central nervous system (CNS) and occur as a rapid proliferation or abnormal growth of cells normally found within the CNS.

● Secondary tumors occur as a result of metastasis from other areas of the body, such as the lungs, breast, kidney, or gastrointestinal tract.

● Secondary tumors occur as malignant cells from tumors outside the CNS and metastasize to the brain.

● Malignant tumors include

1. *Gliomas*, which arise from the neuroglial cells and infiltrate and invade surrounding brain tissue
2. *Astrocytoma*, grades 2–4, which are found anywhere within the cerebral hemispheres
3. *Oligodendrogliomas*, which are generally located within the temporal lobes of the brain and are slow growing
4. *Glioblastomas*, which are highly malignant, rapidly growing, invasive astrocytomas
5. *Ependymomas*, which arise from the lining of the ventricles and are difficult to treat because of their location

- Benign tumors include
  1. *Grade I astrocytoma* (may undergo changes and become malignant)
  2. *Meningiomas*, which are highly vascular and arise from the meninges; although complete removal is possible, they tend to reoccur
  3. *Pituitary tumors*, which result in a wide variety of symptoms caused by their effect on the pituitary gland
  4. *Acoustic neuromas*, which arise from the sheath of Schwann's cells in the peripheral portion of cranial nerve VIII; they compress brain tissue and tend to surround adjacent cranial nerves (V, VII, IX and X)
- The remainder of adult tumors are of miscellaneous origin.

COLLABORATIVE MANAGEMENT

Assessment

- The nurse records the client's
  1. Headache, which is generally more severe upon awakening
  2. Vomiting shortly after awakening that is not accompanied by nausea (The client may eat a full breakfast after vomiting without further episodes of emesis.)
  3. Double vision, decreased visual acuity, and visual field deficit
- The nurse elicits the following information concerning each symptom
  1. When the symptom first occurred
  2. Whether the symptom has increased or decreased in severity
  3. Pattern of occurrence
  4. Triggering event(s)
  5. Actions taken to relieve the symptom
- The nurse assesses for changes in neurologic status
  1. Decreased level of consciousness, stupor, or coma
  2. Pupils that are large or pinpoint and nonreactive to light; papilledema; VI cranial nerve palsy
  3. Decreased motor strength, hemiparesis, hemiplegia
  4. Inability to follow commands, disorientation
  5. Diminished sensation, hyperesthesia, astereognosis, agnosia, apraxia, agraphia
  6. Broca's or Wernicke's aphasia, dysarthria
  7. Cranial nerve dysfunction

8. Ataxic gait
9. Seizure activity
10. Personality and behavior changes
11. Indication of anxiety and fear

Planning and Implementation

NDx: ALTERED (CEREBRAL) TISSUE PERFUSION

B

Nonsurgical Management

- The nurse
    1. Performs a neurologic assessment every 4 hours or more often if clinically indicated
        a. Verbal response, orientation
        b. Eye opening, pupil size and reaction to light
        c. Motor response
        d. Vital signs
    2. Elevates the head of bed 30 to 45 degrees
    3. Administers analgesic for headache, as ordered
    4. Administers dexamethasone (Decadron) to control cerebral edema, as ordered
    5. Administers phenytoin (Dilantin) to prevent seizures, as ordered
    6. Administers cimetidine (Tagamet) or ranitidine (Zantec) to prevent stress ulcers, as ordered
    7. Administers prochlorperazine (Compazine) or other antiemetics for nausea, as ordered

- Radiation therapy is used alone or in combination with surgery and chemotherapy.

- The radiation dose is based on tumor type and location, as well as the client's response or toleration of the treatment.

- Radiation often causes the skin to be reddened and irritated.

- The nurse
    1. Never uses alcohol, powder, oils, or creams without the written permission of the physician because these products can cause severe burns during the next treatment
    2. Does not wash the marks off the skin that outline the area of radiation
    3. Observes and reports side effects of radiation, including nausea, vomiting, anorexia, dry mouth, and mild temporary increase in intracranial pressure
    4. Offers small frequent meals and hard candy for dry mouth
    5. Encourages fluid unless contraindicated

- Chemotherapy may be given alone or in combination with surgery and radiation therapy.

- The medications are usually injected intrathecally; a reservoir is inserted into the ventricles to give intraventricular medications.
- The nurse
  1. Observes for side effects of chemotherapy, including nausea, vomiting, diarrhea, alopecia, irritation of the oral mucosa, and anorexia
  2. Administers antiemetics prior to chemotherapy, as ordered, and as often as needed at the completion of the treatment
  3. Monitors complete blood count (CBC) since chemotherapeutic agents may cause bone marrow suppression

Surgical Management

- Conventional dissection, laser, or a stereotaxic approach may be used depending on the tumor type, size, and location.
- The nurse provides preoperative care
  1. Provides routine preoperative care
  2. Informs the client that all or part of his or her hair will be shaved
  3. Provides information about the intensive care unit (ICU) if the client will go there after surgery
- The nurse provides postoperative care
  1. Monitors vital signs every hour until stable
  2. Monitors neurologic signs every hour until stable
  3. Records strict intake and output every hour; checks urine specific gravity every hour or with every voiding
  4. Implements cardiac monitoring while in the ICU
  5. Does not position on operative site
  6. Monitors serum electrolytes, CBC, and osmolarity
  7. Applies thigh-high antiembolism stockings
  8. Turns, coughs, and deep breathes the client every 2 hours
  9. Elevates the head of bed 30 to 45 degrees
  10. Checks the head dressing for drainage
  11. Measures output from the surgical (Hemovac) drain every 8 hours
  12. Observes for and reports complications of cranial surgery (craniotomy)
      a. Increased intracranial pressure (ICP) includes
         (1) Change in level of consciousness, restlessness, or irritability
         (2) Pupils large or pinpoint and nonreactive to light

  (3) Decreased or absent motor movement
  (4) Decerebrate or decorticate posturing
  (5) Seizure activity
  (6) Bradycardia and hypertension with
    widened pulse pressure

 b. Epidural or subdural hematoma includes the
  same complications as for increased ICP plus

  (1) Severe headache
  (2) Bleeding into the posterior fossa, which
    may cause cardiac and respiratory arrest

 c. Hydrocephalus includes the same
  complications as for increased ICP plus

  (1) VI cranial nerve palsy
  (2) Urinary incontinence

 d. Wound infection

  (1) Incision is reddened, puffy
  (2) Incision may separate
  (3) Sensitive to touch, feels warm
  (4) Client may be febrile
  (5) Treatment based on severity of
    symptoms
   —Cleanse with alcohol and apply antiseptic
    ointment
   —Systemic antibiotics

NDx: PAIN

- The nurse

 1. Assesses the severity, location, and extent of the
  pain
 2. Administers analgesics, such as codeine
  phosphate and acetaminophen, as ordered
 3. Recognizes that severe pain may indicate
  increased ICP or other complications

NDx: POTENTIAL FOR INJURY

- The nurse

 1. Implements seizure precautions (see Epilepsy)
 2. Orients the client to time, place, and event
 3. Maintains a structured, repetitive schedule
 4. Has the family bring in pictures and other
  familiar objects
 5. Restrains only if necessary; uses seat belt when up
  in chair
 6. Maintains normal day-night cycle

NDx: ANXIETY AND FEAR

- The nurse

 1. Encourages the client and family to discuss their
  concerns regarding the diagnosis and treatment

2. Provides preoperative and postoperative teaching
3. Advises the physician of client concerns to enable the surgeon to plan sufficient time to answer these questions
4. Helps the client/family to develop a list of questions to ask the physician

Discharge Planning

- The nurse
  1. Identifies and suggests corrections of hazards in the home prior to discharge
  2. Ensures that the client can correctly use all assistive-adaptive devices ordered for home use
  3. Provides a detailed plan of care at the time of discharge for clients to be transferred to a rehabilitation or long-term-care facility (rehabilitation may be a lengthy process) (see Rehabilitation)
  4. Provides drug information as needed
  5. Teaches seizure precautions
  6. Obtains a dietary consult to ensure adequate caloric intake for the client receiving radiation or chemotherapy
  7. Emphasizes the importance of follow-up visits with the physician(s) and other therapists

For more information on brain tumors, see *Medical-Surgical Nursing: A Nursing Process Approach,* **pp. 947–956.**

Breast Cancer

OVERVIEW

- The most common type of breast cancer is infiltrating *ductal carcinoma*, which originates in the epithelial cells lining the mammary ducts; the cancer remaining in the duct is noninvasive.
- Cancer is classified as invasive when it penetrates the

tissue surrounding the duct and grows in an irregular pattern.

- The mass is irregular and poorly defined; fibrosis develops around the cancerous tumor and contributes to dimpling, which is characteristically seen in advanced disease.
- The tumor invades the lymphatic channels, blocking skin drainage and causing edema and an orange peel appearance of the skin (peau d'orange).
- Invasion of the lymphatic channels carries tumor cells to the lymphatic nodes in the axilla.
- The tumor replaces the skin, and ulceration of the overlying skin occurs.
- Common sites of metastatic disease are the bone, lungs, brain, and liver.
- The stages of breast cancer are
  1. Stage I: smaller than 2 cm without lymph node involvement
  2. Stage II: 2 to 5 cm without lymph node involvement
  3. Stage III: larger than 5 cm with no lymph node involvement; smaller than 2 cm with axillary nodes or 2 to 5 cm with supraclavicular or intraclavicular nodes
  4. Stage IV: any size, with or without lymph node involvement but distant metastasis is present

COLLABORATIVE MANAGEMENT

Assessment

- The nurse records the client's
  1. Age, sex, and race
  2. Marital status
  3. Height and weight
  4. Personal and family history of breast cancer
  5. Hormonal history
  6. Age at first menarche
  7. Age at menopause
  8. Age at first child's birth
  9. Number of children
  10. History of breast mass discovery and medical care intervention
  11. Health maintenance, including regularity of breast self-examination and mammography history
  12. Diet history, including alcohol intake
  13. Medications
- The nurse assesses for
  1. Mass location, size, shape, consistency, and fixation to surrounding tissues

2. Skin changes, such as dimpling, peau d'orange, increased vascularity, nipple retraction, or ulceration
3. Enlarged axillary and supraclavicular lymph nodes
4. Breast pain or soreness

Planning and Implementation

NDx: ANXIETY

Nonsurgical Management

- The nurse
  1. Assesses the client's perceptions and personal level of anxiety concerning the possible diagnosis
  2. Allows the client to ventilate feelings, even if a diagnosis has not been established
  3. Encourages the client to seek information and outside resources
  4. Contacts resource people, if needed

NDx: POTENTIAL FOR INJURY

Nonsurgical Management

- Radiation may be used in conjunction with chemotherapy for late-stage breast cancer.

Surgical Management

- Conservative surgical management of breast cancer is used for early disease and usually involves *lumpectomy with lymph node dissection*, in which only the tumor and lymph nodes are removed, leaving the breast tissue intact, or a *simple mastectomy*, in which breast tissue and usually the nipple are removed, but the lymph nodes are left intact, followed by radiation.

- In a *modified radical mastectomy*, the breast tissue, nipple, and lymph nodes are removed, but muscles are left intact.

- In a *radical radical mastectomy*, the breast tissue, nipple, underlying muscles, and lymph nodes are removed.

- Preoperative care focuses on psychologic preparation, as well as usual preoperative measures. (See Preoperative Care.)

- The nurse provides postoperative care
  1. Places the client on the back or unaffected side, with the arm on the surgical side elevated on a pillow
  2. Assesses drains and dressings for constriction, position, and functioning
  3. Records amount of and reports excess postoperative drainage

4. Assesses operative site for swelling or presence of fluid collection under skin flaps
5. Consults with the physical therapist to recommend and teach the client appropriate postmastectomy exercises (with the physician's consent)
6. Reviews the exercise program with the client
7. Assesses for signs and symptoms of infection
8. Provides routine postoperative care

- The nurse teaches the client to

1. Avoid having blood pressures taken, blood drawn, or injections on the affected arm
2. Avoid injury to the affected arm, such as burns, scratches, and scrapes
3. Treat injuries immediately to avoid infection

- The decision to follow the original surgical procedure with chemotherapy, radiation, or hormonal therapy is based on the stage of the breast cancer, the age and menopausal state of the client, client preference, and hormonal receptor status.

Discharge Planning

- The nurse teaches the client/family

1. Measures to optimize positive body image following mastectomy
2. Information to enhance interpersonal relationships and roles
3. Postmastectomy exercises to regain full range of motion
4. Measures to prevent infection of the incision
5. Measures to avoid injury, infection, and swelling of the affected arm, including no blood pressure measurements, injections, or venipunctures; wearing mitts or gloves for protection when appropriate; and treating cuts and scrapes quickly
6. The importance of avoiding deodorant, lotion or ointment on the affected arm
7. The importance of reporting signs of swelling, redness, increased heat, and tenderness to the physician

- The nurse refers the client to community resources, including Reach for Recovery and Encore.

For more information on breast cancer, see *Medical-Surgical Nursing: A Nursing Process Approach*, **pp. 1667–1685.**

Breast Fibroadenoma

- A breast fibroadenoma is the most common breast lump that occurs during the teenage years.
- The fibroadenoma is a solid, benign mass of connective tissue that is unattached to the surrounding breast tissue.
- The lump is characteristically firm, hard but not cystic, easily movable, and clearly delineated from surrounding tissue, and it is usually located in the upper outer quadrant of the breast.
- A needle aspiration is performed to establish whether the lump is cystic or solid.
- Solid lumps are usually excised on an outpatient basis by local anesthesia.

For more information on breast fibroadenomas, see *Medical-Surgical Nursing: A Nursing Process Approach*, **p. 1665.**

Bronchitis, Acute

OVERVIEW

- Acute bronchitis is an inflammation of the bronchi associated with increased mucus production.
- Chemical agents or microorganisms assault conducting airways, inducing an inflammatory response that causes vasoconstriction, followed by vasodilation and transudation of fluid into interstitial spaces and airway lumen.
- Migration of polymorphonuclear white blood cells into the mucus exudate changes sputum to a yellow-green color.

• Bloody sputum occurs from ulceration of the mucosa with exfoliation of bronchial epithelial cells.

COLLABORATIVE MANAGEMENT
Assessment

• The nurse records the client's
  1. Age
  2. Presence of chronic lung disease
  3. Medication use (steroids, bronchodilators, antibiotics)
  4. Use of cigarettes and alcohol
  5. Activity and rest
  6. Recent viral episode or infection
  7. Exposure to environmental pollution
  8. Respiratory symptoms
• The nurse assesses for
  1. Dyspnea
  2. Breathing patterns
  3. Color
  4. Position
  5. Adventitious lung sounds
  6. Abnormal dullness on percussion
  7. Amount, color, quantity, and quality of sputum
  8. Frequency of coughing
  9. Fever
  10. Tachycardia
  11. Mental status changes

Planning and Implementation
NDx: INEFFECTIVE AIRWAY CLEARANCE AND IMPAIRED GAS EXCHANGE

• The nurse
  1. Monitors respiratory status, including blood gas results
  2. Assists the client with learning coughing and breathing techniques
  3. Teaches the client to conserve energy due to increased coughing episodes
  4. Provides chest physical therapy and postural drainage
  5. Increases oral fluid intake
  6. Provides room humidification
  7. Administers humidified aerosol treatments, as ordered
  8. Uses care when administering cough suppressants, as ordered
  9. Administers antibiotic therapy, as ordered
  10. Administers inhaled bronchodilators, as ordered

Discharge Planning

- The nurse teaches the client/family to
  1. Increase activity gradually to avoid fatigue
  2. Avoid crowds, chilling, and exposure to others with respiratory tract infections or viruses
  3. Avoid smoking
  4. Follow medication instructions for antibiotics, bronchodilators, inhaled bronchodilators, and/or inhaled steroids, including prescriptions
  5. Maintain adequate hydration to liquefy secretions
  6. Use coughing and breathing techniques, as instructed
  7. Keep follow-up visits with the physician(s)

For more information on acute bronchitis, see *Medical-Surgical Nursing: A Nursing Process Approach*, **pp. 1986–1988.**

Buerger's Disease

- Buerger's disease, or thromboangiitis obliterans, is an uncommon occlusive arterial vascular disease limited to medium and small arteries and veins in the body; larger arteries become involved in the late stages of disease.

- The distal upper and lower limbs are most frequently affected.

- The disease often extends to the perivascular tissue, resulting in fibrosis and scarring that binds the artery, vein, and nerve firmly together.

- The cause of the disease is unknown.

- There is a strong incidence associated with smoking, familial or genetic predisposition, and autoimmune etiologies.

- Smoking cessation arrests the disease process; persistence in smoking causes occlusion in more proximal vessels.

- Clinical manifestations include
  1. Claudication (pain in muscles resulting from an inadequate blood supply) of the arch of the foot
  2. Intermittent claudication in the lower extremities
  3. Ischemic pain occurring in the digits while at rest
  4. Increased sensitivity to cold
  5. Complaints of coldness and numbness
  6. Diminished pulses in the distal extremities
  7. Cool extremities
  8. Red or cyanotic extremities in dependent position
- Interventions include
  1. Complete abstinence from alcohol and smoking
  2. Prevention of extreme or prolonged exposure to cold
  3. Vasodilator drugs

For more information on Buerger's disease, see *Medical-Surgical Nursing: A Nursing Process Approach*, **pp. 2225–2226.**

Bulimia Nervosa

OVERVIEW

- Bulimia nervosa ia an eating disorder characterized by secret episodes of binge eating that recur, are uncontrolled, and involve the ingestion of large amounts of food in a short time.
- Binge eating is usually followed by some form of purging behavior, such as vomiting and/or the excess use of laxatives or diuretics.
- Purging behavior is an attempt to regain a sense of control and to eliminate the ingested calories; it may be precipitated by a variety of factors, such as hunger, boredom, anger, anxiety, or depression.
- An intense fear of fatness distinguishes the bulimic from individuals who binge-eat for pleasure or stress reduction.

- DSM-III-R diagnostic criteria include
  1. Recurrent episodes of binge eating (rapid consumption of a large amount of food in a discrete period of time)
  2. A feeling of lack of control over eating behavior during the eating binges
  3. Regular self-induced vomiting, use of laxatives or diuretics, strict dieting or fasting, or vigorous exercise to prevent weight gain
  4. A minimum average of two binge-eating episodes a week for at least 3 months
  5. Persistent overconcern with body shape and weight.

COLLABORATIVE MANAGEMENT

Assessment

- The nurse records the client's
  1. Sequelae of vomiting and laxative abuse, including cardiac, renal, or gastrointestinal tract problems
  2. History of seizures
  3. Use of ipecac syrup to induce vomiting
  4. Weight history, including highest, lowest, and fluctuations
  5. Sexual activity and/or abuse
  6. Attitudes and behaviors related to food and weight
  7. Specific information about binges
  8. Method of purging
  9. Activity
  10. Previous episodes of psychiatric illness
  11. Family history
- Also see Anorexia Nervosa ("Assessment").
- The nurse assesses for
  1. Normal, healthy body (usually)
  2. Weakness and tiredness
  3. Constipation
  4. Depression
  5. Irregular heartbeat
  6. Signs of urinary tract infection
  7. Seizures and peripheral paresthesias
  8. Dry swelling and swelling of the parotid glands
  9. Loss of tooth enamel and color change
  10. Gastrointestinal tract disturbances, such as esophagitis, gastric dilation, or loss of bowel reactivity
  11. Dehydration alternating with rebound fluid retention
  12. Irregular menses or amenorrhea

Planning and Implementation

NDx: ALTERED NUTRITION: MORE THAN BODY REQUIREMENTS

• Tranylcypromine sulfate, a monoamine oxidase inhibitor, is used to decrease the client's urge to binge.

• Based on the client's basal metabolic rate, caloric requirements may be low for the bulimic (1000 to 1200 kcal per day).

• The nurse
  1. Stresses that correct food portions and eating patterns are emphasized rather than calorie counting
  2. Encourages the client to eat slowly
  3. Teaches the importance of increased activity level and a regular exercise program
  4. Cautions the client to avoid exercise extremes

NDx: POTENTIAL FOR DECREASED CARDIAC OUTPUT

• The nurse
  1. Administers oral potassium supplements, as ordered, to treat potassium levels of 3.0 to 3.4; decreased potassium levels may cause cardiac dysrhythmias, which can lead to sudden cardiac arrest
  2. Administers intravenous sodium chloride and potassium, as ordered, for more serious electrolyte imbalances
  3. Monitors vital signs and assesses for irregular pulse rate and rhythm
  4. Monitors cardiac status
  5. Monitors for recurrent purging behaviors

NDx: FLUID VOLUME EXCESS

• The nurse
  1. Provides a low-sodium diet (2g/day) to minimize fluid retention
  2. Limits fluid intake to 1000 mL daily when edema is severe
  3. Elevates the client's extremities
  4. Suggests comfortable, nonrestricting clothing and shoes
  5. Teaches the client to avoid wearing rings
  6. Applies cool compresses over the eyes to decrease facial edema

NDx: CONSTIPATION

• The goal of therapy is to establish a regular pattern of elimination without the use of laxatives.

NDx: Ineffective Individual Coping/Self-Esteem Disturbance

- Antidepressants are indicated for depression; otherwise medication is not indicated.
- The nurse
    1. Arranges for individual therapy with a psychiatrist, psychologist, or psychiatric nurse specialist as an inpatient and after discharge
    2. Initiates a supportive, behavioral therapy program
    3. Teaches the client/family about groups that provide support during periods of stress and on an ongoing basis

NDx: Potential for Noncompliance

- The nurse
    1. Monitors behavior and provides support combined with client motivation
    2. Instructs the client/family with specific information related to the illness and treatment plan, emphasizing the consequences of noncompliance
- If the client is treated with a monoamine oxidase inhibitor, noncompliance is particularly serious because foods with high tyramine levels, including aged cheese or chianti wine, may precipitate hypertensive crisis.

Discharge Planning

- Educational efforts are focused on teaching the client/family to recognize and understand the physical, behavioral, and emotional characteristics of bulimia.
- The nurse
    1. Teaches the client/family to recognize the physical manifestations of bulimia that require medical interventions
    2. Develops an individualized teaching plan to identify client-specific problems to move toward wellness
    3. Stresses the importance of continued individual client therapy and family therapy
    4. Emphasizes the importance of follow-up visits with the physician(s) and psychotherapist

For more information on bulimia nervosa, see *Medical-Surgical Nursing: A Nursing Process Approach*, **pp. 1434–1443.**

Burn Injury

OVERVIEW

- A burn is an injury to the skin and other epithelial tissues caused by exposure to temperature extremes, radiation, electrical current, mechanical abrasion, or chemical abrasion.
- Burns are classified according to their depth:
  1. *Partial-thickness* injuries damage only part of the skin, with remaining tissue capable of stimulating regeneration and successful wound healing.
     a. *First-degree* burns are superficial partial-thickness injuries (epidermis is the only portion of the skin injured or destroyed).
     b. *Second-degree* burns are deep partial-thickness injuries
        (1) Superficial second-degree burns reach only the upper layers of the dermis.
        (2) Deep second-degree burns reach the deeper layers of the dermis and destroy structures within the dermis, such as nerves and hair follicles.

  2. *Full-thickness* burns involve damage to all layers of the skin and do not heal spontaneously.
     a. *Third-degree* burns damage the entire dermal layer down to and sometimes including the subcutaneous fat; all dermal appendages are destroyed, and the regeneration function of the skin is absent.
     b. *Fourth-degree* burns occur when damage extends beyond the subcutaneous level and includes muscle and bone; usually the wounds contain a thick, dry, charred eschar, which is black and always without sensation.
- The expected course of illness is as follows
  1. *Emergent* period
     a. Begins at the time of injury and is characterized by vascular changes
     b. Most life-threatening complications are shock and respiratory failure
     c. Lasts between 24 and 48 hours
  2. *Acute* phase
     a. Continues until all wounds are closed
     b. Client is at high risk for infection
     c. Lasts from 1 week to several months

3. *Rehabilitation* stage
   a. Period of intense effort to regain or compensate for functions lost as a result of the burn
   b. May last for several years
- Typical types of burns and emergency interventions limiting the extent of injury include
  1. *Thermal*: The client should Stop, Drop, and Roll to smother flames; clothes that are on fire or saturated with hot liquids should be removed.
  2. *Chemical*: Treatment depends on the type of chemical involved but generally should be flushed with copious amounts of water; agents containing sodium or potassium are covered with mineral oil and are not flushed with water.
  3. *Electrical*: The client should be separated from the electric current by shutting off the source of electricity or using a nonconductive implement, such as wooden poles or ropes made of plant fiber.
  4. *Radiation*: Treatment depends on whether the source is sealed or not sealed (self-contained).

COLLABORATIVE MANAGEMENT

Assessment

- The nurse records
  1. Time of injury
  2. Source of heat or injurious agent
  3. Detailed description of how the burn occurred
  4. Whether the influence of alcohol or drugs may have been a factor
  5. A description of the place/environment where the burn occurred
  6. Events occurring from the time of the burn to admission
  7. Any other events or circumstances contributing to the injury
- The nurse records the client's
  1. Past medical history
  2. Current medications
  3. Smoking history and history of drug or alcohol use
  4. Weight
- The nurse assesses for
  1. Direct airway injury, including
     a. Changes in the appearance and function of the mouth, nose, pharynx, trachea, and pulmonary mechanisms

    b. Facial injury or singed hair on the head, eyebrows, eyelids, and nasal mucosa
    c. Blisters and soot on the lips and oral mucosa
    d. Alterations in breathing patterns (progressive hoarseness, expiratory wheeze, crowing, and stridor)

2. Carbon monoxide poisoning, including

    a. Headache
    b. Decreased cerebral function and visual acuity, coma
    c. Tinnitus
    d. Nausea
    e. Irritability
    f. Pale to reddish-purple skin

3. Smoke poisoning, including

    a. Atelectasis and pulmonary edema
    b. Hemorrhagic bronchitis 6 to 72 hours after injury

4. Pulmonary parenchymal failure, including

    a. Shortness of breath, hypoxia
    b. Moist breath sounds and crackles

5. Cardiovascular dysfunction, including

    a. Hypovolemic and/or cardiogenic shock
    b. Rapid thready pulse
    c. Hypotension and a wide pulse pressure
    d. Diminished peripheral pulses
    e. Slow or absent capillary refill
    f. Edema
    g. Complications that generally develop 48 hours after injury, such as fluid overload, heart failure, and pulmonary edema

6. Renal dysfunction, including

    a. Decreased urinary output
    b. Renal failure

7. Integumentary changes, including

    a. Size and depth of injury
    b. Color and appearance of skin

8. Gastrointestinal (GI) dysfunction, including

    a. Paralytic ileus
    b. Gastric dilation and vomiting
    c. GI ulceration
    d. Occult blood in the stool

9. Neuroendocrine dysfunction, including

    a. Hypothermia
    b. Weight loss and subsequent negative nitrogen balance

    c. Pseudodiabetes, which causes hyperglycemia and ketosis

10. Immune system dysfunction, including

    a. Infections
    b. Sepsis

11. Musculoskeletal dysfunction, including

    a. Problems that develop secondary to immobility, healing process, treatment, and other injuries
    b. Decreased range of motion (ROM)

12. Body image changes
13. Grieving
14. Anxiety and fear

Planning and Implementation

NDx: DECREASED CARDIAC OUPUT; FLUID VOLUME DEFICIT; ALTERED TISSUE PERFUSION

- The client receives extensive infusion of intravenous fluids; commonly used fluids include Ringer's lactate, normal saline, colloids, and glucose in water.

- The nurse

  1. Follows facility fluid resuscitation formula/protocol
  2. Monitors vital signs to determine adequate fluid resuscitation, including
     a. Clear mentation
     b. Normal blood pressure and pulse for the client
     c. Central venous pressure (CVP) between 6 and 9
     d. Urinary output equal to 1 mL of urine per kilogram of body weight (or 30 to 100 mL) per hour
  3. Records strict measurement of intake and output
  4. Adjusts fluid intake to maintain urinary output between 30 and 100 mL per hour
  5. Does not administer diuretics as they decrease circulating volume and cardiac output and may lead to a dangerous reduction in perfusion to other vital organs; however, diuretics may be given to the client with an electrical burn, as ordered
  6. Provides intensive cardiac monitoring such as CVP, pulmonary artery pressures, and cardiac output
  7. Monitors for cardiac dysrhythmias such as atrial fibrillation

- An escharotomy may be performed to incise but not remove the eschar, if present.

NDx: INEFFECTIVE BREATHING PATTERN

- The nurse
  1. Performs a respiratory assessment every hour
     a. Auscultates the lung fields for quality and depth of respirations
     b. Loosens tight dressings if necessary to facilitate chest expansion
  2. Turns and encourages the client to cough and deep breathe at least every 2 hours
  3. Has intubation equipment readily available (crowing, stridor, and dyspnea are indications for immediate intubation)
  4. Suctions client as clinically indicated; obtains sputum culture to determine if an infection is contributing to breathing problems
  5. Performs chest physiotherapy and incentive spirometry
  6. Administers aerosol treatments, as ordered
  7. Obtains arterial blood gases and chest x-rays, as indicated
  8. Administers oxygen therapy; intubation and mechanical ventilation are indicated if the PaO_2 is less than 60 mmHg
  9. Administers antibiotics, as ordered, for pneumonia or other pulmonary infections

- Extracorporeal membrane oxygenation (ECHMO) may help the client with severe lung damage.

NDx: PAIN

- The nurse
  1. Assesses the client's pain tolerance, coping mechanisms, and physical status
  2. Administers narcotic and nonnarcotic analgesics such as morphine, meperidine (Demerol), and pentazocine (Talwin), as ordered
  3. Monitors the client receiving anesthetic agents such as ketamine (Ketalar), pentobarbital sodium (Nembutal), and nitrous oxide
  4. Teaches relaxation techniques, meditative breathing, guided imagery, and music therapy
  5. Increases the client's sleep and rest periods to reduce the adverse effects of sleep deprivation, replenish catecholamine stores, and restore the diurnal effects of endorphins
  6. Provides tactile stimulation through frequent position changes and massages; maintains a comfortable room temperature
  7. Allows the client participation in pain control (e.g., patient-controlled analgesia)

NDx: Impaired Skin Integrity

- The health care team performs an in-depth assessment of burned and nonburned skin areas to determine the degree of skin integrity, adequacy of circulation, presence of infection, and effectiveness of therapy.

- Wound débridement procedures include
  1. *Mechanical*: using hydrotherapy (immersion in tub, shower on a specially designed table, successively washing only small areas of the wound); forceps and scissors are used to remove loose, nonviable tissue
  2. *Enzymatic*: can occur naturally by autolysis (spontaneous disintegration of tissue by the action of the client's own cellular enzymes) or artificially by application of proteolytic agents such as sutilains (Travase)
  3. *Surgical*: excising the burn wound by either a tangential or a fascial excision technique and covering it with a skin graft or temporary covering. The procedure, done within the first 5 days after injury, reduces the number of hydrotherapy treatments that are needed, but risks include massive blood loss and complications associated with anesthesia.

- Types of dressings typically used are
  1. *Standard*: involve the application of topical antibiotics on the burn wound, followed by sterile application of multiple layers of gauze. The number of gauze layers used depends on the depth of injury, the amount of drainage expected, the client's mobility, and the frequency of dressing changes.
  2. *Biological*: contain some amount of viable tissue or are derived from once-living tissue.
     a. Used to débride untidy wounds after eschar separation, to promote reepithelialization of deep second-degree burns, to cover a burn temporarily after wound excision, and to protect granulation tissue between autografts.
     b. *Heterograft* dressing is skin from another species such as a pig. Rejection occurs after 24 to 72 hours, and the pigskin is replaced on a continuous basis until closure with an autograft is complete.
     c. *Homograft* is skin from another human, usually a cadaver. Rejection can occur after 24 hours, but in some cases the graft has remained adherent for up to 90 days.

3. *Synthetic* and *biosynthetic*, such as Op Site, Vigilon, Biobrane, and Tegaderm; usually in place for 2 to 5 days.

NDx: POTENTIAL FOR INFECTION

- The nurse
  1. Monitors for signs of sepsis, including altered sensorium, increased respiratory rate, hypothermia or hyperthermia, oliguria, elevated serum glucose, glycosuria, decreased platelet count, and increased white blood cell count with a left shift
  2. Observes the wound for pervasive odor, exudate, changes in texture, purulent drainage, color changes, and redness at the wound edges

- Aggressive surgical débridement of the wound may be necessary if the colony count approaches 105 colonies/g of tissue.

- Tetanus toxoid is given; additional administration of tetanus immune globulin is recommended when the history of tetanus immunity is questionable.

- Topical antibiotics/antimicrobials are administered using the open technique (ointment is applied without further dressing of the wound) or closed technique (burn is covered with a dressing after the ointment is applied).

- Topical agents commonly used in the treatment of burns include
  1. Silver sulfadiazine (Silvadene)
     a. Adverse side effects include local allergic reactions and leukopenia.
     b. Not consistently effective for burns covering more than 60% of the client's body
  2. Mafenide acetate (Sulfamylon)
     a. Causes severe pain if used on partial-thickness burns
     b. Adverse side effects include metabolic acidosis and superinfection.
     c. Effective against *Pseudomonas*
  3. Silver nitrate
     a. Applied with the use of wet dressings that are bulky and uncomfortable and restrict the client's mobility; inexpensive
     b. Adverse reactions include electrolyte imbalance and difficulty with core body temperature maintenance
     c. Stings when applied; penetrates wound only 1 to 2 mm, so acts only on surface organisms

4. Sodium hypochlorite solution (Dakin's)
   a. Helps dry wounds that have become soupy and aids débridement
   b. As a side effect, dissolves blood clots and may inhibit clotting; may cause electrolyte imbalance
5. Povidone-iodine (Betadine)
   a. Effective against many infections not well controlled by silver sulfadiazine
   b. May cause electrolyte imbalance and metabolic acidosis and form crust if burns are not properly cleaned
6. Nitrofurazone (Furacin)
   a. Effective against *Staphylococcus aureus* and some antibiotic-resistant organisms
   b. May cause contact dermatitis; messy to apply
   c. May cause renal problems if used in clients with extensive burns
7. Gentamicin sulfate (Garamycin)
   a. Effective against many organisms, including *Pseudomonas*, and does not cause pain when applied
   b. Adverse reactions include ototoxicity and nephrotoxicity
8. Neomycin sulfate (Myciguent) bactericide used to reduce numbers of organisms before débriding and grafting burn
9. Bacitracin with polymyxin B sulfate (Polysporin)
   a. Bactericidal for gram-positive and gram-negative organisms; aesthetically suitable for use on face
   b. May cause itching, burning, or inflammation; cannot be used for full-thickness burns
10. Sutilains ointment (Travase)
    a. Digests necrotic tissue; aids in initial débridement before client can tolerate surgical débridement
    b. Adverse reactions include bleeding, increased fluid loss, and wound irritation
11. Bismuth tribromophenate (Xeroform)
    a. Débrides and protects donor sites and grafts; nontoxic and nonsensitizing
    b. Sticks to wound; removal is painful

• Systemic drugs used to treat infections include amikacin (Amikin), gentamicin (Apogen, Cidomycin, Garamycin), and tobramycin (Nebcin).

1. A higher dose than normal is required to maintain therapeutic serum levels; dosage is determined by peak and trough serum levels.
2. Adverse reactions include ototoxicity and nephrotoxicity.
- The nurse ensures isolation therapy
   1. Proper and consistent hand washing is the single most effective technique to prevent the transmission of infection.
   2. The client is isolated according to specific organism and facility procedure.
   3. Special isolation procedures may be needed if the organism becomes resistant to antibiotic therapy.
   4. Visitors are restricted while the client is immunosuppressed; ill persons and small children should be restricted.
- The nurse
   1. Wears gloves whenever coming in contact with the burn; changes gloves when handling wounds on different areas of the body
   2. Uses disposable equipment as much as possible and does not share equipment between clients

NDx: ALTERED NUTRITION: LESS THAN BODY REQUIREMENTS

- Total parenteral nutrition (TPN) may be needed until the client has sufficient gastric motility for oral or tube feedings
- The nurse
   1. Provides a high-calorie and high-protein diet and offers supplemental feedings as needed
   2. Collaborates with the dietitian and client to plan alternatives to conventional nutritional patterns
   3. Encourages the client to order food whenever the client feels he or she can eat, not just at the scheduled mealtime

NDx: IMPAIRED PHYSICAL MOBILITY

- The nurse
   1. Maintains the client in a neutral body position with minimal flexion
   2. Uses splints and other conforming devices according to the prescribed schedule
   3. Performs ROM exercises at least three times per day
   4. Begins ambulation as soon as possible
   5. Applies pressure dressings to prevent formation of contractures and tight hypertrophic scars, including
       a. Ace bandages

b. Custom -fitted elasticized clothing items (Jobst garments), which are worn 23 hours per day, every day, until the scar tissue is mature

- See Appendix D-1, p. 670, Guidelines for Positioning Burn Victim.

NDx: Body Image Disturbance

- The nurse
  1. Reassures the client that feelings of grief, loss, anxiety, anger, fear, and guilt are normal
  2. Collaborates with other health team members (e.g., psychiatrist, social worker) to address these problems
  3. Accepts the client's physical and psychological characteristics
  4. Provides information and support
  5. Engages the client in decision making and independent activities
  6. Provides information on and resources for reconstructive and cosmetic surgery, if needed

Discharge Planning

- The nurse begins the discharge process early by assessing the client's and family's readiness for discharge and care requirements.
- The nurse
  1. Identifies and suggests correction of hazards in the home prior to discharge
  2. Ensures that the client can correctly use all assistive-adaptive devices prior to discharge
  3. Provides a detailed plan of care for clients transferred to a rehabilitation or long-term-care facility
  4. Obtains a dietary consultation to help the client select personal food preferences appropriate for healing
  5. Provides drug information as needed
  6. Teaches wound care/dressing changes, including
     a. Use of correct technique
     b. How to dispose of soiled dressings
     c. Methods to prevent contamination
     d. Signs and symptoms of infection
  7. Teaches the proper use of prosthetic and positioning devices
  8. Teaches how to apply pressure garments correctly
  9. Refers to home health care as needed
  10. Helps the client to deal with the reactions of others to the sight of healing wounds and disfigurement

11. Emphasizes the importance of follow-up visits with the physician(s) and other members of the health care team

For more information on burns, see *Medical-Surgical Nursing: A Nursing Process Approach,* **pp. 361–401.**

Cancer, General

OVERVIEW

- Cancer is the second leading cause of death in the United States.
- Lung, colon, rectal, and prostate cancer are associated with the highest mortality in men.
- Breast, lung, colon, and rectal cancer are the leading cause of death in women.
- The danger of cancer is that it invades and destroys normal tissue, compromising physiological function in that tissue.
- Pathological alterations can occur as a result of treatment regimens and are referred to as secondary effects.
- Physiological dysfunction due to cancer may lead to
  1. Impaired immune and hematopoietic function
  2. Malnutrition
  3. Alteration in the structure and function of the gastrointestinal tract
  4. Motor and sensory dysfunction
  5. Altered mechanical and chemical defense mechanisms
  6. Infection and altered respiratory function
  7. Pain
  8. Organic sexual dysfunction.

COLLABORATIVE MANAGEMENT
Assessment
- The nurse records the client's
    1. Family history of cancer
    2. Exposure to known carcinogenics
    3. History of smoking
- The nurse assesses for
    1. The seven warning signs of cancer
        a. A change in bowel or bladder habits
        b. A sore that does not heal
        c. Unusual bleeding or discharge
        d. Thickening or lump in the breast or elsewhere
        e. Indigestion or difficulty swallowing
        f. An obvious change in a wart or mole
        g. Nagging cough or hoarseness
    2. Manifestations of infection
    3. Indications of metastasis to other organs
    4. Signs of bleeding such as petechiae, ecchymosis, and hematomas
    5. Anemia (shortness of breath, tachycardia, fatigue, and chest pain)
    6. Alterations in nutritional status
    7. Pain
    8. Changes potentially or actually affecting sexual functioning
    9. Anxiety, fear, stress
    10. Body image and self-concept changes

Planning and Implementation
NDx: POTENTIAL FOR INJURY

- Therapeutic decisions are determined by the type, grade, stage, and known or usual pattern of growth and spread of the cancer.

- *Primary* therapy refers to the initial or major form of therapy offered.

- *Adjuvant* therapy refers to modalities provided as an addition to the primary therapy.

- *Palliative* therapy refers to modalities that attempt to make the client more comfortable.

Surgical Management
- Surgery may be a treatment option with curative, control, palliative, and prophylactic goals.

- *En bloc dissection* is the total removal of the tumor and surrounding structures or tissues with nodal drainage.

- *Debulking* procedures remove as much of the tumor

as possible; minimal tumor remains to be controlled by adjuvant treatment.

- The extent of surgery is determined by the type of cancer and its growth pattern.
- *Electrosurgery* involves application of electrical current directly to cancer cells.
- *Cryosurgery* involves application of liquid nitrogen directly to tumor tissue; this procedure freezes and destroys cancer cells.
- *Chemosurgery* combines the application of cytotoxic chemicals and surgical excision of cancer cells.
- *CO_2 laser* is used for local excision of cancer cells.

Nonsurgical Management

- *Radiation therapy* is used as a primary, adjuvant, or palliative modality. It involves therapeutic application of high-energy rays to tumors.
- The action of ionizing radiation is essentially the same on both normal and malignant cells; normal cells that survive an initial, sublethal dose usually recover in 24 hours.
- Damage to normal cells is the primary cause of side effects and toxicities.
- The biological effects of radiation can be modified, which expands the range of therapeutic approaches.
- The type and method of delivery of radiation is determined by
    1. Location, depth, and stage of the cancer
    2. Field size needed
    3. Radiosensitivity of the cancer
    4. Client history and physical condition
- *External* radiation is delivered from an external source.
- *Intraoperative* radiation is delivered directly to the tumor site during a surgical procedure.
- *Intracavity implants* involve the temporary insertion of a sealed source into a body cavity, such as the vagina or uterus.
- *Radioactive isotopes* that are "sealed" are placed inside wires, needles, catheters, or seeds in interstitial implants to position the radioactive source directly into the tumor and surrounding tissue.
- Regulations for exposure to radiation are based on the concepts of *time, distance,* and *shielding.*
- The nurse
    1. Organizes tasks to minimize exposure
    2. Recognizes that most clients require minimal nursing care

3. Provides direct care from the head, foot, or side of the bed depending on the source of the radiation

• The nurse observes for and reports acute side effects of radiation therapy, including
1. Erythema, skin changes
2. Change and/or loss of taste, dry mouth
3. Pain, esophagitis
4. Nausea, vomiting, diarrhea
5. Cystitis
6. Diminished white blood count and platelets
7. Pneumonitis
8. Pericarditis, myocarditis (rare)
9. Edema and inflammation of the brain, spinal cord, or peripheral nerves

• Chemotherapeutic agents are used as primary, adjuvant, or palliative therapy.

• The nurse observes for and reports adverse effects of chemotherapy
1. Bone marrow suppression
2. Somatitis, mucositis
3. Nausea, vomiting, and anorexia
4. Alopecia
5. Skin reactions
   a. Hyperpigmentation, erythema, desquamation of the palms of the hands and soles of the feet (antimetabolites)
   b. Acne (Actinomycin D)
   c. Photosensitivity and hyperpigmentation of skin, and nails and along injected veins (methotrexate)
   d. Generalized urticaria (doxorubicin)
   e. Extravasation and subsequent local necrosis (actinomycin, daunomycin, doxorubicin, mithramycin, mitomycin, vinblastine, and vincristine)
6. Cardiomyopathy (doxorubicin [Adriamycin] and daunomycin)
7. Pneumonitis, interstitial fibrosis (bleomycin, busulphan, and carmustine)
8. Hematologic cystitis (cyclophosphamide [Cytoxan])
9. Acute tubular necrosis (cisplatin)
10. Paresthesia of the hands and feet, constipation, weakness, or impotence (vincristine)
11. Cerebral dysfunction (L-Asparaginase)

• Laboratory and other diagnostic tests are done to rule out renal, cardiac, and pulmonary disease before the following drugs are given:
1. Bleomycin: chest x-ray, pulmonary function tests

2. Cisplatin: creatine clearance, intravenous (IV) fluid hydration followed by diuretics to keep the kidneys flushed and to prevent accumulation of the drug in renal tubules, serum magnesium levels

- Other drugs are sometimes used in conjunction with chemotherapeutic agents to protect normal tissue.
    1. Mesna (Mesenex): used with ifosfamide (Iflex) to protect against renal toxicity
    2. Leucovorin (Citrovorum): given with methotrexate to prevent bone marrow toxicity
- The route of chemotherapy administration is determined by
    1. Pharmacokinetics of the drug
    2. Therapeutic goals
    3. Specific tumor factors
    4. Client's clinical status
- The routes for drug administration include
    1. Oral
    2. IV
    3. Intra-arterial
    4. Intrapleural
    5. Intraperitoneal
    6. Intrathecal
- Most chemotherapeutic agents are excreted in body fluids. Therefore, the nurse
    1. Properly handles and disposes of body fluids
    2. Dons gowns and gloves when handling blood, vomitus, or body excreta for 48 hours after drug administration
    3. Dons gowns, gloves, and eye protection when cleaning cytotoxic drug spills
- Most biological response modifiers (BRM) are still experimental.
- The actions of BRM include
    1. Modifying the host's biological responses to tumor cells
    2. Augmenting the host's defenses
    3. Increasing differentiation of tumor cells
    4. Increasing the host's ability to tolerate damage from other cytotoxic agents
- The classification of BRM includes
    1. Immunomodulating agents
    2. Interferon
    3. Interferon inducers
    4. Thympsins
    5. Lymphokines
    6. Cytokines

C

- The nurse observes for side effects of BRM, including
  1. Headache, fever, chills, myalgia, and flulike symptoms
  2. Fatigue, weakness
  3. Orthostatic blood pressure changes
  4. Cognitive changes and/or mood changes
  5. Nausea, vomiting and/or diarrhea
  6. Abnormal laboratory studies, including
     a. Complete blood count, differential, and platelet count
     b. Prothrombin time and partial thromboplastin time
     c. Lactate dehydrogenase, alanine aminotransferase, alkaline phosphatase, and aspartate aminotransferase
     d. Bilirubin level
     e. BUN, creatinine, and electrolyte levels

NDx: POTENTIAL FOR INFECTION

- Strict attention is given to prevention of infection in the client with cancer.
- The nurse
  1. Instructs the client to avoid large crowds and persons with upper respiratory infections when the leukocyte and granulocyte counts are low (generally between 7 and 14 days after administration of chemotherapeutic agents)
  2. Avoids invasive procedures, such as insertion of a Foley catheter
  3. Takes additional precautions for clients with granulocyte counts between 500 and 1000/mm^3, including
     a. A private room
     b. Strict attention to hand washing required by all staff and visitors
     c. No fresh flowers
     d. Proper nutrition and oral hygiene
  4. Is alert for subtle signs of infection and reports them to the physician
     a. Obtains urine, sputum, and blood cultures and a wound culture if appropriate
     b. Obtains a chest x-ray, as ordered
     c. Administers broad-spectrum antibiotics, as ordered, which are generally started after cultures are obtained and include cephalosporin, synthetic penicillin, and an aminoglycoside; may be changed based on culture results
     d. Monitors the client for response to antibiotics

5. Monitors for indications of septic shock

NDx: Potential for Altered (Cardiopulmonary) Tissue Perfusion

- The client with cancer is at risk for thrombocytopenia.
- The nurse
  1. Observes for bleeding
  2. Teaches the client how to assess for bleeding, risk factors, implications of bleeding, self-care measures, and other actions should bleeding occur
  3. Minimizes the number of venipunctures, injections, and suctionings
  4. Avoids rectal temperatures, rectal suppositories, enemas, and douches
  5. Applies pressure to venipuncture sites for 5 minutes
  6. Provides oral care using a soft toothbrush or sponge tooth swabs; avoids floss or toothpicks
  7. Instructs the client to use an electric razor for shaving

NDx: Activity Intolerance

- The nurse
  1. Instructs the client to
     a. Allow time for rest
     b. Utilize stress management and energy conservation techniques
     c. Eat a balanced diet
  2. Assesses the need for oxygen or a blood transfusion and notifies the physician

NDx: Altered Nutrition: Less Than Body Requirements

- Many clients report that one particular mealtime is better than another (often breakfast); as many of the daily requirements for nutrients as possible and tolerated by the client are incorporated into this meal.
- The nurse
  1. Administers vitamin supplements, as ordered
  2. Provides small, frequent meals for clients who experience early satiety
  3. Consults with the dietitian to vary spices in meals and marinates food in sweet sauces, sweet wines, or fruit juice, which may be helpful for clients with alterations in taste
  4. Provides oral hygiene before and after meals
  5. Does *not* use lemon glycerin swabs for mouth care; glycerin is an ideal bacterial medium

6. Makes a copy of the National Cancer Institutes (NCI) book *Eating Hints: Tips for Better Nutrition During Cancer Treatment* available (free of charge from the NCI)
7. Provides enteral feeding, as ordered; parenteral nutrition if the digestive system is not functional
8. Gives medications as ordered for nausea and vomiting; documents their effectiveness
9. Administers lidocaine (Xylocaine) liquid, as ordered, for stomatitis

NDx: DIARRHEA

- The nurse
  1. Provides a low-residue diet
  2. Encourages the client to drink at least 2000 mL of fluid per day unless contraindicated
  3. Records all episodes of diarrhea
  4. Administers antidiarrheal drugs, as ordered, such as loperamide (Imodium) or diphenoxylate with atropine (Lomotil)

NDx: CONSTIPATION

- Interventions depend on the frequency and cause of constipation.
- The nurse
  1. Provides a high-fiber diet
  2. Administers prophylactic laxatives as ordered, such as senna (Senokot), milk of magnesia, mineral oil, or magnesium citrate

NDx: IMPAIRED PHYSICAL MOBILITY

- The nurse
  1. Encourages the client to ambulate as much as possible
  2. Evaluates the need for an assistive device, such as a cane or walker
  3. Teaches muscle-strengthening exercises
- Radiation therapy may be used to control bone pain.
- Pathological fractures may occur secondary to hypercalcemia.

NDx: PAIN

- The nurse collaborates with other members of the health care team to develop a pain management program.
- An etiological diagnosis for each type of pain is established.
- An adequate analgesic dosage is used and titrated individually.
- Oral preparations are used when possible and may be administered prophylactically to prevent pain.

- Mild and moderate pain are treated with salicylate, acetaminophen, and nonsteroidal anti-inflammatory drugs.
- Severe pain is treated with narcotics such as codeine; meperidine, morphine, and hydromorphine are added as needed.
- Continuous IV and subcutaneous infusions of narcotic analgesics are individually titrated and often provide superior pain control.
- The nurse
  1. Anticipates side effects of medications
  2. Monitors the client for both side effects of the medication and indications of drug tolerance
  3. Administers anticonvulsant agents, phenothiazines, butyrophenones, tricyclic antidepressants, antihistamines, amphetamines, steroids, and levadopa, as ordered (have provided analgesic effects according to anecdotal reports)
- The nurse
  1. Teaches relaxation techniques (progressive muscle relaxation and guided imagery)
  2. Consults with a therapist to teach hypnosis
  3. Consults with a therapist to teach biofeedback
  4. Provides music, art, and recreation for diversion
  5. Applies transcutaneous electrical stimulation (TENS), as ordered
  6. Applies heat or cold
- Temporary or permanent nerve blocks may be used.
- Neurosurgical techniques such as a cordotomy or placement of epidural, intrathecal, and intraventricular catheters for drug delivery may be performed.

NDx: POTENTIAL FOR IMPAIRED SKIN INTEGRITY

- The nurse
  1. Prevents extravasation through meticulous attention to policies and procedures when administering chemotherapeutic agents
  2. Instructs clients receiving external radiation to avoid or reduce lotion, oil, temperature extremes, chemical irritants, tapes, and dressings on treatment sites
  3. Applies cornstarch, baby powder, baby oil, anhydrous lanolin, and other alcohol and menthol-free moisturizers for dry skin and erythema
  4. Applies moisture vapor–permeable and hydrocolloid dressing for moist desquamations
     a. Uses topical antibiotics, only if proved infection

    b. Applies topical steroid to relieve itching, but medications may increase susceptibility to injury

NDx: Impaired Gas Exchange

- Treatment of malignant pleural effusions includes
    1. Palliation of symptoms
    2. Systemic chemotherapy, hormonal treatment, or irradiation
    3. Evacuation of pleural fluid, reexpanding the lung, and obliterating the pleural space
    4. Sclerosing agents added to the pleural cavity through a chest tube immediately or after a period of drainage
        a. Agents used include antineoplastic agents (nitrogen mustard, 5-fluorouracil, bleomycin, and triethylenethiophosphoramide), radioisotopes of gold or phosphorus, and tetracycline
        b. Chest tube is clamped for a period of time after the agent is inserted
- Malignant tumors without pleural effusions are treated with external radiation to relieve dyspnea.

NDx: Sexual Dysfunction

- The nurse
    1. Provides counseling for clients who may experience sexual dysfunctions as a result of treatment
    2. Informs the client that he or she can consider depositing sperm in a sperm bank or making egg or embryo donations prior to treatment
    3. Informs the client that many clinicians recommend the use of birth control during and for 2 years after cancer treatment
    4. Provides information that may assist in changing or adding approaches to sexual expression and refers clients to an appropriate resource for specific intervention

NDx: Ineffective Individual Coping

- The nurse
    1. Assesses past experiences and coping strategies or skills that can be implemented
    2. Facilitates open communication
    3. Encourages the client to participate in the decision-making process
    4. Promotes acknowledgment of possible outcomes of the cancer
    5. Avoids forcing details on the client

6. Encourages sharing of fears and anxieties
7. Promotes the quality of life as well as the prolongation of life
8. Emphasizes what the client has instead of what was lost
9. Facilitates acceptance of the limitations imposed by cancer
10. Facilitates implementation of relaxation and meditation techniques

EMERGENCY CARE

- Hypercalcemia
  1. Seen most frequently in clients with cancer of the breast, lung, or multiple myeloma
  2. Manifested by lethargy, anorexia, nausea, vomiting, constipation, polyuria, nocturia, and dehydration
  3. Treatment
     a. Hydration with IV fluids followed by IV administration of furosemide (Lasix)
     b. Mithramycin (Mithracin) for severe hypercalcemia
     c. Diphosphanates such as etidronate (Didronel)
- Syndrome of inappropriate antidiuretic hormone (SIADH)
  1. Seen most often in small-cell lung cancer
  2. Manifested by hyponatremia, serum hyposmolality, and urinary hyperosmolality; weakness, muscle cramps, anorexia, and fatigue
  3. Treatment
     a. Fluid restriction
     b. Diuretics may be tried
     c. Hypertonic saline may be cautiously administered
     d. Strict measurement of intake and output
     e. Daily weights
- Spinal cord compression
  1. Associated with lung, prostate, breast, and colon cancers
  2. Manifested by back pain, numbness, tingling, loss of urethral, vaginal, and rectal sensation, and motor weakness
  3. Treatment
     a. Radiation therapy
     b. IV steroids
     c. Decompression laminectomy
- Disseminated intravascular coagulation (DIC)
  1. Associated with leukemia, adenocarcinomas of

the lung, pancreas, stomach, and prostate, and metastatic lesions to the liver
   2. Manifested by concurrent bleeding, bleeding from multiple sites, and thrombosis, pain, neurological alterations (syncope, hemiplegia, paresthesia), dyspnea, tachycardia, oliguria, and bowel necrosis
   3. Treatment
      a. Treat underlying cause such as sepsis
      b. Fresh frozen plasma, platelets, or red blood cells
- Superior vena cava syndrome
   1. Related to bronchogenic cancers, but lymphoma, metastatic breast, and GI cancers can also cause this syndrome
   2. Manifested by distended neck veins, venous engorgement of the anterior chest wall, or cough; later symptoms include edema of the face and hands, severe dyspnea, cerebral anoxia, hemorrhage, and strangulation from edema of the glottis and the airways
   3. Treatment
      a. Radiation to site of compression
      b. Chemotherapy
- Cardiac tamponade
   1. Seen more often in lymphoma, leukemia, and melanoma
   2. Manifested by high central venous pressure, arterial hypotension, distant muffled heart sounds, shortness of breath with normal breath sounds, weakness, diaphoresis, and alterations in mental status
   3. Treatment includes
      a. Corticosteroids
      b. Diuretics
      c. Pericardiocentesis

Discharge Planning

- The nurse assists in making arrangements for transportation for follow-up treatments.
- Educational needs depend on the specific type of cancer and the treatment plan.
- The nurse provides drug information
   1. Taking all medications in the correct dosage, at the right time, and by the right route
   2. What to do if a dose is missed or if complications or side effects occur
   3. What to do if pain medications are ineffective
- The nurse teaches the client/family

1. How to use any home care equipment or adaptive-assistive devices ordered for home use
2. How to contact the American Cancer Society and other local support groups
3. The importance of follow-up visits with the physician(s) and other health care providers

For more information on cancer, see *Medical-Surgical Nursing: A Nursing Process Approach,* **pp. 564–603.**

Cancer, Nasal and Sinus

● Tumors of the nose and sinuses are uncommon; they may be benign or malignant.

● Carcinomas metastasize early, with progressive invasion of the neck and cervical lymph nodes and spread to the lung and liver.

● Symptoms mimic respiratory tract illnesses and include persistent nasal obstruction, drainage, bloody discharge, and pain.

● Treatment includes
  1. Surgical resection (possible nasal prosthesis)
  2. Radiation therapy
  3. Chemotherapy

For more information on cancer of the nose and sinuses, see *Medical-Surgical Nursing: A Nursing Process Approach,* **pp. 1955–1956.**

Cardiogenic Shock

- Cardiogenic shock is defined as circulatory failure resulting from severe depression of myocardial contractility in which cardiac output is markedly depressed.
- Cardiogenic shock is produced by any condition that causes the heart to fail; the most common cause is myocardial infarction.
- Cardiogenic shock also results from dysrhythmias, severe heart failure, cardiomyopathy, pulmonary embolism, papillary muscle rupture, and cardiac tamponade.
- Clinical manifestations include
    1. Hypotension
    2. Decreased urinary output
    3. Tachycardia
    4. Cool, moist skin
    5. Impaired state of consciousness
    6. Metabolic acidosis
- Medical management includes
    1. Determining and eliminating the cause
    2. Treating the underlying condition precipitating the heart failure
    3. Improving pump performance
- Cardiogenic shock is a severe form of heart failure. See Heart Failure for nursing management.

For more information on cardiogenic shock, see *Medical-Surgical Nursing: A Nursing Process Approach,* **p. 2184** and **Chapter 17.**

Cardiomyopathy

OVERVIEW

- Cardiomyopathy is a heart muscle disease of unknown cause.
- Cardiomyopathies are divided into two etiologic categories

  1. *Primary* cardiomyopathy, a disease of the heart muscle without a known cause
  2. *Secondary* cardiomyopathy, a disease of the heart muscle with a known cause, including infectious processes, metabolic disorders, immunologic disorders, pregnancy and postpartum disorders, toxic processes, and infiltrative processes.

COLLABORATIVE MANAGEMENT

- The disease is classified based on abnormalities in structure and function into three categories.
- *Dilated cardiomyopathy*, the most common type, involves extensive damage to the myofibrils and interference with myocardial metabolism and is characterized by dilation of both ventricles and impairment of systolic function.

  1. Signs and symptoms of dilated cardiomyopathy include

     a. Fatigue and weakness
     b. Left-sided heart failure
     c. Dysrhythmias or heart block
     d. Systemic or pulmonary emboli
     e. S_3 or S_4 gallops
     f. Moderate to severe cardiomegaly

  2. Treatment for dilated cardiomyopathy includes

     a. Symptomatic treatment of heart failure
     b. Vasodilator drugs
     c. Control of cardiac dysrhythmias
     d. Heart transplantation

- Massive ventricular hypertrophy and small ventricular cavities are typical in *hypertrophic cardiomyopathy*. Left ventricular (LV) hypertrophy leads to a hypocontractile left ventricle with rigid ventricular walls. Obstruction in the LV outflow results from movement of the anterior leaflet of the mitral valve against the hypertrophied cardiac septum during systole, decreasing the amount of ejected blood.

1. Signs and symptoms of hypertrophic cardiomyopathy include
   a. Dyspnea
   b. Angina
   c. Fatigue
   d. Syncope
   e. Palpitations
   f. Mild cardiomegaly
   g. S_4 gallop
   h. Ventricular dysrhythmias or atrial fibrillation
   i. Heart failure
   j. Sudden death
2. Treatment for hypertrophic cardiomyopathy involves
   a. Symptomatic treatment
   b. Beta-blocker drugs
   c. Conversion of atrial fibrillation
   d. Ventriculomyotomy or muscle resection with mitral valve replacement

• *Restrictive cardiomyopathy*, the least common type, which involves restriction of ventricular filling, is caused by endocardial or myocardial disease, or both, and produces a clinical picture similar to constrictive pericarditis.

1. Signs and symptoms of restrictive cardiomyopathy include
   a. Dyspnea
   b. Fatigue
   c. Right-sided heart failure
   d. Mild to moderate cardiomyopathy
   e. S_3 and S_4 gallops
   f. Heart block
   g. Emboli
2. Interventions include
   a. Supportive measures
   b. Treatment of hypertension
   c. Conversion of dysrhythmias
   d. Exercise restrictions
   e. Treatment of acute pulmonary edema

For more information on cardiomyopathy, see *Medical-Surgical Nursing: A Nursing Process Approach*, **pp. 2182–2184.**

Carpal Tunnel Syndrome

OVERVIEW

- Carpal tunnel syndrome (CTS) is a condition in which the median nerve in the wrist is compressed, causing pain and numbness.

COLLABORATIVE MANAGEMENT

Assessment

- The nurse records the client's
  1. Occupation
  2. Family history of the problem
  3. Concurrent medical conditions, such as rheumatoid arthritis
  4. History of recent wrist fracture or burn
  5. Usual exercise routine
- The nurse assesses for
  1. Nature, location, and intensity of the pain and numbness
  2. Time of day pain usually occurs
  3. Paresthesia
  4. Positive Phalen's test, which produces paresthesia in the median nerve distribution within 60 seconds (the client is asked to relax the wrist into flexion or place the backs of both hands together and flex both wrists simultaneously.)
  5. Positive Tinel's sign, which is the same response as for the Phalen's test (elicited by tapping lightly over the area of the median nerve)
  6. Weak pinch, clumsiness, and difficulty with fine movements
  7. Muscle weakness and wasting
  8. Wrist swelling
  9. Autonomic changes manifested by skin discoloration, nail changes such as brittleness, and increased or decreased swelling
  10. Fear that the symptoms are related to a spinal problem or that job or life-style changes may have to be made

Planning and Implementation

NDx: PAIN

Nonsurgical Management

- The nurse
  1. Administers analgesics such as aspirin and nonsteroidal anti-inflammatory drugs, as ordered

2. Administers diuretics if edema is present, as ordered
3. Assists the physician with direct injection of corticosteroids into the carpal tunnel to relieve inflammation
4. Administers pyridoxine hydrochloride (vitamin B_6) when CTS is not related to systemic disease

Surgical Management

• Wrist immobilization is tried before surgical intervention.

• Surgery is done to relieve compression on the median nerve.

• If CTS is a complication of rheumatoid arthritis, a *synovectomy*, or removal of excess synovium, may resolve the problem.

• The nurse provides routine preoperative care.

• The nurse provides postoperative care
  1. Checks pressure dressing carefully for drainage and tightness
  2. Elevates the hand and arm for 1 or 2 days
  3. Checks neurovascular status every hour for the first 12 hours
  4. Encourages the client to move all fingers of the affected hand frequently

NDx: SENSORY/PERCEPTUAL (TACTILE) ALTERATION

• The nurse
  1. Teaches the client to check the temperature of bath water
  2. Teaches the client that mild exercises may be helpful to improve circulation to the hand as long as they do not increase pain
  3. Encourages the client to ask for help in performing activities he or she is no longer able to do

NDx: ALTERED (PERIPHERAL) TISSUE PERFUSION

• The nurse
  1. Assesses the circulation in the affected hand and wrist
  2. Elevates the arm if edema is present

Discharge Planning

• The nurse teaches the client/family
  1. Restriction on lifting heavy objects for 4 to 6 weeks after surgery
  2. Assessment of neurovascular status

3. Importance of follow-up visits with the physician(s)

For more information on carpal tunnel syndrome, see *Medical-Surgical Nursing: A Nursing Process Approach,* **pp. 768–772.**

Cataract

OVERVIEW

- A cataract is an opacity of the lens that distorts the image projected onto the retina.
- Types of cataracts include
  1. *Age related,* generally over 65 years of age
  2. *Traumatic,* caused by blunt trauma, penetrating blows, or overexposure to excessive heat, x-rays, or radioactive material
  3. *Toxic,* seen after ingestion of or exposure to certain chemicals, such as extended use of corticosteroids, chlorpromazine, or miotic agents
  4. *Associated,* seen with other diseases, such as diabetes mellitus, hypoparathyroidism, Down's syndrome, and atopic dermatitis
  5. *Complicated,* which develops as a result of ocular disorders such as retinitis pigmentosa, glaucoma, or retinal detachment

COLLABORATIVE MANAGEMENT

Assessment

- The nurse records the client's
  1. Age
  2. History of trauma
  3. Exposure to radioactive materials or x-rays
  4. Current medical problems

5. Medication history
6. History of intraocular disease
- The nurse assesses for
  1. Blurred vision
  2. Decrease in color vision; blue, green, and purple appear gray
  3. Diplopia
  4. Reduced visual acuity progressing to blindness
  5. Presence of white pupil
  6. Anxiety and fear

Planning and Implementation

NDx: SENSORY/PERCEPTUAL ALTERATIONS (VISUAL)
Nonsurgical Management
- The nurse
  1. Assesses and documents baseline visual acuity
  2. Elicits a functional description of what the client can and cannot see
  3. Adapts the environment to the client's visual needs
     a. Orients the client to the environment
     b. Places frequently used articles within the client's view and in a consistent location
     c. Provides appropriate lighting; avoids glare
     d. Uses the "clock hour" system to orient client to the location of food on a plate
  4. Assesses the amount and type of stimuli that are preferred by the client, such as radio, TV, and audiotapes
  5. Refers the client to services that provide aids such as talking books and large-print books

Surgical Management
- Two extraction procedures are commonly performed
  1. *Extracapsular*, removal of the anterior portion of the capsule
  2. *Intracapsular*, removal of the lens completely within the capsule
- The nurse provides preoperative care
  1. Provides routine preoperative care
  2. Allows the client who may be anxious to talk about losing his or her sight
  3. Reviews the procedure for local and retrobulbar anesthesia, which is usually used
  4. Administers preoperative medications, as ordered
     a. Oral acetazolamide (Diamox) or methazolamide (Neptazane) to reduce intraocular pressure

b. Sympathomimetic drugs such as phenylephrine (Neo-Synephrine) to achieve vasoconstriction and mydriasis

c. Parasympatholytic drops such as tropicamide (Mydricyl) or cyclopentolate hydrochloride (Cyclogyl) to induce paralysis and render the ciliary muscles unable to move the lens

- The nurse provides postoperative care

1. Provides routine postoperative care

2. Administers antibiotics such as gentamicin, as ordered, which is administered immediately after surgery subconjunctivally, as well as an antibiotic plus steroid ointment; both are used for several days after surgery

3. Maintains a semi-Fowler's position or keeps the client on the unoperative side, as ordered

4. Reports visual drainage on the eye pad to the surgeon

5. Applies cool compresses if the eye itches

6. Administers analgesics such as acetaminophen, as ordered

7. Restricts the client's coughing, bending at the waist, sneezing, lifting objects that weigh more than 15 pounds, and sleeping or lying on the operative side (which increases intraocular pressure)

8. Recommends eyeglasses, sunglasses, or an eye shield during the day and an eye shield at night

9. Observes for and reports complications of surgery, including

a. Increased intraocular pressure, manifested by severe pain, nausea, and vomiting

b. Infection

c. Bleeding into the anterior chamber of the eye, manifested by a change in vision

d. Secondary membrane or secondary cataract formation, manifested by the posterior lens's becoming cloudy

e. Retinal detachment, manifested by seeing dark spots, an increased number of floaters, or bright flashes of light and losing all or part of the visual field

- Rehabilitation options depend on the severity of the problem, client's age, and the type of surgery.

1. Eyeglasses called aphakic spectacles

a. Distort images by as much as 25% to 33% and cause vertical lines, such as doorways and lampposts, to look curved

b. Cause peripheral vision to be lost

c. May cause the two eyes not to function

together, resulting in diplopia, if only one eye has been operated on

d. Are the least expensive option

2. Contact lenses

a. Chief advantage over glasses is that image size with the contact lens is only 7% larger than normal size so both eyes function together

b. Visual field is not distorted or constricted

c. Disadvantages include that an adequate amount of tears must be present; requires manual dexterity for insertion and removal; potential for infection and corneal abrasion

3. Intraocular lens implant

a. Minimal 1% to 3% distortion of the image produced

b. Immediate return to binocular vision

c. Disadvantages include a higher rate of complications, the possibility of rejection of the lens, and higher cost

NDx: POTENTIAL FOR INJURY (FALL)

- The nurse
  1. Advises the client that covering an eye with a patch and/or shield causes monocular vision, which changes depth perception and narrows the field of vision
  2. Eliminates potential hazards in the environment
  3. Monitors the room for spills and loose objects on the floor, such as tissues, pencils, pens, and needle caps
  4. Teaches the client to change position slowly and to avoid reaching for objects for stability when ambulating
  5. Encourages the client to use adaptive equipment (cane) for ambulation as needed
  6. Advises the client to go up and down stairs one step at a time
  7. Reinforces the importance of wearing an ocular shield when participating in high-risk activities such as ambulating at night or playing with children or pets

NDx: IMPAIRED HOME MAINTENANCE MANAGEMENT

- The nurse
  1. Discusses the current ability of the client to meet self-care needs and activities of daily living
  2. Evaluates how the client's current functional ability will be affected by activity restriction and postoperative needs

112

3. Helps the client to decide on a realistic site for recovery
4. Teaches the client required self-care activities, including
   a. Personal care
   b. Shield application
   c. Eyedrop instillation
   d. Activities permitted and restricted
   e. Medications
   f. Monitoring for complications
5. Identifies and suggests ways to correct hazards in the home prior to discharge

Discharge Planning

● See "Impaired Home Health Maintenance Management."
● The nurse
  1. Teaches the client that hair washing may be done several days after surgery if this can be performed with the head tilted back, such as in a hair salon
  2. Advises the client to stand in the shower with the face turned away from the shower head
  3. Advises the client not to drive, operate machinery, and participate in sports until given specific permission to do so
  4. Emphasizes the importance of follow-up visits with the physician(s)

For more information on cataracts, see *Medical-Surgical Nursing: A Nursing Process Approach,* **pp. 1037–1046.**

Cerebral Vascular Accident

OVERVIEW

- Cerebral vascular accident (CVA), commonly referred to as a *stroke*, is a disruption in the normal blood supply to the brain.
- CVAs may be classified as
  1. *Ischemic*, caused by the occlusion of a cerebral artery by either a thrombus or embolus
     a. Types of ischemic CVA include
        (1) *Thrombolic*, commonly associated with the development of atherosclerosis of the blood vessel wall. The artery becomes occluded, blood flow to the area is markedly diminished, causing transient ischemia and then complete ischemia and infarction of brain tissue. Signs and symptoms occur gradually.
        (2) *Embolic*, caused by an embolus or group of emboli that travel to the cerebral arteries via the carotid artery and block the artery, causing ischemia. Sudden and rapid development of focal neurologic deficits occurs. Cerebral hemorrhage may result if the vessel wall is damaged.
     b. Ischemic CVA may be preceded by warning signs, including
        (1) *Transient ischemic attack* (TIA), a transient focal neurological deficit such as vertigo or blurred vision
        (2) *Reversible ischemic neurologic deficit* (RIND), which lasts longer than a TIA.
  2. *Hemorrhagic*, in which the integrity of the vessel wall is interrupted and bleeding occurs into the brain tissue or subarachnoid space. Causes include hypertension, ruptured aneurysm, or arteriovenous malformation (AVM).
     a. *Aneurysm* is an abnormal ballooning or blister on the involved artery, which may become stretched or thinned and ruptures.
     b. *AVM* is a tangled or spaghettilike mass of malformed, thin-walled, dilated vessels, which form an abnormal communication between the arterial and venous systems.

COLLABORATIVE MANAGEMENT
Assessment

- The nurse records the client's
  1. Activity at onset of CVA
  2. Progression and severity of symptoms, including the presence of a TIA or RIND
  3. Level of consciousness, orientation
  4. Motor status (gait, balance, reading and writing abilities)
  5. Sensory status (speech, hearing, vision)
  6. Past medical history
  7. Social history, with attention toward identifying risk factors
  8. Current medications and nonprescribed drugs. (The nurse should be alert for anticoagulants, aspirin, vasodilators, and illegal drug use.)

- The nurse assesses for changes in the client's
  1. Level of consciousness, orientation, cognition, memory, judgment, and problem-solving and decision-making abilities
  2. Ability to concentrate and attend to tasks
  3. Motor status: muscle strength, muscle tone, range of motion, proprioception, head and trunk control, balance, gait, coordination, bowel and bladder control
  4. Sensory status: response to touch and painful stimuli; ability to distinguish between two tactile stimuli presented simultaneously; ability to read, write, and follow verbal directions; ability to name objects and/or use objects correctly
  5. Visual system: pupil size and reaction to light, visual field deficits (homonymous hemianopsia, bitemporal hemianopsia)
  6. Cranial nerve function, especially V, VII, IX, X, and XII
  7. Cardiac system such as hypertension and murmurs
  8. Body image and self-concept disturbance
  9. Coping mechanisms or personality changes
  10. Emotional lability
  11. Impact of hospitalization on financial status and occupation and client's reaction

Planning and Implementation
NDx: Altered (Cerebral) Tissue Perfusion
Nonsurgical Management

- The nurse
  1. Performs a neurologic assessment at a minimum of every 2 to 4 hours, checking
     a. Verbal response, orientation

    b. Eye opening, pupil size, and reaction to light

    c. Motor response

2. Monitors vital signs with neurologic checks

    a. Asks the physician for acceptable limits for blood pressure

    b. Performs a cardiac assessment

3. Elevates the head of the bed 30 to 45 degrees

4. Avoids activities that may increase intracranial pressure

    a. Positions the client to avoid extreme hip or neck flexion

    b. Avoids clustering nursing procedures

    c. Provides a quiet environment

• Occlusive CVA is treated with anticoagulant therapy (contraindicated in clients with a history of ulcers, uremia, and hepatic failure). Sodium heparin subcutaneously or via continuous intravenous drip is commonly used.

• The nurse obtains a baseline prothrombin time and partial thromboplastin time before initiating therapy, 6 to 8 hours after the start of the drug, and every morning thereafter.

• Anticoagulation therapy may cause bleeding. The nurse observes for blood in the urine and stool and easy bruising.

• Phenytoin (Dilantin) may be used to prevent seizures.

• Enteric-coated or other forms of aspirin or dipyridamole (Persantine) may be used to forestall thrombotic and embolic strokes.

• Calcium channel blockers (nimodipine) may be given to treat vasospasm or chronic spasm of the vessel, which inhibits blood flow to the area.

• Epsilon-aminocaproic acid (Amicar) may be used to stabilize a clot over the site of ruptured aneurysm.

• The nurse implements aneurysm/AVM precautions, including

1. Complete bed rest in a quiet, darkened room

2. Head of bed elevated 30 to 45 degrees

3. Restriction on TV, radio, reading, and visitors

4. No hot or cold beverages and no caffeine products

5. No straining or vigorous coughing

Surgical Management

• Two surgical procedures may be used for *occlusive CVA* (both under scrunity since some studies indicate medical management may be equally effective)

1. Carotid *endarterectomy* to remove atherosclerotic plaque
2. Superior temporal artery–middle cerebral artery *anastomosis* to bypass the occluded area and reestablish blood flow to the affected area

- The surgical procedures to treat *AVM* include
    1. Injecting small silicone beads into the carotid artery, which travel to involved vessels, become lodged, and cause the vessels to thrombose
    2. Surgically removing involved vessels

- The surgical procedures to treat *aneurysm* include
    1. Placing a clip or clamp at the base or neck of the aneurysm
    2. Wrapping the aneurysm with muscle, muslin, or plastic coating

- The nursing care for these procedures is similar to that discussed under Brain Tumor, "Surgical Management."

NDx: Sensory/Perceptual Alteration

- The nurse
    1. Uses frequent verbal and tactile cues to help the client perform activities of daily living
    2. Breaks tasks down into small steps when cueing
    3. Approaches the client from the nonaffected side
    4. Teaches the client to scan with eyes and turn the head side to side (when visual impairments occur)
    5. Places objects within the client's field of vision
    6. Places a patch over the affected eye if diplopia is present
    7. Removes clutter from the room
    8. Orients the client to time, place, and event
    9. Provides a structured, repetitious, and consistent routine or schedule
    10. Presents information in a clear, simple, concise manner
    11. Uses a step-by-step approach
    12. Places pictures and other familiar objects in the room

NDx: Impaired Physical Mobility; Self-Care Deficit

- The nurse
    1. Performs active and passive range-of-motion exercises at least daily
    2. Carefully positions the client in proper body alignment
    3. Maintains correct use of splints and braces

4. Uses antiembolism stockings; frequently positions and mobilizes the client as soon as possible to prevent deep-vein thrombosis or pneumonia
5. Measures thighs and calves daily and checks for positive Homan's sign (indicative of possible deep-vein thrombosis)

NDx: Total Urinary Incontinence; Bowel Incontinence

- The nurse
  1. Establishes the cause of the problem and type (bowel/bladder)
  2. Determines the client's usual voiding or bowel movement pattern
  3. Implements an individualized bladder training program (see Rehabilitation for a thorough discussion)
     a. Uses an intermittent catheterization program if urinary incontinence is due to upper motor lesion
     b. Places the client on a bedpan or commode every 2 hours; encourages fluids to 2000 mL per day unless contraindicated
  4. Implements an individualized bowel training program (see Rehabilitation for a thorough discussion)
     a. Determines the normal time or routine for bowel elimination
     b. Places the client on a bedpan or commode at the same time each day; uses a suppository or stool softener if needed
     c. Provides a diet high in bulk or fiber (may need a dietary consult)

NDx: Impaired Verbal Communication

- The nurse
  1. Gives repetitive, simple directions; breaks each task into simple steps
  2. Faces the client and speaks slowly and distinctly
  3. Allows sufficient time for the client to understand the direction
  4. Uses pictures or a communication board if necessary

NDx: Impaired Swallowing

- The nurse
  1. Positions the client to facilitate swallowing
     a. Places the client in a chair or sitting straight up in bed

b. Positions the client's head and neck slightly forward and flexed

2. Provides foods that are soft or semisoft and thick fluids (e.g., milkshakes)
3. Maintains a quiet room with few distractions from visitors or TV

Discharge Planning

- The nurse
  1. Identifies and suggests corrections of hazards in the home prior to discharge
  2. Ensures that the client can correctly use all assistive-adaptive devices ordered for home use
  3. Arranges follow-up appointments, as ordered
  4. Provides a detailed plan of care at the time of discharge for clients to be transferred to a rehabilitation center or long-term-care facility (rehabilitation can be a lengthy process; see Rehabilitation.)
  5. Provides drug information as needed
  6. Reinforces mobility skills (in collaboration with other therapists)
     a. How to safely climb stairs, transfer bed to chair, get into and out of a car
     b. How to use adaptive equipment

For more information on cerebral vascular accident, see *Medical-Surgical Nursing: A Nursing Process Approach,* **pp. 876–891.**

Cervical Cancer

OVERVIEW

- Cervical cancer can be preinvasive or invasive.
- Preinvasive cancer is limited to the cervix and usually originates in the area called the transformation zone.

- Invasive cancer is in the cervix and other pelvic structures.

- Squamous cell cancers spread by direct extension to the vaginal mucosa, the lower uterine segment, the parametrium, the pelvic wall, the bladder, and the bowel.

- Metastasis is usually confined to the pelvis but distant metastases occur through lymphatic spread.

- Premalignant changes can be described from dysplasia, the earliest change, to *carcinoma in situ* (CIS), the most advanced premalignant change.

- Preinvasive cancers can also be described using the term *cervical intraepithelial neoplasia* (CIN).

COLLABORATIVE MANAGEMENT

Assessment

- The nurse records the client's
    1. Age
    2. Race
    3. Socioeconomic status
    4. Parity status
    5. History of sexually transmitted disease
    6. History of long-term birth control pill use
- The nurse assesses for
    1. Painless vaginal bleeding
    2. Watery, blood-tinged discharge that may become dark and foul smelling as the disease progresses
    3. Leg pain or unilateral leg swelling (late sign)
    4. Weight loss
    5. Pelvic pain
    6. Dysuria
    7. Hematuria
    8. Rectal bleeding
    9. Chest pain
    10. Coughing

Planning and Implementation

NDx: ANXIETY AND FEAR

Nonsurgical Management (for CIN)

- Laser therapy is used when all boundaries of the lesion are visible during colposcopic examination.

- Cryosurgery involves placing a probe against the cervix to cause freezing of the tissues and subsequent necrosis

Nonsurgical Management (for invasive cervical cancer)

- Intracavitary and external radiation therapy are used in combination, depending on the extent and location of the lesion.
- For nursing management of clients having radiation, refer to Cancer, General.
- Chemotherapy has generally performed poorly for cervical cancers.

Surgical Management

- Conization may be used therapeutically for CIN in women who desire childbearing.
- A vaginal hysterectomy is commonly performed.
- A radical hysterectomy and bilateral lymph node dissection is as effective as radiation for cancer that has extended beyond the cervix but not to the pelvic wall.
- For preoperative and postoperative care, see Uterine Leiomyoma.
- *Pelvic exenteration* is a radical surgical procedure, used for recurrent cancers if there is no lymph node involvement; there are three types

  1. *Anterior* exenteration is the removal of the uterus, ovaries, fallopian tubes, vagina, bladder, urethra, and pelvic lymph nodes.
  2. *Posterior* exenteration is the removal of the uterus, ovaries, fallopian tubes, descending colon, rectum, and anal canal.
  3. *Total* exenteration is a combination of the anterior and posterior procedures, with urinary diversion created by an ileal conduit and a colostomy for passage of feces.

- The nurse provides preoperative care

  1. Assesses anxiety, concerns about sexual functioning, and the ability to adjust to altered body image
  2. Assists in selection of stoma sites
  3. Provides extensive bowel preparation
  4. Provides routine preoperative care

- The nurse informs the client to expect the following after surgery

  1. Transfer to a critical care unit
  2. Multiple intravenous lines
  3. Other invasive lines and monitoring, such as an arterial line
  4. Nasogastric tube

- Refer to Colorectal Cancer for preoperative and postoperative care for the client undergoing colostomy, and Urothelial Cancer for preoperative and postoperative care for the client undergoing ileal conduit.
- The nurse assesses for (after surgery)
  1. Cardiovascular complications, such as hemorrhage and shock
  2. Pulmonary complications, such as atelectasis and pneumonia
  3. Fluid and electrolyte imbalances, such as metabolic acidosis or alkalosis
  4. Renal complications
  5. Gastrointestinal complications, such as paralytic ileus
  6. Pain
  7. Wound infection, dehiscence, or evisceration
- The nurse provides postoperative care
  1. Assists with coughing and deep breathing
  2. Observes for dehydration
  3. Monitors urinary output
  4. Administers narcotic analgesics, as ordered
  5. Administers and monitors total parenteral nutrition, as ordered
  6. Administers prophylactic heparin and applies antiembolism, as ordered; stockings to prevent deep-vein thrombosis
  7. Administers antibiotics, as ordered
  8. Performs perineal irrigations, if ordered
  9. Provides sitz baths, as ordered

Discharge Planning
- The nurse implements a teaching plan for the client undergoing exenteration
  1. Colostomy and/or ileal conduit care
  2. Care for perineal drainage (for several months to a year)
  3. Use of sanitary pads, such as Maxipads
  4. Dietary adjustment to maintain high nutritional intake
  5. Medication effects, dosages, and side effects
  6. Sexual counseling about alternatives to intercourse
  7. Activity modification; walking
  8. Information about complications, including infection and bowel obstruction
  9. Emotional support about changes in body image

10. Importance of follow-up visits with the physician(s)

For more information on cervical cancer, see *Medical-Surgical Nursing: A Nursing Process Approach*, **pp. 1720–1726.**

Cervical Polyp

- Cervical polyps are pedunculated tumors arising from the mucosa and extending to the cervical os.
- The polyps result from hyperplastic condition of the endocervical epithelium or inflammation and are the most common neoplastic growth of the cervix.
- Clinical findings include
  1. Premenstrual or postmenstrual bleeding
  2. Postcoital bleeding
  3. Small, single, or multiple bright-red polyps that are soft with fragile consistency and may bleed when touched
- Polyps are easily removed in the physician's office.
- Immediate postprocedure instructions include avoidance of
  1. Tampons
  2. Douching
  3. Sexual intercourse

For more information on cervical polyps, see *Medical-Surgical Nursing: A Nursing Process Approach*, **p. 1715.**

Cervicitis

- Cervicitis is an infection of the endocervix, most often caused by sexually transmitted diseases, particularly chlamydiosis, gonorrhea, trichoniasis, and herpes simplex virus infection.
- Physical findings include
  1. Mucopurulent discharge from the endocervix
  2. Pelvic pain; postcoital, intermenstrual bleeding
  3. Inflamed cervix that may bleed when touched
- Treatment is dependent on the underlying cause.

For more information on cervicitis, see *Medical-Surgical Nursing: A Nursing Process Approach*, **pp. 1700–1701.**

Chalazion

- A chalazion is a sterile, granulomatous inflammation of the meibomian gland of the eye.
- It is characterized by gradual, painless swelling at the gland; eye fatigue; sensitivity to light; and excessive tearing.
- When fully developed, no inflammatory signs are present.
- An untreated chalazion may press on the cornea or globe and cause astigmatism.
- Treatment consists of warm compresses.
- Excision may be necessary.
- After excision, an antibiotic ointment is applied, and the client is instructed to notify the physician of

infection, redness, purulent drainage, or reduced
vision.

For more information on chalazion, see *Medical-
Surgical Nursing: A Nursing Process Approach,*
pp. 1024–1026.

For more information on chalazion, see *Medical-
Surgical Nursing: A Nursing Process Approach,*
pp. 1024–1026.

Chancroid

- Chancroid is most common in tropical and
subtropical countries.
- Recent spread of the causative organism
Haemophilus ducreyi has made chancroid an
important sexually transmitted disease in the United
States.
- The incubation period varies from 1 to 14 days.
- A tender papule appears at the site of inoculation.
- The lesion rapidly breaks down to form an
irregularly shaped, deep ulcer with purulent discharge
that bleeds easily.
- Complications include inguinal adenopathy,
balanitis, phimosis, and urethral fistulas.
- Transmission is through contact with the ulcer or
with discharge from the infected local lymph glands
during sexual intercourse.
- Treatment includes antibiotics such as erythromycin
for 7 days or a single dose of intramuscular ceftriaxone.
- Sexual contacts must be treated with antibiotics
whether or not they are symptomatic.

For more information on chancroid, see *Medical-
Surgical Nursing: A Nursing Process Approach,*
p. 1782.

Chemical Burn, Ocular

- Acids and alkaline compounds are most commonly involved in chemical burns of the eye.
- Treatment includes
  1. Irrigating eye(s) with a large amount of clean liquids such as water or irrigating solution for 15 to 20 minutes, with no attempt to neutralize the chemical, as this generates heat and causes further damage
  2. Assessing the client's visual acuity and checking for ability to perceive light
  3. Obtaining a sample of the chemical involved
  4. Transporting the client to the hospital as soon as possible
  5. Anesthetizing the eye with a drop of proparacine hydrochloride (ophthetic), repeating as needed (a piece of litmus paper should be dabbed onto the conjunctiva to determine the acid or alkali nature of the irritant)
  6. Applying an antibiotic-steroid ointment such as neomycin sulfate, polymyxin B sulfate, or dexamethasone

For more information on chemical burns of the eye, see *Medical-Surgical Nursing: A Nursing Process Approach,* **pp. 1068–1069.**

Chlamydia

- *Chlamydia trachomatis* is the most commonly transmitted bacteria in the United States, with 4 million acute infections estimated annually.
- *C. trachomatis* invades columnar epithelial tissues in the reproductive tract and causes clinical manifestations similar to gonorrhea.

- The incubation period ranges from 1 to 3 weeks, although the pathogen may be present in the genital tract for months or years without producing symptoms.
- Clinical manifestations include
  1. Men: urethritis, dysuria, frequency of urination, mucoid discharge that is more watery and less copious than gonorrheal discharge
  2. Women: 75% are asymptomatic, mucopurulent cervicitis, change in vaginal discharge, dysuria, urinary frequency, soreness in the affected area
- Complications include
  1. Men: epididymitis, prostatitis, infertility, and Reiter's syndrome
  2. Women: salpingitis, pelvic inflammatory disease, ectopic pregnancy, and infertility
- Assessment includes
  1. Sexual history
     a. History of sexually transmitted diseases (STDs)
     b. Sexual partner with history of STDs
     c. Sexual partner with suspicious symptoms
  2. Risk factors associated with *C. trachomatis*
     a. Pregnancy
     b. Sexual activity during adolescence
     c. Use of nonbarrier method of birth control
     d. History of multiple sexual partners
  3. Exclusion of gonorrhea on Gram's stain and culture
  4. Diagnostic tests such as enzymelike immunoassay and a direct fluorescent antibody test
- The treatment of choice is doxycycline or tetracycline.
- Client education includes
  1. Transmission and treatment
  2. Signs and symptoms
  3. Complications of untreated chlamydial infections
  4. Avoid sexual activity
  5. Partner treatment
  6. Use of condoms

For more information on chlamydia, see *Medical-Surgical Nursing: A Nursing Process Approach*, **pp. 1785–1787.**

Cholecystitis

OVERVIEW

• Cholecystitis is defined as an inflammation of the gallbladder that may occur as an acute or chronic process.

• *Acute* inflammation is usually associated with gallstones (cholelithiasis).

• *Chronic* cholecystitis results when inefficient bile emptying and gallbladder muscle wall disease contribute to a fibrotic and contracted gallbladder, with decreased motility and deficient absorption.

• *Acalculous* cholecystitis occurs in the absence of gallstones and is due to bacterial invasion via the lymphatic or vascular systems.

COLLABORATIVE MANAGEMENT

Assessment

• The nurse records the client's
  1. Height and weight
  2. Sex, age, race, and ethnic group
  3. History of pregnancies, menopause or use of birth control pills, estrogen, or other hormone supplements
  4. Food preferences, including excess fat and cholesterol intake
  5. Food intolerances and related gastrointestinal (GI) symptoms, including flatulence, dyspepsia (indigestion), eructation (belching), anorexia, nausea, vomiting, or abdominal pain in relation to fatty food intake
  6. Exercise routine or daily activities
  7. Family history of gallbladder disease
• The nurse assesses for
  1. Abdominal pain of varying intensities, including radiation to the scapula, and asks the client to describe the intensity, duration, precipitating factors, and relief measures
  2. Other GI symptoms including nausea, vomiting, dyspepsia, flatulence, eructation, or feelings of abdominal heaviness
  3. Guarding, rigidity, and rebound tenderness
  4. Sausage-shaped mass in the right upper quadrant
  5. Late symptoms seen in chronic cholecystitis such as jaundice, clay-colored stools, and dark urine
  6. Steatorrhea (fatty stools)

7. Elevated temperature with tachycardia and dehydration

Planning and Implementation

NDx: PAIN

Nonsurgical Management

• Food and fluids are withheld during nausea and vomiting episodes; nasogastric decompression is initiated for severe vomiting.

• Clients with chronic cholecystitis are encouraged to consume low-fat meals more frequently in smaller amounts.

• The nurse administers

1. Narcotic analgesics, as ordered, such as meperidine to relieve pain and reduce spasm
2. Antispasmodic agents such as anticholinergics (e.g., Pro-Banthine), as ordered, to relax the smooth muscle
3. Antiemetics, as ordered, to provide relief from nausea and vomiting

Surgical Management

• *Cholecystectomy* (removal of the gallbladder) is the usual surgical treatment to remove the cause of discomfort.

• A T tube drain is surgically inserted when the common bile duct is explored to ensure patency of the duct.

• The nurse provides preoperative care

1. Stresses the importance of deep breathing, coughing, and turning, as well as early ambulation after surgery
2. Teachs the use of sustained maximal inspiration (SMI) devices
3. Teaches how to use a folded bath blanket or pillow as a splint for the abdomen to prevent jarring during coughing
4. Provides routine preoperative care

• The nurse provides postoperative care

1. Administers intramuscular meperidine (Demerol), as ordered, for pain relief
2. Administers antiemetics, as ordered, for relief of postoperative nausea and vomiting
3. Ensures that the client receives nothing by mouth (NPO) for 24 to 48 hours
4. Maintains nasogastric suction
5. Advances the diet from clear liquids to solid foods, as tolerated by the client
6. Maintains the client's T tube

a. Assesses the amount, color, consistency, and odor of the drainage
b. Collects and administers the excess bile output to the client via the nasogastric tube or administers synthetic bile salts, such as dehydroccolic acid (Decholin), as ordered
c. Reports sudden increases in bile output to the physician
d. Assesses for foul odor and purulent drainage and reports changes in drainage to the physician
e. Inspects the skin around the T tube insertion site for signs of inflammation
f. Keeps the drainage system below the level of the gallbladder
g. Positions the client in a semi-Fowler's position
h. Avoids the irrigation, aspiration, or clamping of the T tube without a physician's order
i. Assesses the drainage system for pulling, kinking, or tangling of the tubing
j. Assists the client with early ambulation
k. Observes the client's stools for brown color

Discharge Planning

• If surgery is performed, the nurse supplies written postoperative instructions

1. Inspection of the abdominal incision for redness, tenderness, swelling, and drainage
2. Dressing change, wound care, and T tube drain care instructions
3. Pain management, including prescriptions
4. Signs and symptoms of infection, including when to call the physician (elevated temperature and increased pain)
5. Activity limitations

• The nurse provides diet therapy instructions based on the client's tolerance of fats, including a low-fat diet and foods to avoid; small, more frequent feedings; and weight reduction if indicated.

For more information on cholecystitis, see *Medical-Surgical Nursing: A Nursing Process Approach*, **pp. 1447–1456.**

Cholelithiasis

OVERVIEW

- Cholelithiasis (calculous cholecystitis) is a condition in which calculi, or gallstones, lodge in the neck of the gallbladder or in the cystic duct, interfering with or totally obstructing normal bile flow from the gallbladder to the duodenum.
- Vascular congestion results from impeded venous return, with edema and congestion.
- Trapped bile is reabsorbed, acting as a chemical irritant and producing a toxic effect, resulting in tissue sloughing with necrosis and gangrene.
- Contributing factors include supersaturation of bile with cholesterol, excess bile salt losses, decreased gallbladder emptying rates, and changes in bile concentration or bile stasis in the gallbladder.
- Stones may lie dormant or migrate within the biliary tree, causing obstruction.
- Stones are typically composed of cholesterol, bilirubin, bile salts, calcium, and various proteins and designated as cholesterol, mixed, or pigment stones.
- *Cholangitis*, associated with choledocholithiasis (common bile duct stones), involves infection of the bile ducts.

COLLABORATIVE MANAGEMENT

Assessment

- The nurse records the client's
  1. Height and weight
  2. Sex, age, race, and ethnic group
  3. History of pregnancies, menopause or use of birth control pills, estrogen, or other hormone supplements
  4. Food preferences, including excess fat and cholesterol intake
  5. Food intolerances and related gastrointestinal (GI) symptoms, including flatulence, dyspepsia, eructation, anorexia, nausea, vomiting, or abdominal pain in relation to fatty food intake
  6. Exercise routine or daily activities
  7. Family or previous history of gallbladder disease
- The nurse assesses for
  1. Abdominal pain, including severity (based on whether the stone is stationary or mobile, size and

location of the stone, degree of obstruction, and the presence and extent of inflammation)
2. Severe pain of biliary colic accompanied by tachycardia, pallor, diaphoresis, and prostration
3. Other GI symptoms, including nausea, vomiting, dyspepsia, flatulence, eructation, or feelings of abdominal heaviness
4. Guarding, rigidity, and rebound tenderness
5. Sausage-shaped mass in the right upper quadrant
6. Jaundice in acute ductal obstruction

Planning and Implementation

NDx: Pain

Nonsurgical Management

- The nurse
  1. Provides a low-fat diet to prevent further pain of biliary colic
  2. Replaces fat-soluble vitamins (A, D, E, and K) and bile salts, as ordered, if gallstones cause obstruction, to facilitate digestion and vitamin absorption
  3. Withholds food and fluids if nausea and vomiting occur
  4. Administers narcotic analgesia with meperidine hydrochloride (Demerol), as ordered (not morphine, which interferes with biliary flow)
  5. Administers antispasmodic or anticholinergic drugs, as ordered, to relax smooth muscles and decrease ductal tone and spasm
  6. Administers antiemetics, as ordered, to control nausea and vomiting
  7. Administers bile acid therapy, as ordered, to dissolve gallstones; Chenodiol (chenodeoxycholic acid [CDCA]; Chemix) reduces cholesterol stones by maintaining normal cholesterol solubility in bile
  8. Administers cholestyramine (Questran), as ordered, which binds with bile salts in the intestine, removing excess bile salts, and reduces itching (administered in powder form with fruit juices or milk)

- Extracorporeal shock wave lithotripsy involves the use of a lithotriptor to generate powerful shock waves to shatter gallstones when conservative measures are unsuccessful.

- Percutaneous insertion of a transhepatic biliary catheter to decompress obstructed extrahepatic ducts may be performed.

Surgical Management

- Surgical intervention includes

132

1. *Cholecystotomy*, an incision into the gallbladder
2. *Choledocholithotomy*, an incision into the common bile duct to remove stones with common bile duct exploration and T tube placement
3. *Cholecystectomy*, gallbladder removal for stones confined to the gallbladder.

• The nurse provides routine preoperative care and instructions (see Cholecystitis for preoperative instructions).

• The nurse provides postoperative care
    1. Provides routine postoperative care and instructions and T tube care (see Cholecystitis for postoperative instructions)
    2. Administers hydrocholeretic drugs such as Decholin, Cholin, or Neocholin to increase cholesterol solubility and promote drainage of bile through the T tube drainage system

Discharge Planning

• The nurse provides verbal and written postoperative instructions including
    1. Inspection of abdominal incision for redness, tenderness, swelling, and drainage
    2. Dressing change, wound care, and T tube drain care instructions
    3. Pain management, including prescriptions
    4. Signs and symptoms of infection, including when to call the physician (elevated temperature and increase in pain)
    5. Activity limitations
    6. Symptoms of postcholecystectomy syndrome (recurring calculi), including jaundice of skin or sclera, dark urine, light-colored stools, pain, fever, and chills

• Dietary instructions are based on the client's tolerance of fats, including a low-fat diet and foods to avoid; small, more frequent feedings and weight reduction may be indicated.

For more information on cholelithiasis, see *Medical-Surgical Nursing: A Nursing Process Approach*, **pp. 1456–1461.**

Cholesteatoma

- A cholesteatoma is a benign growth of squamous cell epithelium.
- It appears as a grayish-white, shiny mass behind or involving the tympanic membrane and is often described as having a cauliflowerlike appearance.
- Clinical management is dependent on structures that are damaged by the tumor and include decreased hearing, chronic otitis media, vertigo, and possibly facial paralysis.
- Treatment includes
  1. Antibiotics if an infection is present
  2. Surgical removal of the tumor
     a. Myringoplasty to repair the tympanic membrane
     b. Tympanoplasty to repair or replace the ossicles to improve conductive hearing
     c. Mastoidectomy for more extensive growths

For more information on cholesteatoma, see *Medical-Surgical Nursing: A Nursing Process Approach,* **pp. 1120–1121.**

Chronic Obstructive Pulmonary Disease

OVERVIEW

- Chronic obstructive pulmonary disease (COPD) is a group of diseases including emphysema, chronic bronchitis, and asthma.

- COPD is also known as chronic obstructive lung disease (COLD) and chronic airflow limitation (CAL).

- These chronic conditions are characterized by progressive airflow limitations into and out of the lungs, elevated airway resistance, irreversible lung distention, and arterial blood gas (ABG) imbalance.

- COPD leads to pulmonary insufficiency, pulmonary hypertension, and cor pulmonale.

- *Emphysema*, identified by altered lung architecture and characterized by destruction of alveolar walls by elastin, resulting in hyperinflation of air spaces and limited airflow out of the lung, is classified according to patterns of destruction and dilation of the lung's acini (gas exchange unit):

    1. *Pancinar* or *panlobar* emphysema (PLE) involves destruction of the alveoli in the acinus; diffuse disease is usually more severe in the lower lung.
    2. *Centriacinar* or *centrilobar* emphysema (CLE) involves fenestrations in respiratory bronchioles, allowing spaces to develop as tissue walls disintegrate; diffuse disease affects the upper portions of the lung.

- *Chronic bronchitis* involves increased secretions, edema, bronchospasm, and impaired mucociliary clearance, causing diffuse airway obstruction because of inflammatory changes in the thickened bronchial wall lumen; the disease hinders airflow and gas exchange.

- *Asthma* is defined as intermittent airway narrowing caused by constriction of bronchial smooth muscle, excess production of mucus, and mucosal edema.

- Asthma characteristically occurs as attacks but may occur continuously.

- Overreactive airways, stimulated by changes in the environment, exercise, fog, odors, smoke, aerosols, dust, pollen, mold spores, animal danders, or emotional excitement, may aggravate wheezing.

COLLABORATIVE MANAGEMENT

Assessment

- The nurse records the client's
    1. Chief complaint
    2. Breathlessness
    3. Cough, dyspnea, and wheezing
    4. Cigarette use
    5. Activity tolerance
    6. Nutritional intake
    7. Medications

- The nurse assesses for
  1. Breathing rate and pattern
  2. Respiratory muscle fatigue
  3. Abdominal paradox
  4. Barrel chest
  5. Use of accessory muscles
  6. Cyanosis
  7. Capillary refill
  8. Nail clubbing
  9. Diminished airflow
  10. Cardiac dysrhythmias
  11. Ankle edema
  12. Decreased coping mechanisms

Planning and Implementation

NDx: Impaired Gas Exchange/Ineffective Airway Clearance

- The nurse administers drug therapy, as ordered,
  1. Bronchodilators—oral, intravenous, or inhalant
     a. Methylxanthines (theophylline and aminophylline)
     b. Sympathomimetics (metaproterenol, terbutaline, albuterol)
  2. Corticosteroids—oral, intravenous, or inhalants (prednisone, methylprednisolone, beclomethasone, cromolyn sodium) to reduce inflammation
  3. Mucolytic therapy (Mucomyst) to thin and expectorate secretions
- The nurse
  1. Monitors oxygen therapy by pulse oximetry
  2. Maintains the endotracheal tube and mechanical ventilation, which are indicated when the client is unable to maintain adequate ventilation, oxygenation, or effective breathing pattern
  3. Assists the physician in performing a tracheostomy for prolonged intubation, airway obstruction, obstructive sleep apnea, facilitation of weaning process, airway clearance, laryngectomy, or prophylaxis against airway obstruction
  4. Performs suctioning to clear the airway and prevent infection; includes nasopharyngeal, endotracheal tube, or tracheostomy
  5. Provides bronchial and oral hygiene to promote a patent airway and prevent infections
  6. Repositions the client for breathing comfort and to mobilize secretions

7. Assists with ambulation out of bed, observing energy conservation
8. Refers to the pulmonary rehabilitation department, as ordered
9. Provides chest physical therapy
10. Provides nutritional support via parenteral or enteral routes; increased calories and electrolyte replacements are essential
11. Consults with the dietitian
12. Provides adequate fluid hydration
13. Teaches diaphragmatic or abdominal and pursed-lip breathing techniques

Discharge Planning

● The nurse provides a structured pulmonary rehabilitation program
1. Disease process education
2. Exercise conditioning
3. Energy conservation
4. Breathing retraining
5. Bronchial hygiene
6. Psychologic counseling
7. Vocational rehabilitation

● The nurse teaches the client/family how to manage the disease
1. Medications
2. Diet
3. Activity progression
4. Stress avoidance
5. Techniques of breathing, including pursed-lip and diaphragmatic breathing, positioning, relaxation therapy, coughing and deep breathing, and energy conservation
6. Home oxygen therapy
7. Airway care, including tracheostomy care, if indicated
8. Importance of follow-up visits with the physician(s)

For more information on COPD, see *Medical-Surgical Nursing: A Nursing Process Approach*, **pp. 1988–2040.**

Circumcision

- Circumcision is the surgical removal of the prepuce from the penis.
- In the adult male, circumcision is usually done for medical reasons, such as to correct phimosis, a condition in which the prepuce is constricted, and to eliminate the infections that frequently occur as a result of this condition.
- When circumcision is performed on the adult male, one of two surgical procedures is used:
  1. Method I: pulling the prepuce forward and clamping it distal to the tip of the glans. The prepuce is then excised, the clamp is removed, and sutures are applied in the foreskin around the base of the glans to prevent bleeding.
  2. Method II: incising and dissecting away the outer and inner surfaces of the prepuce without cutting the larger blood vessels in the prepuce. The two surfaces are approximated and sutured.
- The nurse
  1. Instructs the client to soak in a warm bath and allow the penile dressing to float off
  2. Tells the client not to replace the dressing if it falls off
  3. Informs the client that the sutures will be absorbed and do not need to be removed
  4. Instructs the client to resume normal activities within 1 week and sexual activity after 1 or 2 weeks
  5. Advises the client to take barbiturate sleeping medication, as ordered, which suppresses the rapid eye movement phase of sleep, so that normal nocturnal erections do not occur
  6. Instructs the client to notify the physician for any wound complication

For more information on circumcision, see *Medical-Surgical Nursing: A Nursing Process Approach*, **p. 1768.**

Cirrhosis

OVERVIEW

- Cirrhosis is a chronic, progressive liver disease characterized by diffuse fibrotic bands of connective tissue that distort the liver's normal architectural anatomy.
- Extensive degeneration and destruction of hepatocytes occur.
- Vascular, lymphatic, and bile drainage flow alterations result from compression caused by proliferation of fibrous tissue.
- Cirrhosis is classified as
    1. *Micronodular* cirrhosis: the liver is enlarged; it is seen in conditions with a persistent damaging agent, such as alcohol; and it is characterized by small, regular, thick bands of connective tissue. Every liver lobule is involved, and nodules do not vary in size.
    2. *Macronodular* cirrhosis: the liver is small, shrunken, not palpable, irregular in shape, multilobular, and characterized by bands of connective tissue of varying thickness; nodules vary in size.
    3. *Mixed* cirrhosis: has features of both micronodular and macronodular disorganizational patterns of connective tissue.
- The four main types of cirrhosis are
    1. *Laennec's cirrhosis* (also known as alcohol-induced, nutritional, or portal cirrhosis)
        a. Alcohol has a direct toxic effect on liver cells, causing liver inflammation (alcoholic hepatitis).
        b. Metabolic changes lead to fatty infiltration of the hepatocytes and scarring between the liver lobules.
        c. The liver becomes enlarged with cellular infiltration by fat, leukocytes, and lymphocytes.
        d. Early scar formation is caused by fibroblast infiltration and collagen formation.
        e. Damage to the hepatic parenchyma progresses, and widespread scar tissue forms with fibrotic infiltration of the liver as a result of cellular necrosis.
    2. *Postnecrotic cirrhosis*
        a. Occurs after massive liver cell necrosis,

139

resulting as a complication of acute viral hepatitis or after exposure to industrial or chemical hepatotoxins.

   b. Broad bands of scar tissue cause destruction of liver lobules and entire lobes.

3. *Biliary cirrhosis*

   a. Develops from chronic biliary obstruction, bile stasis, and inflammation, resulting in severe obstructive jaundice.

   b. Primary biliary cirrhosis results from intrahepatic bile stasis.

   c. Secondary biliary cirrhosis is caused by obstruction of the hepatic or common bile ducts, producing hepatic bile stasis, which causes progressive fibrosis, hepatocellular destruction, and regenerated nodules.

4. *Cardiac cirrhosis*

   a. Associated with severe right-sided congestive heart failure, it results in an enlarged, edematous, congested liver.

   b. The liver serves as a reservoir for a large amount of venous blood that the failing heart is unable to pump into circulation.

   c. The liver becomes anoxic, resulting in liver cell necrosis and fibrosis.

- Complications of cirrhosis include

1. *Portal hypertension*: a persistent increase in pressure within the portal vein developing as a result of increased resistance or obstruction to flow

2. *Ascites*: the accumulation of free fluid containing almost pure plasma within the peritoneal cavity; increased hydrostatic pressure from portal hypertension results in venous congestion of the hepatic capillaries, causing plasma to leak directly from the liver surface and portal vein; other contributing factors include reduced circulating plasma protein and increased hepatic lymphatic formation

3. *Bleeding esophageal varices*: fragile, thin-walled, distended esophageal veins that are irritated and rupture; varices occur in the lower esophagus most frequently and also occur in the proximal esophagus and stomach

4. *Coagulation defects*: decreased synthesis of bile fats in the liver that prevent the absorption of fat-soluble vitamins; without vitamin K, and clotting factors II, VII, IX, and X, the client is prone to bleeding

5. *Jaundice,* caused by one of two mechanisms:
    a. Hepatocellular jaundice: The liver is unable to metabolize bilirubin.
    b. Intrahepatic obstruction: Edema, fibrosis, or scarring of the hepatic bile duct channels and bile ducts interfere with normal bile and bilirubin excretion.
6. *Portal systemic encephalopathy* (hepatic encephalopathy and hepatic coma): end-stage hepatic failure and cirrhosis; manifested by neurologic symptoms, characterized by altered level of consciousness, impaired thinking processes, and neuromuscular disturbances
7. *Hepatorenal syndrome:* progressive, oliguric renal failure associated with hepatic failure resulting in functionally impaired kidneys; manifested by a sudden decrease in urinary flow and elevated serum urea nitrogen and creatinine levels, with abnormally decreased urine sodium excretion and increased urine osmolarity

COLLABORATIVE MANAGEMENT

Assessment

- The nurse records the client's
    1. Age, sex, and race
    2. Employment history, including working conditions exposing the client to harmful chemical toxins
    3. History of individual and family alcoholism
    4. Previous medical conditions, including acute viral hepatitis, biliary tract disease, viral infections, recent blood transfusions, or history of heart disease or respiratory disorders
- The nurse assesses for
    1. Generalized weakness
    2. Weight loss
    3. Gastrointestinal symptoms, including loss of appetite, early morning nausea and vomiting, dyspepsia, flatulence, and changes in bowel habits
    4. Abdominal pain or tenderness
    5. Jaundice of the skin and sclera
    6. Dry skin, rashes
    7. Petechiae or ecchymosis
    8. Palmar erythema
    9. Spider angiomas on the nose, cheeks, upper thorax, and shoulders
    10. Hepatomegaly palpated in the right upper quadrant

11. Ascites revealed by bulging flanks and dullness on percussion of the abdomen
12. Protruding umbilicus
13. Dilated abdominal veins (caput medusae)
14. Presence of blood in vomitus or nasogastric drainage
15. Fetor hepaticus, the fruity, musty breath odor of chronic liver disease
16. Amenorrhea and testicular atrophy
17. Gynecomastia (enlarged breasts)
18. Impotence
19. Asterixis (liver flap), a coarse tremor characterized by rapid, nonrhythmic extension and flexions in the wrist and fingers

Planning and Implementation

NFDx: FLUID VOLUME EXCESS

Nonsurgical Management

- The nurse
  1. Provides a low-sodium diet initially, restricting sodium to 200 to 500 mg daily
  2. Suggests alternative flavoring additives
  3. Consults the dietitian
  4. Restricts fluid intake to 1500 mL/day
  5. Supplements vitamins with thiamine, folate, and multivitamin preparations, as ordered
  6. Gives diuretics, as ordered
  7. Monitors intake and output carefully
  8. Weighs the client daily
  9. Measures abdominal girth daily
  10. Monitors electrolyte balance
  11. Administers low-sodium antacids, as ordered
  12. Assists the physician with paracentesis to remove ascitic fluid
  13. Elevates the head of the bed to minimize shortness of breath

Surgical Management

- A peritoneovenous shunt, or surgical bypass shunting procedure, such as a LeVeen's or Denver shunt, may be performed for severe ascites. Ascites is drained through a one-way valve into a silicone rubber tube that terminates in the superior vena cava.
- Preoperative care is aimed at optimizing the client's physical state.
- The nurse provides preoperative care
  1. Administers fresh frozen plasma, as ordered
  2. Administers vitamin K, as ordered
  3. Ensures that packed red cells are available for surgery

4. Provides routine preoperative care
- The nurse provides postoperative care
  1. Provides routine postoperative care
  2. Assesses for fluid volume excess and hemodilution
  3. Administers diuretics, as ordered, for volume excess
  4. Monitors coagulation results
  5. Performs daily abdominal girth measurements
  6. Records accurate intake and output
  7. Weighs the client daily

NDx: POTENTIAL FOR INJURY
Nonsurgical Management
- The nurse
  1. Maintains gastric intubation to assess bleeding
  2. Maintains esophagogastric balloon tamponade with a Sangstaken-Blakemore or Minnesota tube to control bleeding varices, as ordered
  3. Administers blood products (red blood cells and fresh frozen plasma), as ordered
- Vasopressin is given intra-arterially or intravenously to lower pressures in the portal venous system to decrease bleeding.
- The nurse assesses for
  1. Abdominal cramping
  2. Pallor
  3. Cardiac dysrhythmias
  4. Chest pain
- Injection sclerotherapy is done to sclerose bleeding esophageal varices.

Surgical Management
- Surgical portal-systemic shunting procedures are considered a last-resort intervention for clients with portal hypertension and esophageal varices, to decrease the portal hypertension:
  1. The *portocaval shunt* diverts the portal venous blood flow into the inferior vena cava to decrease portal pressure.
  2. The *splenorenal shunting* procedure involves a splenectomy with anastamosis of the splenic vein with the left renal vein.
  3. In the *mesocaval shunt*, the superior mesenteric vein is anastamosed to the inferior vena cava.
- Preoperative care includes correcting bleeding and clotting deficits by administering fresh frozen plasma and packed cells.

- After surgery the client is admitted to a critical care unit.
- The nurse provides postoperative care
  1. Provides routine postoperative care
  2. Closely monitors the client's hemodynamic status
  3. Maintains mechanical ventilation and the artificial airway
  4. Carefully administers narcotic analgesia for pain and sedation, as ordered
  5. Closely monitors urinary output
  6. Monitors for rebleeding from esophageal varices or from shunting procedure anastamosis sites
  7. Observes for postshunt encephalopathy
  8. Administers total parenteral nutrition, as ordered
  9. Administers albumin, as ordered

NDx: POTENTIAL FOR ALTERED THOUGHT PROCESSES
Nonsurgical Management
- The nurse
  1. Assesses for neurologic changes
  2. Limits protein intake in the diet to reduce excess protein breakdown by intestinal bacteria
  3. Consults with the dietitian to limit dietary protein to 50 to 60 g/day
  4. Initiates total parenteral nutrition (TPN), as ordered, if GI bleeding precipitates hepatic encephalopathy
  5. Gives lactulose, as ordered, to promote excretion of fecal ammonia
  6. Administers neomycin sulfate, as ordered, to act as an intestinal antiseptic
  7. Administers stool softeners, as ordered, to prevent constipation in long-term therapy
  8. Restricts drugs such as narcotics, sedatives, or barbiturates

Discharge Planning
- Client/family education is individualized for the client depending on the etiology of the disease.
- The nurse teaches the client/family to
  1. Consume a diet high in calories, protein, and vitamins
  2. Restrict sodium intake if ascites occurs
  3. Restrict protein if prone to encephalopathy
  4. Take diuretics as prescribed, including reporting symptoms of hypokalemia and consuming foods high in potassium
  5. Take antacids or H_2 antagonists, as ordered, for GI bleeding
  6. Avoid all over-the-counter medications
  7. Avoid alcohol

8. Keep follow-up visits with the physician(s)

For more information on cirrhosis, see *Medical-Surgical Nursing: A Nursing Process Approach*, **pp. 1479–1505.**

Colorectal Cancer

OVERVIEW

- Colorectal cancer is the most common cancer in the United States among men and women when considered as a group.
- The malignant process begins in cells lining the bowel wall.
- Tumors occur in all areas of the colon, and most cancers develop from adenomatous polyps.
- Tumors spread by direct invasion and via the lymphatic and circulatory systems.
- Complications include bowel perforation with peritonitis, abscess and/or fistula formation, frank hemorrhage,and complete intestinal obstruction.

COLLABORATIVE MANAGEMENT

Assessment

- The nurse records the client's
  1. Diet history
  2. Family history of colorectal cancer
  3. Personal history of ulcerative colitis, familial polyposis, or adenomas
  4. Weight loss
  5. Change in bowel habits with or without blood in stool

- The nurse assesses for
  1. Rectal bleeding (the most common manifestation)
  2. Cachexia (a late sign)
  3. Guarding or abdominal distention
  4. Abdominal mass (a late sign)

Planning and Implementation

NDx: POTENTIAL FOR INJURY

Nonsurgical Management

- Radiation therapy aids in creating more definite tumor margins, facilitating surgical resection.

- Radiation is also used postoperatively to decrease the risk of recurrence or palliatively to reduce pain, hemorrhage, bowel obstruction, or metastasis.

- Chemotherapy is used postoperatively to assist in control of metastatic symptoms and spread of the disease.

- The chemotherapeutic drug typically used is 5-fluorouracil in conjunction with Leucovirin.

- Intrahepatic arterial chemotherapy is given with liver metastasis.

Surgical Management

- Surgical intervention is the primary treatment method for tumors located in the colon or rectum.

- The bowel segment containing the tumor is resected (removed) along with several inches of bowel beyond the tumor margin, and an end-to-end anastamosis is performed; a temporary or permanent colostomy may be performed.

- Right-sided colon tumors require a right hemicolectomy for smaller lesions, a right-ascending colostomy or ileostomy for large, widespread tumors, or a cecostomy (opening into the cecum with intubation to decompress the bowel).

- Left-sided colon tumors require a left hemicolectomy for smaller lesions or a left-descending colostomy for larger lesions (e.g., Hartmann's colostomy).

- Sigmoid colon tumors require a sigmoid colectomy for smaller lesions, a sigmoid colostomy for larger lesions (e.g., Hartmann's colostomy), or an abdominal-perineal resection for large low sigmoid tumors (near the anus) with colostomy (the rectum and anus are completely removed, leaving a perineal wound).

- Rectal tumors require resection with anastamosis or pull-through procedure (preserves anal sphincter and normal elimination patterns), a colon resection with permanent colostomy, or an abdominal-perineal (A-P) resection (the entire rectum and support structures are removed, and the anus is closed) with permanent colostomy.

- The nurse provides preoperative care
  1. Reinforces the physician's explanation of the procedure
  2. Consults the enterostomal therapist to assist in identifying optimal placement of the ostomy and to instruct the client about the rationale and general principles of ostomies
  3. Instructs the client to eat a low-residue diet for a day or longer before bowel surgery to minimize colonic contents
  4. Prepares the client for general anesthesia
  5. Administers laxatives or enemas, if ordered, the morning of surgery or the day before surgery if the client is hospitalized
  6. Administers antibiotics preoperatively, as ordered; intravenous cephalothin (Keflin) or oral erythromycin (E-Mycin) and kanamycin (Kantrex) are typically given the night before surgery
- The nurse provides postoperative care
  1. Places a petroleum gauze over the stoma to keep it moist, followed by a dry, sterile dressing, if a pouch system is not in place immediately postoperatively
  2. Places a pouch system on the stoma as soon as possible
  3. Observes the stoma for
     a. Necrotic tissue
     b. Unusual amount of bleeding
     c. Color changes (the normal color is red pink, indicating high vascularity; pale pink indicates low hemoglobin and hematocrit levels, and purple black indicates compromised circulation)
     d. Size
  4. Checks the pouch system for proper fit and signs of leakage
  5. Assesses for functioning of the colostomy 2 to 4 days postoperatively; stool is liquid immediately postoperatively but becomes more solid
  6. Empties the pouch for excess gas collection and when it is one-third to one-half stool
  7. Irrigates the perineal wound, if ordered
  8. Changes the perineal wound dressing, as directed
  9. Provides comfort measures for perineal itching and pain, such as antipruritic medications (benzocaine) and sitz baths

10. Assesses for signs of infection, abscess, or other complications
11. Instructs the client regarding activities such as assuming a side-lying position, avoiding sitting for long periods, and using a foam pad or pillow when in a sitting position
12. Administers cephalosporin antibiotics such as cefalothin (Keflin) intravenously, as ordered
13. Administers pain medication, as ordered

Discharge Planning
• The nurse provides verbal and written postoperative instructions
1. Inspection of the abdominal incision (and perineal wound if an A-P resection was done) for redness, tenderness, swelling, and drainage
2. Dressing change and wound care procedures
3. Colostomy care, including care of the stoma, application of the pouch system, skin protection, and gas and odor control
4. Pain management, including medications
5. Dietary control and foods that cause excess gas formation and odor
6. Tips on how to resume normal activities, including work, travel, and sexual intercourse
7. Signs and symptoms of complications, such as intestinal obstruction and perforation

For more information on colorectal cancer, see *Medical-Surgical Nursing: A Nursing Process Approach*, **pp. 1379–1393.**

Conjunctivitis

• Conjunctivitis is an inflammation or infection of the conjunctiva of the eye.
• Types of conjunctivitis and their treatment include

1. *Allergic* conjunctivitis
   a. Associated with a sensitivity to pollens, animal protein, feathers, certain foods or materials, insect bites, and/or drugs
   b. Manifested by edema of the conjunctiva, burning and itching sensation, excessive tearing, and engorgement of blood vessels
   c. Treatment consists of instillation of vasoconstrictors, corticosteroid for severe cases, and teaching the client to instill the eye medication
2. *Bacterial* conjunctivitis
   a. Referred to as "pink eye" and is easily transmitted
   b. Manifested by blood vessel dilation, mild conjunctival edema, tearing, and watery discharge, which becomes purulent
   c. Treatment consists of broad-spectrum antibiotic ointment until the causative organism is identified
   d. Client education consists of
      (1) Hygienic principles to prevent spread of the infection
      (2) Importance of hand washing before and after instilling eyedrops
      (3) How to instill eyedrops
      (4) Importance of not rubbing the eye or carelessly disposing of tissues
3. *Viral* conjunctivitis
   a. Results from infection with the human adenovirus or from systemic viral diseases like mumps and mononucleosis
   b. Manifested by enlarged preauricular lymph nodes, photophobia, and a sensation of a foreign body in the eye
   c. Treatment consists of rest and a mild analgesic; antibiotic ointment is used for secondary infection

For more information on conjunctivitis, see *Medical-Surgical Nursing: A Nursing Process Approach,* **pp. 1027–1028.**

Corneal Disorders

OVERVIEW

- There are several types of corneal problems:
  1. *Keratoconus*, a degenerative disease that causes generalized thinning and forward protrusion of the cornea
  2. *Dystrophies*, characterized by the abnormal deposition of substances, cause changes in the corneal structure
  3. *Keratitis*, an inflammation of the cornea, caused by infection or irritation
  4. *Corneal ulcer*, a break in the normally intact corneal epithelium

COLLABORATIVE MANAGEMENT

Assessment

- The nurse assesses for
  1. Location, quantity, quality, timing, and setting
     a. Eye pain
     b. Impaired vision
     c. Drainage
  2. Aggravating or relieving factors
  3. Vision history, photophobia
  4. Associated manifestations
  5. Medication history
  6. Hazy or cloudy-looking cornea
  7. Changes in body image, self-esteem, role identity, and social isolation

Planning and Implementation

NDx: SENSORY/PERCEPTUAL ALTERATIONS (VISION)

Nonsurgical Management

- The nurse
  1. Administers antibiotics, antifungal agents, and antiviral agents, as ordered, depending on the causative organism
  2. Administers steroids, as ordered
  3. Times ophthalmic administration of drugs carefully (If two medications must be administered at the same time, 5 minutes should separate their instillation.)
  4. Uses separate, clearly labeled bottles of medication if the same medication is used for both eyes, one of them infected
  5. Wears gloves if drainage is present

6. Washes hands before and after administration of medication

Surgical Management

- *Keratoplasty*, or corneal transplant, is used to restore vision. One of two procedures is performed:
    1. Lamellar, or partial-thickness keratoplasty
    2. Penetrating, full-thickness keratoplasty
- The nurse provides preoperative care
    1. Provides routine preoperative care
    2. Recognizes that the client often has short notice that a transplant is available and may be anxious upon arrival at the hospital
    3. Informs the client that facial and retrobulbar anesthesia is typically used
    4. Instructs the client in the importance of lying still during the procedure; if unable to lie still, general anesthesia may be used
- The nurse provides postoperative care
    1. Leaves the pressure dressing and eye shield in place until a specific order for removal is written by the surgeon
    2. Notifies the physician of any significant drainage
    3. Implements special measures since the client is unable to see out of the affected eye due to the patch
        a. Reorients the client to the environment
        b. Sets up a tray and explains where food items and beverages are located
        c. Places call bell, telephone, and other necessary items within easy reach
        d. Approaches the client from the unaffected side; knocks on the door before entering the room and announces his or her name and purpose of the visit
        e. Provides sensory stimulation, such as a radio and TV
    4. Observes for and reports complications of surgery
        a. Bleeding
        b. Infection
        c. Graft rejection
        d. Wound leakage

NDx: POTENTIAL FOR INJURY

- The nurse
    1. Assesses the vision in the unaffected eye and provides assistance as needed
    2. Orients the client to the environment
    3. Does not move objects in the room without the client's consent

4. Removes hazards, keeps the bed in the low position, and moves wastebaskets out of the area where the client is likely to walk
5. Places the call bell within easy reach
6. Assists as needed with meals
7. Instructs the client that depth perception will be altered and assists accordingly
8. Informs the client that an eye shield, glasses, or sunglasses are worn during the day and an eye shield at night

NDx: PAIN

• The nurse administers analgesics such as codeine or acetaminophen, as ordered.

• Severe pain or pain accompanied by nausea is indicative of increased intraocular pressure; the nurse notifies the physician immediately and elevates the head of the bed 30 degrees.

Discharge Planning

• The nurse
1. Assists with the identification and correction of hazards in the home prior to discharge
2. Refers the client/family to a home health agency and Meals on Wheels, as needed
3. Instructs the client not to bend over from the waist or rub, bump, or scratch the eye
4. Reviews eyelid care
    a. Moisten the cotton ball with the ophthalmic irrigation solution
    b. Close the eye and wipe gently across the eyelashes from the medial canthus to the lateral canthus
    c. Use a new cotton ball for each wipe
5. Instructs the client about vision checks
    a. Check vision using the same focal point daily
    b. Notify the physician immediately if vision is reduced or if previously clear objects appear to be out of focus
6. Provides drug information
    a. Aseptic instillation of drops
    b. Schedule of administration
7. Emphasizes the importance of follow-up visits with the physician(s)

For more information on corneal disorders, see *Medical-Surgical Nursing: A Nursing Process Approach,* **pp. 1028–1036.**

Coronary Artery Disease

OVERVIEW

- Coronary artery disease (CAD), also known as coronary heart disease or ischemic heart disease, affects the three major coronary arteries (right, left anterior descending, and left circumflex), which provide nutrients and blood to the myocardium.
- When blood flow is blocked, ischemia and infarction of the myocardium occur.
- The most common cause of CAD is atherosclerosis, which is characterized by a fibrous plaque lesion that obstructs blood flow (see Atherosclerosis).
- Other causes include coronary artery spasm and nonatherosclerotic causes, such as hypotension, anemia, hypovolemia, polycythemia, and valvular problems.
- The presence of *angina* (chest pain) indicates ischemia.
- *Myocardial infarction* (MI) results from a sudden interruption in blood supply to the heart from occlusion of a coronary artery, resulting in death of cardiac muscle.

COLLABORATIVE MANAGEMENT

Assessment

- The nurse records the client's
  1. Description of chest discomfort currently and in the past, especially in terms of sensation, location, radiation, and duration
  2. Related pain, including upper back, jaw, or arms
  3. Past hospitalizations for angina or MI
  4. Medications
  5. Family history
  6. Risk factors, including eating habits, life-style, and physical activity levels
- The nurse assesses for
  1. Presence of chest, epigastric, jaw, back, or arm discomfort
  2. Associated symptoms of ischemia, including
     a. Nausea
     b. Vomiting
     c. Diaphoresis
     d. Dizziness
     e. Weakness

f. Palpitations
g. Shortness of breath
3. Blood pressure changes
4. Cardiac dysrhythmias
5. Distal peripheral pulses
6. Skin temperature
7. S_3 gallop
8. Respiratory rate
9. Adventitious breath sounds
10. Psychologic denial of MI or angina

Planning and Implementation

NDx: ALTERED (CARDIOPULMONARY) TISSUE PERFUSION

Nonsurgical Management

- The nurse administers the following drugs, as ordered
    1. Nitrates, including sublingual, oral, intravenous, and topical nitroglycerin agents, which are vasodilators that reduce venous return to the heart (preload), decreasing myocardial oxygen consumption, and also increase coronary artery blood flow and reduce coronary spasm
    2. Beta-blocking agents, such as propranolol (Inderal), which decrease myocardial oxygen consumption by decreasing heart rate and contractility
    3. Calcium channel blockers, which cause coronary artery dilation and peripheral arterial dilation; Verapamil (Calan) and diltiazem (Cardiazem) reduce heart rate
    4. Platelet antiaggregates that modify platelet behavior to prevent adhesion in the coronary arteries
    5. Narcotic analgesia used for chest pain unrelieved by nitroglycerin
    6. Thrombolytic agents, such as Streptokinase and tissue-type plasminogen activator (TPA), which are used in acute MI to lyse or dissolve clots
- The nurse
    1. Maintains the client on bed rest during an acute attack
    2. Provides supplemental oxygen, as ordered
    3. Monitors the heart rate and rhythm continuously
    4. Monitors vital signs frequently to assess hemodynamic effects of drug therapy and tissue perfusion
    5. Controls the environment to minimize anxiety and stress

- *Percutaneous transluminal coronary angioplasty (PTCA)*, an invasive, nonsurgical technique, is done to reduce or eliminate the occluded lesion.
- An *intra-aortic counterpulsation* device, such as the intra-aortic balloon pump (IAPB), is used in an emergency to improve coronary perfusion in acute MI.

Surgical Management

- *Coronary artery bypass surgery (CABG)* is a surgical procedure in which a saphenous vein from a leg or the internal mammary artery is used to bypass an occlusion or lesion in the coronary artery. The vessel is anastamosed proximally and distally to the coronary artery to bypass blood around the occluded artery, improving cardiac tissue perfusion.
- CABG requires that the client undergo cardiopulmonary bypass, which is accomplished by cannulation of the inferior and superior venae cavae. Blood is diverted from the heart to the bypass machine, which oxygenates the blood and returns it through a cannula placed in the ascending aortic arch.
- Emergency CABG is necessary when the client does not respond to medical treatment for angina or when complications occur during PTCA or cardiac catheterization.
- The nurse provides preoperative care
  1. Informs the client to expect the following after surgery
     a. Sternal and graft harvest incisions
     b. One or more chest tubes
     c. A Foley catheter
     d. Multiple intravenous (IV) lines
     e. An endotracheal tube connected to a mechanical ventilator
     f. Sophisticated monitoring devices such as an arterial line or pulmonary artery catheter
  2. Provides the client/family the opportunity to visit the cardiothoracic surgery critical care area to meet the staff and examine the environment
  3. Teaches the client respiratory and leg exercises
- After surgery, the client is transferred to the critical care area. The critical care nurse provides postoperative care
  1. Maintains the endotracheal tube and mechanical ventilator
  2. Connects the chest tubes to water seal drainage/suction systems and monitors for excess bleeding

3. Assesses epicardial pacer wires and tape to the client's chest
4. Connects the arterial and pulmonary artery catheters to the monitoring system
5. Monitors the client's hemodynamic status
6. Assesses for cardiac dysrhythmias, including ventricular ectopic beats or heart block
7. Connects the epicardial pacer wires to a pacemaker box, as indicated, for dysrhythmias
8. Replaces fluid and electrolytes by administering IV fluids with potassium supplements
9. Administers vasoactive drugs, such as dopamine, dobutamine, isuprel, or epinephrine, as ordered, to maintain blood pressure and coronary perfusion
10. Provides routine postoperative care

NDx: Decreased Cardiac Output

• A major objective of treatment is the maintenance of cardiac output to promote circulatory function.

• Control of chest pain associated with decreased cardiac output is managed by administration of nitrates, such as nitroglycerin (Nitrostat, Tridil) and isosorbide dinitrate (Isordil, Iso-Bid), and other vasodilator agents, such as calcium channel blockers, e.g., Nifedipine (Procardia, Adalat).

• Maintenance of normal sinus rhythm is accomplished by administration of antidysrhythmic agents, as needed.

• Inotropic medications, such as dopamine (Intropin) and dobutamine (Dobutrex), are given to increase cardiac output.

• Pacemaker insertion may be necessary for heart block rhythms.

NDx: Activity Intolerance

• The nurse assists the client in following a cardiac rehabilitation program
1. Phase 1, acute illness phase, promotes rest yet ensures some limited mobilization.
2. Phase 2 begins after discharge and continues through home convalescence.
3. Phase 3 refers to long-term conditioning.

Discharge Planning

• The nurse implements the cardiac teaching plan
1. Normal cardiac anatomy and physiology
2. Pathophysiology of angina and MI
3. Risk factor modification
   a. Smoking cessation

   b. Changing dietary habits by reducing total fat intake, reducing sodium intake, and maintaining ideal body weight

   c. Exercising regularly

   d. Controlling high blood pressure

   e. Controlling diabetes

   f. Reducing stress

4. Cardiac medications, including type and benefit of drug prescribed, potential side effects, and correct dosing

5. Activity and exercise protocols

- The nurse reinforces
1. Activities specified in the cardiac rehabilitation program
2. The basic tenets of a stress-reduction program
3. Postoperative instructions for the client undergoing CABG

   a. Incisional care for the sternal wound and leg graft harvest site

   b. Reporting signs and symptoms of infection to the surgeon, including wound erythema, swelling, drainage, and fever

3. Elevating the donor site leg
4. Importance of follow-up visits with the physician(s)

For more information on coronary artery disease, see *Medical-Surgical Nursing: A Nursing Process Approach*, **pp. 2149–2163.**

Crohn's Disease

OVERVIEW

- Crohn's disease, or regional enteritis, occurs anywhere in the gastrointestinal (GI) tract but most often affects the terminal ileum with patchy lesions that extend through all bowel layers.

- This inflammatory bowel disease is similar to ulcerative colitis and is characterized by remissions and exacerbations.

- Chronic pathologic changes within the colon and small bowel include thickening of the bowel wall and narrowing of the lumen.

- In advanced disease, the bowel mucosa has nodular swelling intermingled with deep ulcerations, which contribute to fistula formation.

COLLABORATIVE MANAGEMENT
Assessment
- The nurse records the client's
    1. Family history of inflammatory bowel disease
    2. Previous and current therapy for illnesses
    3. Diet history, including usual patterns and intolerance to milk products and greasy, fried, or spicy foods
    4. History of diarrheal stools, anorexia, and fatigue
- The nurse assesses for
    1. Right lower quadrant abdominal pain or periumbilical pain before and after bowel movements
    2. Diarrhea with steatorrhea (the stool does not usually contain blood)
    3. Low-grade fever
    4. Weight loss

Planning and Implementation
NDx: Impaired Skin Integrity
- The care of the client with Crohn's disease is similar to that for the client with ulcerative colitis (see Ulcerative Colitis).

- Impaired skin integrity results from fistula formation; the degree of associated problems is related to the location of the fistula, the client's general health status, and the character and amount of fistula drainage.

- The nurse
    1. Replaces fluid loss with oral fluids as well as ordered intravenous fluids
    2. Recognizes that the client requires at least 3000 kcal/day to promote fistula healing
    3. Provides high-calorie, high-protein meals with supplements
    4. Applies a pouch to the fistula to prevent skin irritation and to measure the drainage
    5. Covers the area around the fistula with skin barriers such as Stomahesive or DuoDerm, and

applies a wound drainage system over the fistula, securing it to the protective barriers
6. Cleanses adjacent skin and keeps it dry
7. Consults an enterostomal therapist for skin management plan

Discharge Planning
- See Ulcerative Colitis, "Discharge Planning."

For more information on Crohn's disease, see *Medical-Surgical Nursing: A Nursing Process Approach*, **pp. 1362–1365.**

Cushing's Syndrome

OVERVIEW

- Cushing's syndrome (hypercortisolism) results from the production of excess amounts of glucocorticoids, causing widespread abnormalities.
- The disorder may be caused by bilateral adrenal hyperplasia secondary to a pituitary or nonendocrine tumor that produces excess adrenocorticotrophic hormone (ACTH) or the use of exogenous glucocorticoids or ACTH in the therapy of clinical entities such as organ transplantation, adjunct to chemotherapy, or treatment of neurologic or cardiothoracic disease.

COLLABORATIVE MANAGEMENT
Assessment
- The nurse records the client's
  1. Change in activity or sleep pattern
  2. Past medical history
     a. Steroid or alcohol abuse

    b. Frequency of infections
    c. Easy bruising
- The nurse assesses for
  1. Fatigue
  2. Muscle weakness
  3. Bone pain, history of fractures
  4. Characteristic physical changes
     a. Buffalo hump
     b. Centripetal obesity
     c. Supraclavicular fat pads
     d. Round or moon face
     e. Large trunk
     f. Thin arms and legs
     g. Generalized muscle wasting and weakness
  5. Characteristic skin changes
     a. Bruises
     b. Thin, translucent skin
     c. Wounds that have not healed properly
     d. Reddish-purple striae on the abdomen and upper thighs
     e. Fine coating of hair over the face and body
     f. Acne
  6. Hypertension
  7. Emotional lability, irritability, confusion, depression
  8. Increased plasma cortisol level
  9. Increased urinary 17-ketosteroids and 17-hydroxycorticosteroids

Planning and Implementation

NDx: FLUID VOLUME EXCESS
Nonsurgical Management
- The nurse administers drug therapy, as ordered
  1. Mitotane (Lysodren) for inoperable adrenal tumors
  2. Aminoglutethimide (Elipten, Cytadren) and metyrapone to decrease cortisol production
  3. Metyrapone in combination with mitotane to decrease cortisol production
- Radiation therapy is not always effective and may destroy normal tissue.

Surgical Management
- Transphenoidal removal of the microadenoma is performed if hyperfunction is caused by increased pituitary secretion of ACTH.
- A *hypophysectomy* (surgical removal of the pituitary gland) may be indicated if the microadenoma cannot be located.

- *Adrenalectomy* is indicated if the etiologic agent is an adrenal adenoma or carcinoma.
- A unilateral adrenalectomy is done if only one gland is involved.
- A bilateral adrenalectomy is required for ectopic ACTH-producing tumors that cannot be treated by other means.
- The nurse provides preoperative care
  1. Monitors electrolyte balance
  2. Ensures a high-calorie, high-protein diet
  3. Administers glucocorticoid preparations, as ordered
  4. Monitors for and reports hyperglycemia
- The nurse provides postoperative care
  1. Provides routine postoperative care according to the critical care unit guidelines, including hemodynamic monitoring per protocol
  2. Monitors for signs and symptoms of cardiovascular collapse and shock
  3. Carefully measures intake and output
  4. Weighs the client daily
  5. Monitors serum electrolytes daily
  6. Administer glucocorticoids, as ordered
  7. Identifies the need for and provides pain management

NDx: IMPAIRED SKIN INTEGRITY

- The nurse
  1. Assesses the skin frequently to detect reddened areas, excoriation, breakdown, and edema
  2. Observes venipuncture sites for excessive bleeding
  3. Turns the client frequently (at least every 2 hours)
  4. Pads bony prominences
- The nurse instructs the client
  1. To use a soft toothbrush
  2. To use an electric razor for shaving
  3. To keep the skin clean and dry
  4. To use moisturizing skin lotion

NDx: ACTIVITY INTOLERANCE

- The nurse
  1. Assists the client with activities of daily living, as needed
  2. Provides the client with frequent periods of uninterrupted rest

NDx: POTENTIAL FOR INJURY (FRACTURE)

- Hypercortisolism results in demineralization of bone and may lead to osteoporosis.

- The nurse instructs the client about safety issues and dietary needs
  1. To consume a high-calorie diet, including milk, cheese, yogurt, and green leafy and root vegetables
  2. To avoid caffeine and alcohol
  3. To keep rooms free of hazardous objects
  4. To use ambulatory aids correctly, if necessary

NDx: Body Image Disturbance
- The nurse
  1. Suggests clothing to minimize physical features that may be disturbing to the client
  2. Encourages the client to discuss feelings related to physical changes and refer for further counseling if needed

Discharge Planning
- The nurse teaches the client/family
  1. How to identify and correct hazards in the home prior to discharge
  2. How to care for the surgical wound, if applicable
  3. To report complications of surgery to the physician

For more information on adrenal hyperfunction, see *Medical-Surgical Nursing: A Nursing Process Approach,* **pp. 1550–1555.**

Cyst

- Cysts are firm, flesh-colored nodules containing liquid or semisolid material and characterized by fluctuance and mobility on palpation.
- An *epidermal inclusion* cyst, the most common type,

can be located anywhere on the body but most frequently is found on the head and trunk.

- Cyst removal is rarely indicated.

- A *pilonidal* cyst is a lesion found in the sacral area associated with a sinus tract extending to deeper tissue structures.

- Secondary infection may require surgical incision and drainage.

For more information on cysts, see *Medical-Surgical Nursing: A Nursing Process Approach*, **p. 1207.**

Cystitis

OVERVIEW

- Cystitis is an inflammation of the urinary bladder from infectious causes, such as bacteria, viruses, fungi, or parasites, or noninfectious causes, such as chemical exposure or radiation therapy.

- Cystitis refers to symptomatic lower urinary tract infections (UTI) caused by bacterial invasion.

COLLABORATIVE MANAGEMENT

Assessment

- The nurse records the client's
  1. Age and sex
  2. History of prior UTI
  3. History of renal or urologic problems, such as stones
  4. History of health problems, such as diabetes mellitus

- The nurse assesses for
  1. Pain or discomfort on urination
  2. Urgency to void

3. Difficulty in initiating urination
4. Feelings of incomplete bladder emptying
5. Voiding in small amounts
6. Increased frequency of voiding
7. Complete inability to urinate
8. Changes in urine color, clarity, or odor
9. Abdominal or back pain
10. Confusion or increased confusion in elderly clients
11. Bladder distention
12. Urinary meatus inflammation
13. Prostate gland changes or tenderness

Planning and Implementation

NDx: PAIN

Nonsurgical Management

- The nurse
  1. Administers analgesics, as ordered, to promote comfort
  2. Administers urinary antiseptics, as ordered, such as nitrofurantoin (Furadantin and Macrodantin) and trimethoprim (Proloprim, Trimpex)
  3. Administers anticholinergics, as ordered, to decrease bladder spasm and promote complete bladder emptying
  4. Administers antibiotics, as ordered, for systemic infection
  5. Maintains an adequate caloric intake
  6. Ensures a fluid intake of 2 to 3 L/day
  7. Provides warm sitz baths to relieve local symptoms

Surgical Management

- Surgical interventions for management of cystitis may include endourologic procedures with stone manipulation or pulverization for the management of urinary retention if bladder or urethral calculus is the cause.

Discharge Planning

- The nurse teaches the client to
  1. Complete the prescribed medication regime
  2. Consume liberal fluid intake of at least 2 to 3 L/day
  3. Cleanse the perineum properly after urination
  4. Empty the bladder as soon as the urge is felt
  5. Obtain adequate rest, sleep, and nutrition
  6. Avoid known irritants, such as bubble baths, nylon underwear, and scented toilet tissue
  7. Wear cotton underwear

8. Seek prompt medical care if recurrences are suspected

For more information on cystitis, see *Medical-Surgical Nursing: A Nursing Process Approach*, **pp. 1833–1839.**

c

Cystocele

- A cystocele is a protrusion of the bladder through the vaginal wall due to weakened pelvic structures.
- Causes include obesity, advanced age, childbearing, or genetic predisposition.
- Assessment findings include
  1. Difficulty in emptying the bladder
  2. Urinary frequency and urgency
  3. Urinary tract infections
  4. Stress urinary incontinence
  5. Significant bulging of the anterior vaginal wall during pelvic examination
- Management is conservative with mild symptoms and includes
  1. Use of a pessary for bladder support
  2. Estrogen therapy for the postmenopausal woman to prevent atrophy and weakening of vaginal walls
  3. Kegel exercises to strengthen perineal muscles
- Surgical intervention (anterior colporrhaphy or anterior repair) is recommended for severe symptoms. (Care is similar to other vaginal surgeries).

For more information on cystocele, see *Medical-Surgical Nursing: A Nursing Process Approach*, **p. 1706.**

Death and Dying

OVERVIEW

- Death is the termination of life.
- Brain death is the cessation of brain function; it describes a client whose heart and lungs can be maintained functionally by mechanical life-support apparatus but whose respiratory centers in the brain stem no longer function.
- General brain death criteria (varies among states) include apnea, coma more than 6 hours, loss of all brain stem reflexes, loss of pupillary response to light, loss of corneal reflex, loss of eye movement with doll's eye maneuver or caloric testing, and loss of gag and cough reflex.

COLLABORATIVE MANAGEMENT

- The nurse assesses the client to determine which of the Kübler-Ross stages of dying he or she is experiencing
  1. Shock and disbelief
  2. Denial
  3. Anger
  4. Bargaining
  5. Depression
  6. Acceptance
- Living-dying is a process; although the client is terminally ill, he or she has several months to years to live before death will take place.
- The nurse provides care for the dying client
  1. Keeps the client clean and dry
  2. Gives frequent back rubs and skin care
  3. Provides frequent mouth care
  4. Provides food and fluids according to the client's level of tolerance
  5. Asks the family/significant others if there are any religious or cultural customs that need to be attended to and begins arrangements to ensure compliance within acceptable parameters
  6. Provides accurate information to the client and family; does not attempt to answer questions that have no answers
  7. Helps the client adjust to fear of the
     a. Unknown
     b. Loss of family and friends

    c. Loss of self-control and dependency

    d. Suffering and pain

- The nurse encourages the family to

  1. Engage in normal conversation with the dying client
  2. Touch and gently stroke the client
  3. Play the client's favorite music or television shows
  4. Share their feeling of loss with the client
  5. Discuss with the client, if appropriate

     a. Location of will or other directives

     b. Executor of estate

     c. Medical durable power of attorney

     d. Funeral arrangements and memorial service

- The nurse assesses for signs of impending death

  1. Nausea and gradual refusal of food and fluids
  2. Difficulty swallowing
  3. Sleeping for increasingly longer periods of time
  4. Irregular and possibly noisy breathing
  5. Cold feet, hands, ears, and nose
  6. Mottled and blue hands and feet
  7. Decreased pulse and blood pressure
  8. Fixed and dilated pupils
  9. Emptying of bladder and bowels because of relaxation of sphincters

- The nurse provides care of the client after death

  1. Prepares the body for viewing by the family according to institutional or home policy
  2. Closes the client's eyes
  3. Places dentures (if available) in the mouth
  4. Places the client flat in bed; removes all pillows except one supporting the client's head
  5. Washes the client's body, combs the hair, places a pad around the perineum to absorb fecal material and fluid
  6. Allows the family to say their last words and perform their farewell gestures freely and naturally around the bed
  7. Allows the family and significant others to perform religious or cultural customs
  8. Offers physical and emotional support to the family
  9. Maintains compassionate concern
  10. Validates the family's feelings of loss

For more information on death and dying, see *Medical-Surgical Nursing: A Nursing Process Approach,* **pp. 197–221.**

Degenerative Joint Disease

OVERVIEW

• Degenerative joint disease (DJD), also known as osteoarthritis, is characterized by the progressive deterioration and loss of articular cartilage in peripheral and axial joints.

• Weight-bearing joints, the vertebral column, and the hands are primarily affected.

COLLABORATIVE MANAGEMENT

Assessment

• The nurse records the client's (risk factors)
  1. Occupation and nature of work
  2. Family history of arthritis
  3. Involvement in sports
  4. History of trauma
  5. Age
  6. Weight

• The nurse assesses for
  1. Joint pain, which early in the disease process diminishes after rest and intensifies after activity; later, pain occurs with slight motion or even at rest
  2. Crepitus, a continuous grating sensation
  3. Joint enlargement
  4. If the hands are involved, Heberden's nodes (at the distal interphalangeal joints) or Bouchard's nodes (at the proximal interphalangeal joints)
  5. Intra- and periarticular effusions when the knees are involved
  6. Skeletal muscle atrophy adjacent to the involved area
  7. Compression of the spine manifested by radiating pain, stiffness, and muscle spasms in one or both extremities
  8. Level of mobility
  9. Ability to perform activities of daily living (ADL)
  10. Anger, depression, and body image changes

Planning and Implementation

ND$_x$: CHRONIC PAIN

Nonsurgical Management

• The nurse administers drug therapy, as ordered

1. Nonsteroidal anti-inflammatory drugs such as ibuprofen (Motrin, Advil, Nuprin), naproxen (Naprosyn), or indomethacin (Indocin)
2. Salicylates in small doses
3. Corticosteroid injections into single joints
4. Muscle relaxants for severe muscle spasms

- The nurse
  1. Immobilizes the affected joint with a splint or brace, as prescribed
  2. Recommends 10 hours of sleep at night and a 1- or 2-hour nap in afternoon
  3. Places the affected joints in functional positions
     a. Avoids large pillows under the head or knees
     b. Uses a bed or foot cradle, if needed
     c. Has the client lie prone twice per day
  4. Applies and or teaches the importance of a moist heating pad, a hot shower, hot packs or compresses, paraffin dips, diathermy, and ultrasound
  5. Implements cold applications for acutely inflamed joints
  6. Encourages the obese client to reduce weight
  7. Applies a transcutaneous electrical stimulator (TENS), as ordered
  8. Teaches imagery, music therapy, and relaxation techniques to reduce pain

Surgical Management

- An *osteotomy* is a procedure in which the bone is cut to promote realignment.
- A total joint replacement (TJR) is used when all other measures of pain relief have failed; hips and knees are most commonly replaced. A TJR is contraindicated in the presence of infection, advanced osteoporosis, and severe inflammation.
- *Total hip replacement* (THR)
  1. The nurse provides preoperative care
     a. Reinforces the information concerning the surgery
     b. Obtains urine and sputum cultures and recommends dental examination
     c. Teaches the client to use a povidone-iodine (Betadine) scrub the night before or morning before surgery
     d. Administers intravenous antibiotics, as ordered, which are started before surgery
  2. Intraoperative care includes
     a. A specially cleaned operating room

    b. Laminar airflow units that may be used as an added precaution against infection

    c. A minimum of movement into and out of the operating room

3. The nurse provides postoperative care

    a. Provides routine postoperative care

    b. Places the client in a supine position with the head slightly elevated

    c. Places the affected leg in a neutral position by using a cradle boot

    d. Turns the client toward either side as long as the legs remain abducted

    e. Observes for signs of hip dislocation, including increased pain, shortening of the affected leg, and leg rotation

    f. Observes for signs of infection and bleeding

    g. Performs frequent neurovascular assessments

    h. Follows the physician's orders regarding activities, mobilization, and weight bearing

    i. Applies thigh-high antiembolism stockings, elastic stockings, or sequential compression devices (e.g., Venodyne)

    j. Administers anticoagulants such as aspirin, warfarin, or heparin to prevent thrombi

    k. Teaches leg exercises, including plantar flexion and dorsiflexion, circumduction of the feet, gluteal and quadriceps setting, and straight leg raises (SLR)

    l. Assesses respiratory status for signs of pulmonary emboli, atelectasis, and pneumonia

    m. Teaches the use of incentive spirometry every 1 to 2 hours for the first 2 or 3 days

    n. Provides follow-through on the exercise program developed by the physical therapist

    o. Assists the client to use assistive-adaptive devices

- *Total knee replacement* (TKR)

1. The nurse provides preoperative care
2. The nurse provides postoperative care

    a. Provides routine postoperative care

    b. Provides care similar to that for hip replacement

    c. Monitors and maintains the continuous passive motion (CPM) machine, which is often applied immediately after surgery and used intermittently for 8 to 20 hours per day (to provide passive flexion and extension)

    d. Observes for bleeding, especially if the CPM machine is used

- *Total shoulder replacement*
    1. Not as successful as other replacement surgeries; the Neer prosthesis is the most commonly used
    2. The nurse provides postoperative care
        a. Maintains the affected arm in a sling and swathe for 2 or 3 days until an exercise program begun
        b. Monitors the CPM machine, which may be used instead of the sling
        c. Performs frequent neurovascular assessments
- *Total elbow replacement*
    1. Successful in increasing range of motion
    2. Infection is a frequent complication.
    3. The CPM device is often used.
- *Finger and wrist replacements*
    1. Bulky dressing for 3 to 5 days after surgery followed by a dynamic splint, brace, or cast
    2. The arm is elevated as much as possible.
    3. A splint or short arm cast may be applied.
- *Total ankle and toe replacement*
    1. When an ankle is replaced, an arthrodesis, or bone fusion, is usually performed for added stability.
    2. Treatment involves one or more osteotomies and fusions, which are immobilized by wires and a cast.

NDx: Impaired Physical Mobility

- The nurse reinforces the exercise program developed by physical therapy
    1. Encourages consistency
    2. Teaches the client to stop if pain is increased with exercise
    3. Teaches the client to decrease the number of repetitions when inflammation is severe
    4. Teaches that exercises should be active rather than passive
    5. Teaches that ADL or household tasks do not substitute for an exercise program

Discharge Planning

- The nurse
    1. Helps the client/family to identify and correct hazards in the home prior to discharge
    2. Ensures that the client can correctly use all assistive-adaptive devices prior to discharge
    3. Provides a detailed plan of care at the time of discharge for clients to be transferred to a rehabilitation or long-term-care facility (Also see Rehabilitation.)

4. Reviews the prescribed exercise regimen and ensures client mastery by observing correct performance on return demonstration
5. Teaches joint protection techniques
   a. Turning doorknobs counterclockwise
   b. Using two hands instead of one to hold objects
   c. Sitting in a chair with a high, straight back
   d. Not bending at the waist; bending the knees instead while keeping the back straight
   e. Using a small pillow only
6. Provides drug information, as necessary
7. Instructs the client to check with the Arthritis Foundation about "new" treatments that propose to cure the disease
8. Stresses the importance of follow-up visits with the physician(s) and other therapist(s)

For more information on degenerative joint disease, see *Medical-Surgical Nursing: A Nursing Process Approach,* **pp. 675–691.**

Dehydration

OVERVIEW

● Dehydration is a state in which the body's fluid intake is not sufficient to meet the needs of the body, resulting in a fluid volume deficit.

● Dehydration may represent an actual decrease in total body water (inadequate fluid intake, excessive fluid loss), or it may be present without an actual decrease in total body water, such as when water shifts from the vascular space (plasma volume) into the interstitial space.

● Types of dehydration include
   1. Isotonic, the most common type, which involves general depletion of isotonic fluids from the

extracellular fluid (ECF) compartment (both the vascular and interstitial space). Causes of isotonic dehydration include

a. Hemorrhage
b. Vomiting, diarrhea
c. Profuse salivation
d. Fistulas, abscesses
e. Ileostomy, cecostomy
f. Frequent enemas
g. Profuse diaphoresis
h. Burns
i. Severe wounds
j. Long-term nothing-by-mouth status
k. Diuretic therapy
l. Gastrointestinal suction, nasogastric suction

2. Hypotonic, relatively rare and usually associated with chronic illness; involves the loss of solutes from the ECF in excess of water loss. Causes of hypotonic dehydration include

a. Chronic illness
b. Excessive fluid replacement
c. Renal failure
d. Chronic or severe malnutrition

3. Hypertonic dehydration, which occurs when water loss from the ECF exceeds solute loss; loss of any body fluid that is hypotonic. It is caused by

a. Hyperventilation
b. Watery diarrhea
c. Renal failure
d. Ketoacidosis
e. Diabetes insipidus
f. Excessive fluid replacement (hypertonic)
g. Excessive sodium bicarbonate administration
h. Tube feedings, dysphagia
i. Impaired thirst
j. Unconsciousness
k. Fever
l. Impaired motor function
m. Systemic infection

COLLABORATIVE MANAGEMENT

Assessment

- The nurse records the client's
  1. Past medical history
     a. Chronic or recent acute illness
     b. Recent surgery
     c. Medication history
  2. Age: The very young and the elderly are prone to

dehydration in response to relatively small fluid losses.
3. Height and weight: A weight change of 1 pound corresponds to a fluid volume change of 475 to 500 mL
4. Changes in degree of tightness of clothing, rings, and shoes: A sudden decrease in tightness may indicate dehydration; an increase in tightness may reflect a fluid shift to the interstitial space with an accompanying deficit in the vascular space.
5. Urinary output
   a. Frequency and amount of voidings
   b. Usual fluid intake and intake during the previous 24 hours
   c. Type of fluids ingested
6. Amount of strenuous physical activity
- The nurse assesses for
  1. Cardiovascular changes
     a. Increased pulse rate
     b. Thready pulse quality
     c. Decreased blood pressure
     d. Postural hypotension
     e. Flat neck and hand veins in dependent positions
     f. Diminished peripheral pulses
  2. Respiratory changes
     a. Increased respiratory rate
     b. Increased depth of respirations
  3. Neuromuscular changes
     a. Decreased central nervous system activity (lethargy to coma)
     b. Fever
  4. Renal changes
     a. Decreased urinary output
     b. Increased specific gravity
  5. Integumentary changes
     a. Skin dry and scaly
     b. Turgor poor, tenting present
     c. Mouth dry and fissured; pastelike coat present
  6. Gastrointestinal changes
     a. Decreased motility and bowel sounds
     b. Constipation
     c. Thirst
  7. Manifestations of hypertonic dehydration: skeletal muscle weakness
  8. Manifestations of hypotonic dehydration
     a. Hyperactive deep-tendon reflexes

174

b. Increased sensation of thirst
c. Pitting edema

Planning and Implementation

NDx: FLUID VOLUME DEFICIT

• The nurse replaces fluids orally; intravenous fluid replacement may be necessary for severe dehydration.

• The rate of replacement and type of fluids used is dependent on the degree and type of dehydration and the presence of preexisting cardiac, pulmonary, or renal problems. Commonly used fluids include

1. Isotonic fluids such as 0.9% saline (NS), 5% dextrose in water (D_5W), or Ringer's lactate (RL)
2. Hypertonic fluids such as 0.45% normal saline
3. Hypotonic fluids such as 10% dextrose in water, 5% dextrose in 0.9% saline, 5% dextrose in 0.45% saline, or 5% dextrose in Ringer's lactate

• Protein replacement may be needed in clients who have lost proteins (colloids) from the vascular space.

• The nurse administers drug therapy, as ordered, to ameliorate or correct the underlying cause of the dehydration, such as antidiarrheal medications, antiemetics, or antipyretics.

• The nurse

1. Provides oral fluid replacement of fluids (any substance that is liquid at body temperature is considered in measuring fluid intake such as gelatin, ice pops, and ice cream)
2. Enhances client compliance by using fluids the client enjoys and by timing the intake schedule carefully
   a. Divides the total amount over all shifts
   b. Offers small volumes every hour
3. Recognizes that solid food is not enough to increase the client's fluid volume to normal when dehydration is present

NDx: ALTERED ORAL MUCOUS MEMBRANE

• The nurse

1. Provides mouth care every 2 to 4 hours, including brushing and flossing the client's teeth
2. Moistens the client's lips with a petroleum-based lubricant
3. Rinses the client's mouth frequently
   a. Does not use commercial mouthwashes that contain alcohol or glycerin-containing washes and swabs because these products tend to dry the oral mucosa further and may increase the

discomfort by stinging or burning open fissures in the mucosa
   b. Rinses the mouth no more than two or three times per day with dilute hydrogen peroxide
   c. Uses lukewarm saline or tap water rinses
4. Assists the client with oral hygiene before meals or snacks
5. Teaches the client to avoid foods that are highly spiced or mechanically hard; bland, soft, cool foods are most easily tolerated

Discharge Planning

- The nurse
   1. Teaches the client to determine the electrolyte content of prepared foods and medications by carefully reading labels
   2. Obtains a dietary consult for assistance in providing information on the planning and preparation of palatable meals whenever a specific electrolyte restriction is necessary
   3. Teaches the client about specific food or fluid restriction
   4. Reviews the signs and symptoms of the specific imbalance for which the client is at risk, as well as what specific information should be reported immediately to the primary health care provider
   5. Provides drug information

For more information on dehydration, see *Medical-Surgical Nursing: A Nursing Process Approach,* **pp. 250–260.**

Dermatitis

OVERVIEW

- Cutaneous inflammatory rashes are related to antibody- or cellular-mediated immune responses, resulting in tissue destruction or epidermal alterations.
- Nonspecific eczematous dermatitis (*eczema*) describes inflammatory rashes when the agent is not identified.

• *Contact dermatitis*, an acute or chronic eczematous rash, is caused by either direct contact with an irritant, resulting in toxic injury to the skin, or by contact with an allergen, resulting in a cell-mediated immune reaction.

• *Irritant dermatitis* is due to strong acids, alkalis, solvents, and detergents.

• *Atopic dermatitis* is a chronic rash associated with genetic predisposition to respiratory allergies and atopic skin disease.

• The exact mechanism of atopic dermatitis is unknown, but it is exacerbated by dry or irritated skin, food allergies, chemicals, and stress.

D

COLLABORATIVE MANAGEMENT

Assessment

• The nurse records the client's
   1. Present or past history of allergies to any substances, including medications, foods, topical preparations, and jewelry
   2. Past or present exposure to potential irritants or allergens
   3. Occupational history
   4. Hobbies
   5. Hygiene practices
   6. Factors that worsen or improve the rash
   7. Past or family history of cutaneous inflammation, asthma, or allergic rhinitis
   8. Medication history
   9. Associated symptoms

• The nurse assesses for common clinical manifestations such as
   1. Vesicles
   2. Macules
   3. Papules (weeping)
   4. Oozing
   5. Crusting
   6. Fissuring
   7. Excoriation
   8. Scaling
   9. Pruritis
   10. Dry skin
   11. Erythema
   12. Blisters

Planning and Implementation

NDx: Impaired Skin Integrity

• The nurse teaches the client to
   1. Avoid sensitizing agents

2. Wear protective clothing to provide a barrier
3. Change employment to avoid contact with the offending agent
4. Identify medication, if a drug reaction occurs
5. Try controlled food challenges and elimination diets to confirm food allergen
6. Avoid factors that promote skin drying
7. Avoid woolen clothes

- The nurse

1. Administers topical, intralesion, or systemic steroids to suppress inflammation, as ordered
2. Administers antihistamines, as ordered, to relieve pruritis
3. Applies cool, moist compresses
4. Provides tepid baths with additives such as colloidal oatmeal preparations, tar extracts, oil, or cornstarch
5. Provides pain relief measures, such as skin lubrication and a cool environment
6. Teaches the client to avoid skin scratching; the client may need protective mitts or splints

Discharge Planning

- The nurse

1. Teaches the client to identify substances to avoid
2. Teaches the client to communicate identified allergies
3. Emphasizes skin care and prevention of dry skin
4. Explains drug therapy
5. Demonstrates proper application of topical ointments
6. Explains side effects of prolonged use of steroid preparations and tapering of oral preparations
7. Teaches the client to avoid operating heavy equipment when taking antihistamines
8. Explains the side effects of antihistamines

For more information on dermatitis, see *Medical-Surgical Nursing: A Nursing Process Approach*, pp. 1182–1186.

Diabetes Insipidus

OVERVIEW

- Diabetes insipidus (DI) is a disorder of water metabolism caused by a deficiency of antidiuretic hormone (ADH).

- DI is caused by either a decrease in ADH synthesis or an inability of the kidney to respond appropriately to ADH.

- It is classified into four types:
  1. Nephrogenic, an inherited defect in which the renal tubules do not respond to the actions of ADH, which results in inadequate water absorption by the kidney
  2. Primary, which results from a defect in the pituitary gland related to familial or idiopathic causes
  3. Secondary, which results from tumors in the hypothalamic-pituitary region, head trauma, infectious processes, surgical procedures, or metastatic tumors, usually from the lung or breast
  4. Drug related, which is caused by lithium (Eskalith, Lithobid) and demeclocycline (Declomycim), which can interfere with the renal response to ADH

- The disease is manifested by the excretion of large volumes of dilute urine, dehydration, increased or excessive thirst, and a low urine specific gravity (less than 1.005) and urine osmolality (50 to 200 mOsm/kg).

COLLABORATIVE MANAGEMENT

- The nurse
  1. Administers oral chlorprompamide (Diabinese) or clofibrate (Atromid S) for partial ADH deficiency, as ordered
  2. Administers aqueous vasopressin for short-term therapy or when the dosage must be changed frequently, as ordered
  3. Administers nasal sprays (lypressin, desmopressin), as ordered

- The nurse teaches the client
  1. Side effects of nasal sprays, which include ulceration of the mucous membranes, allergy, sensation of chest tightness, and inhalation of the spray, which precipitates pulmonary problems
  2. If side effects occur or if the client develops an

upper respiratory infection, sustained-action vasopressin (vasopressin tannate in oil) is administered intramuscularly

- The nurse
  1. Monitors strict intake and output
  2. Measures urine specific gravity at least daily
  3. Weighs the client every day
  4. Encourages the client to drink fluids equal to the amount of urinary output; if unable to do so, replaces with intravenous fluids as ordered
  5. Monitors the client carefully for indications of dehydration (dry skin, poor skin turgor, dry or cracked mucous membranes)
  6. Monitors for signs of circulatory collapse (such as vital sign changes)
  7. Provides education on vasopressin preparations for the client who will be discharged
  8. Encourages the client to wear a Medic Alert bracelet or necklace at all times

For more information on diabetes insipidus, see *Medical-Surgical Nursing: A Nursing Process Approach,* **pp. 1539–1540.**

Diabetes Mellitus

OVERVIEW

- Diabetes mellitus is a genetically and clinically heterogeneous group of chronic systemic disorders of various causes, affecting the metabolism of carbohydrates, protein, and fat.
- Insulin, an anabolic hormone made in the beta cells of the islets of Langerhans in the pancreas, plays a key role in allowing body cells to store carbohydrates by affecting several crucial activities that alter cell permeability, allowing entrance of glucose, free fatty acids, and amino acids.

- Insulin also acts as a catalyst to stimulate enzymes and chemicals necessary for cell function and energy production.
- *Type I, Insulin-dependent diabetes mellitus* (IDDM), affects 10% to 15% of the total population of diabetics, and *type II, non–insulin-dependent diabetes mellitus* (NIDDM), affects 85% to 90% of diabetics.

IDDM

1. Associated with deficiency in the amounts of insulin produced, malfunctioning insulin receptor sites, and/or disruption of the glycolytic pathway, which ultimately produces energy for the body to sustain life

2. Formerly known as juvenile-onset and brittle diabetes

3. Frequently associated with destruction of beta cells in the islets of Langerhans attributed to genetic predisposition, an infectious process, or autoimmune response associated with HLA-DR3 gene. Characterized by the following pathophysiology

   a. When insulin is absent, glucose is prevented from entering the cells, producing a state of starvation while excess glucose is present in the body, resulting in overall weight loss.

   b. The body perceives cellular starvation as a crisis and begins to secrete counterregulatory hormones (glucagon, epinephrine, norepinephrine, growth hormone, and cortisol), which attempt to maintain homeostasis by speeding up the available glucose using alternative energy sources.

   c. The presence of *hyperglycemia* (excessive amounts of glucose in the blood) causes a series of fluid and electrolyte imbalances, which result in the classic symptoms

      (1) *Polyuria* (frequent and excessive amount of urination) is a result of an osmotic gradient developed in the kidneys from the presence of glucose.

      (2) *Polydipsia* (excessive thirst) occurs from dehydration stimulating the thirst center.

      (3) *Polyphagia* (excessive eating) results from cellular starvation.

   d. Alternative fuel sources are used when cells are unable to take up glucose as fuel.

   e. The breakdown products of fatty acids, ketone bodies, can be used successfully in small amounts; however, because ketone bodies represent incomplete degradation products of free fatty acids, they are not further metabolized and accumulate in the blood when insulin is unavailable.

  f. Excessive ketone bodies are cleared from the body by kidney filtration, resulting in ketones in the urine, and by evaporation through the exhaled air, resulting in the "fruity" odor of the breath during ketoacidosis (refer to DKA).

  g. Ketone bodies increase the concentration of both hydrogen ions, creating an acidemia; as blood pH decreases, the hydrogen ion concentration and carbon dioxide increase, stimulating the central chemoreceptors in the brain, causing an increased rate and depth of respirations (Kussmaul's respiration).

  h. Potassium shifts from the intracellular to extracellular fluid in response to metabolic acidosis, and excess potassium is lost in the urine; levels may be high or low depending on the state of hydration.

- NIDDM
  1. The beta cells of the pancreas are able to synthesize and release insulin, but the amount may be insufficient compared to the insulin need.
  2. Also referred to as adult-onset or non–ketosis-prone diabetes, it is caused by decreased insulin production, excessive carbohydrate intake, or increased hepatic glucose production.
  3. The basic defect involves an interference with the binding of insulin to the proper cell membrane receptor related to destruction or inactivation of insulin or deficiencies in the amount or activity of receptors.
  4. The body responds to food intake by delayed secretion of insulin, followed by overrelease, causing the person to feel hungry, nervous, and shaky until more food is ingested.

- *Chronic complications* of diabetes include neuropathy, retinopathy, nephropathy, and vascular changes.

COLLABORATIVE MANAGEMENT

Assessment

- The nurse records the client's
  1. Age
  2. Sex
  3. Race
  4. Usual weight and height
  5. Dietary intake
  6. History of diabetes and which type

7. Symptoms
8. History of diabetes medications and other medications
9. Symptoms related to taking medication
10. Type of monitoring (blood and/or urine)
11. Stressors related to home, work, or family
12. Presence of infection or other illness
13. Past history of major illnesses, surgeries, and immunizations
14. Family history of diabetes, heart disease, and stroke
15. History of obesity

- The nurse assesses for

1. Skin turgor to determine dehydration
2. Level of consciousness
3. Vital signs
4. Acetone breath
5. Decreased sensation
6. Decreased reflexes
7. Positional blood pressure changes
8. Circulation deficits
9. Decreased skin temperature

Planning and Implementation

NDx: KNOWLEDGE DEFICIT

Nonsurgical Management

- The nurse provides education about diabetes care that will be integrated into the client's daily life.
- The nurse teaches the client/family to

1. Monitor glucose levels with a blood glucose meter
2. Operate the particular blood glucose monitor that will be used at home
3. Obtain a capillary blood specimen by puncturing the side of the client's finger with a lancet
4. Place the blood droplet on the test strip
5. Read the glucose result following the correct timing by the meter
6. Perform the blood glucose monitoring as ordered, and administer regular insulin according to the physician's recommendations
7. Perform urine testing to identify for the presence of ketones

- The nurse instructs the client/family about nutrition and meal planning

1. Determining the client's activity pattern, finding out what is eaten and when, and coordinating activity and eating patterns with the time the medication is administered and the duration of action of the medication
2. Planning a diet that is 55% to 60% carbohydrates,

30% or less fat, and 12% to 15% protein, utilizing meal planning programs

3. Avoiding concentrated sweets and including a moderate amount of fiber in meals
4. Dividing food intake into three meals and a number of snacks
5. Performing a nutritional assessment in collaboration with the physician and dietitian
6. Recommending that the client decrease salt use and avoid alcohol and caffeine

• The nurse recommends a medically approved exercise program, including guidelines for timing of safe physical activity and food and/or insulin intake adjustments, which may be needed.

• The nurse teaches the client to

1. Notify the physician if pain of any type occurs during exercise
2. Do warm-up and cool-down exercises
3. Avoid exercise at peak insulin times
4. Perform blood glucose monitoring before, during, and after exercise
5. Avoid insulin administration in an exercise extremity
6. Carry a simple sugar, such as hard candy, and take when signs of hypoglycemia occur
7. Wear a Medic Alert bracelet or necklace

• The nurse teaches the client/family methods to deal with stress management

1. Exercise (low-impact aerobic activity)
2. Behavior conditioning
3. Relaxation techniques
4. Problem-solving skills

• The nurse teaches the client/family about the prescribed medication therapy, including

1. Oral hypoglycemic agents—their purpose and side effects
2. Information about and step-by-step guidelines for subcutaneous insulin administration
   a. Wash hands
   b. Inspect the bottle for type of insulin and expiration date
   c. Roll the bottle between the palms of the hands
   d. Wipe the top of the bottle with alcohol
   e. Remove the needle cover and pull back the plunger to draw air into the syringe, equaling the amount of the insulin dose
   f. Draw the correct dose of insulin into the syringe
   g. Tap the syringe to remove any air bubbles

h. Select a site for injection and cleanse with alcohol
i. Pinch up the area and insert the needle at a 90-degree angle
j. Inject the insulin and pull the needle straight out
k. Dispose the uncapped needle into a puncture-proof container

3. Information about site rotation and location
4. How to mix regular and NPH insulin, if both are required
5. Information on insulin storage
6. Information on the insulin pump operation and maintenance, if needed

● The nurse provides information about acute complications such as hypoglycemia and hyperglycemia—their prevention, recognition, and treatment.

● The nurse discusses with the client/family psychosocial adjustments to the illness.

● The nurse emphasizes health habits, including care of the feet, teeth, and skin; avoidance of alcohol, drugs, and tobacco; and regular medical care.

● The nurse teaches the client/family about long-term complications, such as kidney and cardiovascular disease.

Surgical Management

● Pancreas transplants are experimentally being performed for diabetes management to normalize blood glucose levels and reverse pathologic changes.

NDx: POTENTIAL FOR INFECTION

● Diabetics have an increased potential for infection due to hyperglycemia, causing decreased phagocytosis, fibroblastic activity, and increased platelet adhesiveness. The goal is to prevent complications.

● The nurse
1. Encourages daily hygiene, including dental care with flossing, bathing, and inspection of the skin for breakdown
2. Instructs the client to seek early medical intervention and routine follow-up care

NDx: SENSORY/PERCEPTUAL ALTERATIONS

● The nurse provides verbal and written instructions for foot care
1. Inspect feet daily and report cuts, blisters, and

other signs of injury or infection to the health care provider
2. Keep feet clean, dry, and protected from injury
3. Bathe feet in warm water; do not soak for long periods
4. Cut toenails straight across; have ingrown toenails, calluses, or corns treated by a podiatrist only
5. Wear properly fitting shoes and cotton socks
6. Never walk barefoot
7. Use lubricating lotion or cream for dry feet and minimal powder if feet are moist
8. Elevate feet to aid in circulation

NDx: Ineffective Individual Coping; Ineffective Family Coping

- The nurse
  1. Assists the client/family in identifying mechanisms to assist in coping with illness, including organization of equipment, meal planning, and exercise programs
  2. Identifies problem-solving skills of the client and family members
  3. Encourages the family to increase communication
  4. Refers the client/family to a therapist or counselor if needed

NDx: Altered Nutrition: More Than/Less Than Body Requirements

- The nurse
  1. Identifies the desired weight for the client and structures daily dietary intake and exercise program, with dietician consultation
  2. Teaches the client to avoid fad weight-loss programs; standard decrease in caloric intake is 500 kcal less than the daily caloric need
  3. Teaches the client to incorporate an aerobic exercise program
  4. Identifies short- and long-term goals

NDx: Sexual Dysfunction

- The nurse
  1. Obtains a sexual history
  2. Explains that changes in sexuality are normal
  3. Reviews human sexuality and answers questions
  4. Refers for counseling, if needed

Discharge Planning

- The teaching plan includes information provided under "NDx: Knowledge Deficit."

- The nurse
  1. Stresses the importance of monitoring self-care, including routine recording of blood glucose levels, dietary intake, daily exercise, and amount of drug taken
  2. Instructs the client in signs and symptoms of hypo- and hyperglycemia
  3. Teaches the client to record untoward symptoms and report them to the physician
  4. Refers the client to community agencies for additional information on diabetes mellitus
  5. Emphasizes the importance of follow-up visits with the physician(s)

D

For more information on diabetes mellitus, see *Medical-Surgical Nursing: A Nursing Process Approach*, **pp. 1584–1623.**

Diabetic Ketoacidosis

- Diabetic ketoacidosis (DKA), the acute state of type I diabetes mellitus, is characterized by severe hyperosmolarity of body fluids, hypotension, and coma and is triggered by a lack of insulin and excess accumulation of ketones, causing large amounts of circulating glucose and ketones.
- The body attempts to rid itself of excess glucose and ketones by urinary excretion, further perpetuating the hyperosmolar state and intracellular dehydration.
- Excess ketones cause acid buildup, inhibiting metabolic processes and the ability to excrete metabolic by-products.
- Client presentation varies in severity.
- Features of diabetic ketoacidosis include
  1. Gradual or sudden onset
  2. Precipitated by infection, other stressors, stopping insulin

3. Clinical manifestations
    a. Thirst
    b. Nausea and vomiting
    c. Abdominal pain
    d. Fatigue
    e. Polyuria to anuria
    f. Blurred vision
    g. Elevated temperature
    h. Signs of dehydration
    i. Kussmaul's respiration
    j. Fruity breath odor
    k. Flushed face
    l. Rapid, thready pulse
    m. Soft, sunken eyeballs
    n. Hypotension
    o. Coma
4. Laboratory findings
    a. Serum glucose: 400–800 mg/dL
    b. Osmolarity: About 320 mOsm/L
    c. Serum acetone: Large
    d. Serum HCO_3: 10 mEq/L or less
    e. Arterial pH: About 7.07
    f. Serum Na: Low, normal, or high
    g. Serum K: High, normal, or low
    h. Serum P: High, but total is low
    i. Anion gap: Increased
    j. Blood urea nitrogen: Normal to slight elevation

- Goals of treatment include
    1. Rehydration with intravenous fluids at rates of 150 to 200 mL/hr
    2. Restoration of electrolyte imbalance by administering potassium and sodium chloride solution; administration of sodium bicarbonate to correct acidosis if pH is less than 7.0
    3. Reduction of blood glucose levels by administering regular insulin either subcutaneously or intravenously to assist with transport of glucose into the cell

- *Caution in treatment*: If blood glucose levels are lowered too quickly or intravenous fluids are given too rapidly, cerebral edema or hypoglycemia could result.

For more information on diabetic ketoacidosis, see *Medical-Surgical Nursing: A Nursing Process Approach*, **pp. 1594–1595.**

Diabetic Nephropathy

- Diabetic mellitus is the identified cause of end-stage renal disease in 25% or more of clients requiring chronic dialysis or renal transplantation.
- Diabetic nephropathy occurs as a result of type I and type II diabetes mellitus.
- Clients with diabetes mellitus are considered at risk for the development of renal failure, and therefore nephrotoxic agents and dehydration should be avoided.

For more information on diabetic nephropathy, see *Medical Surgical Nursing: A Nursing Process Approach*, **pp. 1856–1857.**

Diabetic Retinopathy

- Diabetic retinopathy, a vascular complication of diabetes that develops in the retina, is a major cause of disability and blindness in the United States.
- Two classes of retinopathy and their treatment include
    1. *Background*, in which the supporting cells of retinal vessels die; treated by controlling blood glucose levels
    2. *Proliferative*, whereby a network of fragile new blood vessels leak blood and protein into the surrounding tissue; treatment includes laser photocoagulation or panretinal photocoagulation to reduce the retina's need for oxygen

- A *vitrectomy* is performed if frequent bleeding occurs into the vitreous and the body is unable to reabsorb it or if fibrin bands threaten to detach the retina.
- The client is referred to agencies for the blind, vocational counseling, and other services for the visually impaired. (See Blindness.)

For more information on diabetic retinopathy, see *Medical-Surgical Nursing: A Nursing Process Approach,* **pp. 1054–1055.**

Disseminated Intravascular Coagulation

- Disseminated intravascular coagulation (DIC) is an acquired, acute coagulation disorder resulting as a complication of other conditions, including septicemia and septic shock.
- Two phases in DIC include
  1. Phase I, characterized by diffuse, abnormal formation of many small clots within microcirculation of organs. The release of tissue factors exposed to endotoxins triggers widespread coagulation, which consumes excess quantities of preformed clotting factors and cofactors. Fibrinogen is degraded to fibrin threads and increased fibrin split products.
  2. Phase II, characterized by an inability to form clots and the presence of overt or hidden hemorrhage. A vicious repeating cycle leads to tissue hypoxia and ischemia, causing necrosis and release of additional tissue factors.
- Treatment in *phase I* includes heparin administration to inhibit excess coagulation and to halt

consumption of vital clotting factors and treatment of the underlying disorder.

- Treatment in *phase II* includes discontinuance of heparin since clotting no longer occurs. Clotting factors are administered, and the underlying disorder is treated.

For more information on disseminated intravascular coagulation, see *Medical-Surgical Nursing: A Nursing Process Approach*, **p. 2277.**

Diverticular Disease

OVERVIEW

- Diverticular disease includes diverticulosis and diverticulitis
  1. *Diverticulosis* is the presence of several abnormal outpouchings or herniations in the wall of the intestine known as diverticula. These outpouchings are caused by significantly high pressures in the lumen of the intestines. They can occur in any part of the intestine but occur most frequently in the sigmoid colon.
  2. *Diverticulitis*, or inflammation of one or more diverticula, results when the diverticulum perforates with local abscess formation. A perforated diverticulum can progress to intra-abdominal perforation with generalized peritonitis.

COLLABORATIVE MANAGEMENT

Assessment

- The nurse records the client's
  1. Report of changes in bowel function, including constipation, diarrhea, and the presence of blood in the stool

2. Recent dietary intake of indigestible roughage or seeds
   3. Known history of diverticulosis
 • The nurse assesses for
   1. Abrupt onset of left lower quadrant abdominal pain, which increases with coughing, straining, or lifting
   2. Generalized abdominal pain (peritonitis)
   3. Temperature elevation with tachycardia
   4. Nausea and vomiting
   5. Abdominal distention and tenderness
   6. Palpable, tender rectal mass
   7. Blood in the stool (microscopic to larger amounts)

Planning and Implementation

NDx: ALTERED (GASTROINTESTINAL) TISSUE PERFUSION

Nonsurgical Management

 • Bed rest is recommended in the acute phase of the disease.
 • The nurse
   1. Teaches the client to refrain from lifting, straining, coughing, or bending to avoid increased intra-abdominal pressure
   2. Provides clear liquids during the acute phase of the disease
   3. Instructs the client that he or she will be restricted to nothing by mouth during severe symptoms
   4. Introduces a fiber-containing diet gradually when the inflammation is resolved
   5. Administers oral broad-spectrum antibiotics, as ordered
   6. Administers intravenous antibiotics, as ordered, for severe diverticulitis
   7. Administers pain medication, as ordered—mild nonopiate drugs for mild cases and narcotic analgesia for severe cases
   8. Avoids administering laxatives

Surgical Management

 • An exploratory laparotomy is performed to determine which extensive intervention is required when conservative measures are ineffective.

 • The recommended surgical approach is a colon resection with primary anastamosis; a temporary or permanent diverting colostomy may be required for increased bowel inflammation. (See "Collaborative Management," Colorectal Cancer, for nursing care of the client with abdominal surgery and colostomy.)

Discharge Planning

- The nurse provides written postoperative instructions
    1. Inspection of the incision for redness, tenderness, swelling, and drainage
    2. Dressing change procedures, if necessary
    3. Avoidance of activities that increase intra-abdominal pressure, including straining at stool, bending, lifting heavy objects, and wearing restictive clothing
    4. Pain management, including prescriptions
- The nurse teaches the client/family
    1. Signs and symptoms of diverticular disease, including fever, abdominal pain, and bloody stools
    2. To avoid enemas and laxatives other than bulk-forming ones such as psyllium hydrophilic mucilloid (Metamucil)
    3. To follow dietary considerations for diverticulosis
        a. Eat a diet high in cellulose and hemicellulose found in wheat bran, whole-grain breads, and cereals
        b. Eat fruits and vegetables with high-fiber content
        c. Avoid foods containing indigestible roughage or seeds
        d. Avoid alcohol due to its irritant effect on the bowel
        e. Avoid gas-forming, hot and cold liquids
        f. Follow a prescribed weight-reduction plan, if necessary

For more information on diverticular disease, see *Medical-Surgical Nursing: A Nursing Process Approach*, **pp. 1371–1379.**

Ductal Ectasia

- Ductal ectasia is a benign breast problem in women approaching menopause, caused by dilation and thickening of collecting ducts in the subareolar area.
- The ducts become distended and filled with cellular debris, which initiates an inflammatory response.
- Clinical signs are a hard, tender mass with irregular borders; greenish-brown nipple discharge; enlarged axillary nodes; redness; and edema over the mass.
- Microscopic examination of nipple discharge is performed for atypical or malignant cells.
- The affected area may be excised.

For more information on ductal ectasia, see *Medical-Surgical Nursing: A Nursing Process Approach*, **p. 1666.**

Dysfunctional Uterine Bleeding

OVERVIEW

- Dysfunctional uterine bleeding (DUB) is abnormal bleeding that is excessive or abnormal in amount or frequency without predisposing anatomic or systemic conditions.
- It occurs in the absence of ovulation related to ovarian function.
- DUB is associated with polycystic ovary disease, stress, extreme weight changes, and long-term drug use, including anticholinergics, reserpine, morphine, and oral contraceptives.

COLLABORATIVE MANAGEMENT
Assessment
- The nurse records the client's
  1. Complete menstrual history
  2. Illnesses
  3. Variations in weight and diet
  4. Exercise patterns
  5. Drug ingestion
  6. Presence of pain
- The nurse assesses for
  1. Symptoms of anemia
  2. Symptoms of systemic disease
  3. Obesity
  4. Undernutrition
  5. Abnormal hair growth
  6. Abdominal pain
  7. Abdominal masses
  8. Abnormalities in external genitalia

Planning and Implementation
NDx: ANXIETY AND FEAR

Nonsurgical Management
- The nurse
  1. Provides reassurance and comfort
  2. Administers hormone therapy for women with anovulatory DUB, which includes medroxyprogesterone or combination oral contraceptives, as ordered
- Treatment for women with ovulatory DUB who have inadequate progesterone levels includes progesterone supplements.

Surgical Management
- Surgical management includes diagnostic dilation and curettage (D&C), which involves the scraping of the endometrial tissue to assess for possible causes of bleeding or to remove bleeding tissue.
- The nurse prepares the client for surgery and provides routine postoperative care, including assessment of vaginal bleeding.

Discharge Planning
- The nurse
  1. Explains the oral contraceptive schedule: one pill per day beginning on the first day of the menstrual cycle; medroxprogesterone is taken on days 16 to 25 of the menstrual cycle
  2. Explains that monthly withdrawal bleeding is expected

3. Reviews postoperative instructions following D&C
   a. Avoid sexual intercourse, tub bathing, and the use of tampons for 2 weeks
   b. Understand that slight bleeding is normal, but if bleeding is as heavy as the normal menstrual period or persists for 2 weeks to notify the physician
   c. Use a hot water bottle or heating pad to relieve abdominal cramping
   d. Take mild analgesics, such as acetaminophen, for abdominal pain, as ordered

For more information on dysfunctional uterine bleeding, see *Medical-Surgical Nursing: A Nursing Process Approach*, **pp. 1696–1698.**

Dysmenorrhea

- Primary dysmenorrhea, or painful menstrual flow, occurs after ovulation is established.
- It is characterized by spasmodic lower abdominal pain beginning with the onset of menstrual flow and lasting for 12 to 48 hours.
- The pain often radiates to the lower back and thighs, and nausea and vomiting frequently occur.
- Researchers believe that the cause is increased uterine prostaglandin production and release, stimulating the myometrium and causing severe spasms, which constrict uterine blood flow, resulting in ischemia and pain.
- Client history includes
  1. Age at menarche
  2. Characteristics of menstruation
  3. Obstetric history
  4. Contraceptive history
  5. Pain characteristics

6. Previous treatment
7. History of pelvic problems
8. Emotional factors, including response to dysmenorrhea

- Interventions include
  1. Pain relief with prostaglandin synthetase inhibitors such as ibuprofen (Motrin), naproxen sodium (Anaprox), and mefenamic acid (Ponstel)
  2. Ovulation inhibitors such as oral contraceptives
  3. Acupressure
  4. Use of sedatives and narcotics
  5. Aerobic exercises
  6. Swimming
  7. Yoga or other meditation
  8. Application of heat or cold
  9. Massage
  10. Orgasm
  11. Biofeedback
  12. Relaxation therapy
  13. Nutritional management to prevent pain, including
     a. Vitamin B_6
     b. Calcium
     c. Magnesium
     d. Protein
     e. Reduced sodium intake

For more information on dysmenorrhea, see *Medical-Surgical Nursing: A Nursing Process Approach*, **pp. 1689–1690.**

Ectropion

- An ectropion is an outward sagging and eversion of the eyelid.
- Types include
  1. *Atonic*, associated with aging

2. *Paralytic*, caused by injury or paralysis of the seventh cranial nerve
3. *Cicatricial*, which results from the scarring produced from trauma, burns, or ulcers

• Treatment consists of outpatient surgery to restore proper alignment.

• Nursing management includes teaching the client how to instill eyedrops and the importance of reporting any drainage or severe pain to the physician.

For more information on ectropion, see *Medical-Surgical Nursing: A Nursing Process Approach,* **pp. 1012–1013.**

Empyema, Pulmonary

OVERVIEW

• Pulmonary empyema is a collection of puss in the pleural space; the fluid is thick, opaque, and foul smelling.

• The most common cause is pulmonary infection or lung abcess, which spreads across the pleura or obstructs lymph nodes and causes a retrograde flood of infected lymph into the pleural space.

• Thoraic surgery or chest trauma are common predisposing conditions where bacteria are introduced directly into the pleural space.

• History findings include recent febrile illnesses, chest pain, dyspnea, cough, and trauma.

• Physical assessment includes diminished chest wall movement on the affected side, decreased breath sounds, decreased or absent fremitus, a flat percussion note, fever, chills, weight loss, and night sweats.

• Therapy is based on emptying the empyema cavity, reexpanding the lung, and controlling the infection.

• Chest tubes are placed in the inferior parts of the

empyema sac to promote drainage and lung expansion, and antibiotics are given.

• An open thoracotomy and lung decortication may be performed for thick pus and marked pleural thickening.

For more information on pulmonary empyema, see *Medical-Surgical Nursing: A Nursing Process Approach*, **pp. 2045–2046**

E

Encephalitis

• Encephalitis, an inflammation of the brain parenchyma (brain tissue) and often the meninges, is most often caused by viral agents
  1. Arboviruses, transmitted through the bite of an infected tick or mosquito
  2. Enteroviruses associated with mumps and chicken pox
  3. Herpes simplex type I
• Ameba such as *Naegleria* and *Acanthamoeba* found in warm freshwater may also be involved.
• The disorder is characterized by severe headache and other symptoms similar to meningitis.
• Supportive nursing care and prompt recognition and treatment of increased intracranial pressure are essential components of treatment.

For more information on encephalitis, see *Medical-Surgical Nursing: A Nursing Process Approach*, **pp. 902–903.**

Endocarditis, Infective

OVERVIEW

• Infective endocarditis (previously called bacterial endocarditis) is an inflammatory process involving the endocardial surface of the heart, including the valves.

• *Acute* infective endocarditis causes tissue sloughing with erosion of valve leaflets, and myocardial damage causes the heart to fail (especially right-sided failure).

• *Subacute* infective endocarditis is more commonly found on the left side of the heart.

COLLABORATIVE MANAGEMENT

Assessment

• The nurse records the client's
  1. Conditions predisposing to endocarditis
     a. Rheumatic heart disease
     b. Congenital heart disease
     c. Mitral valve prolapse
     d. Cardiac surgery
     e. Cardiac defects
     f. Intravenous (IV) drug abuse
     g. Intravascular foreign bodies such as
        (1) IV catheters
        (2) Pacemaker electrodes
        (3) Dialysis shunts
        (4) Hyperalimentation catheters
     h. Immunosuppression
        (1) Diabetes mellitus
        (2) Burns
        (3) Cancer
        (4) Hepatitis
  2. History of recent dental procedure
  3. History of recent infections
  4. Recent invasive procedures or surgery
• The nurse assesses for
  1. Signs of infection, including high fever, chills, malaise, night sweats, and fatigue
  2. Heart murmurs
  3. Right-sided heart failure, evidenced by
     a. Peripheral edema
     b. Weight gain
     c. Anorexia
  4. Left-sided heart failure, evidenced by
     a. Fatigue

b. Shortness of breath
c. Crackles
5. Evidence of arterial embolization
6. Petechiae of the neck, shoulders, wrists, ankles, mucous membranes, or conjunctivae

Planning and Implementation

NDx: DECREASED CARDIAC OUTPUT

- The nurse
  1. Administers IV antibiotic therapy, as ordered (the mainstay of treatment)
  2. Administers prophylactic anticoagulants, as ordered, such as heparin or warfarin (Coumadin)
  3. Monitors the client's tolerance to activity
  4. Applies antiembolism stockings

- Surgical intervention includes removal of the infected valve, removal of congenital shunts, repairing injured valves and chordae tendinae, and abscess drainage.

- Preoperative and postoperative care for the client having surgery involving the valves is similar to that described for clients undergoing a coronary artery bypass grafting or valve replacement described under Coronary Artery Disease.

Discharge Planning

- The nurse teaches the client/family
  1. Information on the cause of the disease and its course, medication regimens, technique for administering IV antibiotics, practices that help avoid future infections, and signs and symptoms of infection
  2. The importance of good personal and oral hygiene
  3. The necessity to inform health care providers and dentists of the history of endocarditis, so prophylactic antibiotics are given prior to treatment
  4. Precautions for anticoagulation therapy, such as reporting unusual bleeding to the physician
  5. The importance of reporting signs and symptoms of reinfection to the primary health care provider

For more information on endocarditis, see *Medical-Surgical Nursing: A Nursing Process Approach*, see **pp. 2178–2181.**

Endometrial Cancer

OVERVIEW

● Endometrial cancer (cancer of the uterus) is the most frequently occurring reproductive organ cancer.

● It is a slow-growing tumor associated with menopause and arises from the glandular component of the endometrial mucosa.

● Its initial growth is within the uterine cavity, followed by extension into the myometrium and cervix.

● The spread occurs through the lymphatics to the ovaries and parametrial, pelvic, inguinal, and para-aortic lymph nodes; by hematagenous metastasis to the lungs, liver, or bone; and by transtubal or intra-abdominal spread to the peritoneal cavity.

COLLABORATIVE MANAGEMENT

Assessment

● The nurse records the client's
  1. Family history of endometrial cancer
  2. History of uterine cancer, diabetes, and hypertension
  3. Age
  4. Race
  5. History of obesity
  6. Childbearing status
  7. Prolonged estrogen use

● The nurse assesses for
  1. Postmenopausal bleeding
  2. Watery, serosanguineous vaginal discharge
  3. Low back pain
  4. Abdominal pain
  5. Low pelvic pain
  6. Enlarged uterus

Planning and Implementation

NDx: ANXIETY AND FEAR

Nonsurgical Management

● Radiation therapy (external and internal) is used alone or in combination with surgery, depending on the stage of the cancer.

● If intracavity radiation therapy (IRT) is done, an applicator is positioned within the uterus through the vagina.

- The nurse
  1. Maintains strict isolation and radiation precautions
  2. Provides bed rest, lying on the back, with head either flat or at less than 20 degrees
  3. Restricts active movement to prevent dislodgement
  4. Inserts a Foley catheter
  5. Assesses for skin breakdown
  6. Provides a low-residue diet
  7. Encourages fluid intake
  8. Administers antiemetics, broad-spectrum anti-infectives, tranquilizers, analgesics, heparin, and antidiarrheal medications
  9. Restricts visitors
- Nurses who are pregnant or attempting pregnancy are usually not assigned clients with IRT.
- The nurse instructs the client undergoing external radiation to
  1. Observe for signs of skin breakdown
  2. Avoid sunbathing
  3. Avoid bathing over the markings outlining the treatment site
  4. Recognize the complications of treatment, including cystitis, diarrhea, and nutritional alterations.
- Chemotherapy is used to treat advanced and recurrent disease. Agents used include doxorubicin (Adriamycin), cisplatin, cyclophosphamide (Cytoxin), 5-fluorouracil, and vincristine. (See discussion of nursing care under Cancer, General.)
- Progesterone therapy may be used for stage I and II cancers, which are estrogen dependent, and for stage IV cancer as palliative treatment. Hormones frequently used are medroxyprogesterone (Depo-Provera) and megestrol acetate (Megace).

Surgical Management
- Total abdominal hysterectomy and bilateral salpingo-oopherectomy is performed for stage I tumors, and a radical hysterectomy is performed for stage II.
- Refer to preoperative and postoperative care for the client undergoing hysterectomy under Cervical Cancer.

NDx: BODY IMAGE DISTURBANCE
- The nurse
  1. Provides emotional support
  2. Creates an atmosphere that encourages the client to ask questions or express fears and concerns

203

3. Recognizes that reactions to radiation therapy vary among clients and that some may feel unclean or radioactive after treatments
4. Provides information about alopecia (loss of hair) with chemotherapy and suggests that wigs, scarves, or turbans be worn until regrowth occurs

Discharge Planning

• The nurse provides the following information if the client undergoes IRT

1. Side effects should be reported to the physician, including vaginal bleeding, rectal bleeding, foul-smelling discharge, abdominal pain or distention, or hematuria.
2. High-dose radiation causes sterility.
3. Vaginal shrinkage occurs.
4. Sexual partners cannot "catch" cancer.
5. The client is not radioactive.
6. Vaginal douching may decrease inflammation.
7. A normal diet may be resumed.

• The nurse teaches the client the following information if the client undergoes an abdominal hysterectomy

1. Avoid or limit stair climbing for 1 month
2. Avoid tub baths and sitting for long periods
3. Avoid strenuous activity or lifting anything weighing more than 10 to 20 pounds
4. Expect physical changes
5. Participate in moderate exercise such as walking
6. Consume foods that aid in healing, such as foods high in protein, iron, and vitamin C
7. Avoid sexual intercourse for 3 to 6 weeks
8. Observe for signs of complications, including infection
9. Expect emotional reactions
10. Keep follow-up visits with the physician(s)

For more information on endometrial cancer, see *Medical-Surgical Nursing: A Nursing Process Approach*, **pp. 1715–1720.**

Endometriosis

OVERVIEW

● Endometriosis is a benign disease of unknown cause characterized by implantation of endometrial tissue outside the uterine cavity.

● The tissue responds to hormonal stimulation and goes through the same cyclic changes.

● Bleeding occurs at the site of implantation, and the blood is trapped in the tissues, causing scarring and adhesions.

● Assessment includes
  1. Menstrual history
  2. Sexual history
  3. Characteristics of bleeding
  4. Lower abdominal pain occurring before the menstrual flow
  5. Rectal pressure
  6. Dysparenuia (painful intercourse)
  7. Painful defecation
  8. Sacral backache
  9. Hypermenorrhea
  10. Infertility

● Management includes
  1. Mild analgesics or prostaglandin synthesase inhibitors for pain relief
  2. Hormonal therapy
     a. Pseudopregnancy induced with oral contraceptives and/or progesterone
     b. Pseudomenopause or ovarian suppression induced by using danzol (Danocrine), an antigonadotropin testosterone derivative
  3. Application of a heating pad to the abdomen or sacrum
  4. Relaxation techniques
  5. Yoga
  6. Biofeedback
  7. Surgical mangement by removing endometrial implants and adhesions with carbon dioxide laser and/or hysterectomy

For more information on endometriosis, see *Medical-Surgical Nursing: A Nursing Process Approach*, **pp. 1694–1695.**

Entropion

- An entropion is an inversion of the eyelid margin, which may result in eyelashes rubbing against the eyeball.
- The client complains of "feeling something in my eye."
- Other manifestations include inward deviation of the eyelid, inflamed conjunctiva, and corneal abrasion.
- Treatment consists of outpatient surgery to correct the position of the eyelid.
- Nursing management includes teaching the client how to instill eyedrops and the importance of reporting any drainage or severe pain to the physician.

For more information on entropion, see *Medical-Surgical Nursing: A Nursing Process Approach,* **p. 1012.**

Epididymitis

- Epididymitis is an infection of the epididymis, which may result from infection of the prostate.
- It occurs as a complication of long-term indwelling catheters, prostatic surgery, and occasionally cystoscopic examination.
- *Chlamydia trachomatis* is the major cause of epididymitis in men under the age of 35.
- Clinical manifestations include
  1. Pain along the inguinal canal and the vas deferens, leading to pain and swelling in the scrotum and groin

   2. Elevated temperature
   3. Pyuria
   4. Bacteriuria
   5. Chills
- Treatment interventions include
   1. Bed rest with scrotal elevation
   2. Antibiotics
   3. Sexual partner treatment if chlamydia or gonorrheal in origin
   4. Comfort measures, including ice packs and sitz baths

For more information on epididymitis, see *Medical-Surgical Nursing: A Nursing Process Approach*, **pp. 1769–1770.**

Epilepsy

OVERVIEW

- Epilepsy is a chronic disorder characterized by recurrent seizure activity.
- A seizure is an abnormal, sudden, excessive discharge of electrical activity within the brain.
- Three major types of epilepsy include
   1. *Generalized*
      a. *Tonic-clonic*, characterized by stiffening or rigidity of the muscles, followed by rhythmic jerking of the extremities. Immediate unconsciousness occurs, and the client may be incontinent of urine or stool and/or frothing of the mouth may occur. This seizure may be referred to as a *grand mal*.
      b. *Absence*, consisting of a brief (often seconds) period of loss of consciousness (as though the client is daydreaming). This type of seizure may be called a *petit mal*.

     c. *Myoclonic*, a brief, generalized jerking or stiffening of the extremities, which may occur singly or in groups

     d. *Atonic*, characterized by sudden loss of muscle tone, which in most cases causes the client to fall

2. *Partial* seizure

     a. Complex, which causes the client to lose consciousness or black out for a few seconds. Characteristic behavior, known as automatism may occur, such as lip smacking and patting

     b. Simple, which consists of a déjà vu phenomenon, perception of an offensive smell, or sudden onset of pain. A *jacksonian* march refers to the spread of seizure activity from one part of the body to the next in a progressive manner (e.g., from the right foot to right leg to left arm).

3. *Idiopathic* or unclassified, which occurs for no known reason

COLLABORATIVE MANAGEMENT

Assessment

- The nurse records the following concerning the seizures

  1. How often they occur
  2. The type of movement or activity and if more than one type occurs
  3. Sequence of progression
  4. How long they last
  5. Presence and description of aura or precipitating events
  6. Postictal status
  7. Length of time before the client returns to preseizure status
  8. If the client is incontinent during the seizure

- The nurse records the client's

  1. Current medications, including dosage, frequency of administration, and the time the medication was last taken
  2. Compliance with the medication schedule and reason(s) for noncompliance, if appropriate

- The nurse assesses for

  1. Any changes in normal neurologic function
  2. Self-concept disturbances
  3. Impaired social interactions or denial of the problem, which may be caused by the client's fear that a seizure may occur at work or in social situations

- During a seizure, the nurse assesses for
  1. Type and progression of seizure activity
  2. Factors that may have precipitated the event
  3. All physical manifestations, including eye fluttering, changes in pupil size, head and eye deviation automatism, changes in level of consciousness, apnea, and cyanosis
  4. Postictal status

Planning and Implementation
NDx: POTENTIAL FOR INJURY
Nonsurgical Management
- The nurse administers drug therapy, as ordered

E

  1. Carbamazepine (Tegretol) is contraindicated if glaucoma, cardiac, renal, or hepatic disease is present.
  2. Clonazepam (Klonopin) is contraindicated if glaucoma is present; the complete blood count (CBC) should be followed.
  3. Diazepam (Valium) is given to stop the motor activity associated with status epilepticus; if given intravenously, the nurse monitors the client closely for respiratory distress.
  4. Ethosuximide (Zarontin) is contraindicated in renal or liver disease; the nurse monitors CBC and liver function tests.
  5. Phenobarbital (Luminal) potentiates phenothiazines; it is potentiated by valproic acid, decreases warfarin absorption, and increases digoxin metabolism.
  6. Phenytoin (Dilantin) is used to control seizures. The nurse monitors CBC and calcium levels. If administered intravenously, the nurse clears the line with saline before and after administering and gives the drug slowly—no more than 50 mg/min IV. Metabolism is inhibited by warfarin, isoniazid, and phenothiazine. Decreased therapeutic blood levels result when given with carbamazepine, clonazepam, prednisone, or digoxin.
  7. Primidone (Myidone) is potentiated by isoniazid; drug interactions are the same as for phenobarbital.
  8. Valproic acid (Depakene) increases serum phenobarbital levels and alters serum phenytoin levels; the nurse monitors CBC.
- The nurse follows institutional policy for the implementation of seizure precautions

  1. Keeps oxygen and suctioning equipment available at the bedside

2. Maintains a heparin lock that may be indicated for clients at risk for tonic-clonic seizures
3. Recognizes that padded tongue blades do NOT belong at the bedside and nothing should be inserted into the client's mouth after a seizure begins
4. Takes action appropriate for the type of seizure, e.g., observes the partial seizure or turns the client with a tonic-clonic seizure on his or her side
5. Applies protective head gear for clients with atonic seizures, as appropriate
6. Keeps the bed in the low position and side rails up at all times

• *Status epilepticus* is a seizure that lasts longer than 4 minutes or occurs in rapid succession. It is a neurologic emergency and must be treated promptly, or brain damage and possibly death from anoxia, cardiac arrhythmias, or lactic acidosis may occur.
• The nurse
  1. Establishes an airway (intubation may be necessary)
  2. Monitors the client's respiratory status carefully
  3. Administers oxygen
  4. Establishes an IV line
  5. Has medications available that are used to treat status epilepticus
     a. Diazepam (Valium)
     b. Phenytoin (Dilantin)
     c. Phenobarbital (Luminal)
     d. Paraldehyde
     e. Thiopental sodium
     f. General anesthesia (treatment of last resort)
  6. Inserts a nasogastric tube, as ordered
  7. Monitors vital signs frequently

Surgical Management
• Two procedures may be performed when traditional methods fail to maintain seizure control
  1. *Corpus callosotomy*, which involves severing the corpus callosum to prevent neuronal discharges from passing through the two hemispheres of the brain
  2. A procedure that involves identifying the seizure focus through elaborate mechanisms involving continuous recording of the client's electroencephalogram, and, when possible, videorecording of the client at all times except during personal care activities. The area of seizure focus is surgically removed if it can be done safely and without affecting vital areas of brain function.

For nursing care for this procedure, see "Surgical Management," Brain Tumor.

NDx: INEFFECTIVE INDIVIDUAL AND FAMILY COPING

- The nurse
  1. Helps the family identify coping strategies used successfully in the past
  2. Provides a complete education program on epilepsy

Discharge Planning

- Most clients are treated on an outpatient basis, and little home-care preparation is needed.
- The nurse provides drug information
  1. Taking all medications in the correct dosage, at the right time, and by the right route
  2. What to do if a dose is missed or if complications or side effects occur
- The nurse teaches
  1. Precautions to take when ill, under stress, fatigued, or when workload or social activities increase
  2. Diet and effects of alcohol
  3. Driving restrictions, if any
  4. Importance of follow-up visits with the physician(s)
  5. Need to wear Medic-Alert bracelet or necklace

For more information on epilepsy, see *Medical-Surgical Nursing: A Nursing Process Approach,* **pp. 891–897.**

Episcleritis

- Episcleritis is a localized inflammation of the episclera, usually close to the corneal margin.
- The disorder is a common finding in clients with rheumatoid arthritis, syphilis, herpes zoster, or tuberculosis.

- Episcleritis is manifested by ocular redness, pain, lacrimation, photophobia, edema of the episclera, hyperemia of the episcleral vessels, and a pink- or purple-appearing eyeball.
- It is usually self-limiting and disappears in 1 to 2 weeks.
- Topical steroids may be used.
- Episcleritis may predispose the client to a corneal ulcer.

For more information on episcleritis, see *Medical-Surgical Nursing: A Nursing Process Approach,* **pp. 1036–1037.**

Epistaxis

- Epistaxis, or nosebleed, is a common problem due to the rich capillary network within the anterior portion of the nose.
- It occurs as a result of trauma, hypertension, blood dyscrasias, inflammation, tumor, decreased humidity, and excessive nose blowing and picking.
- Management includes
  1. Direct pressure to the nose for 3 to 5 minutes
  2. Cold compresses or ice applied directly to the nose and face
  3. Avoidance of nose blowing
  4. Loose nasal packing
  5. Nasal cautery with silver nitrate or electrocautery
  6. Postnasal packing
  7. Humidification

For more information on epistaxis, see *Medical-Surgical Nursing: A Nursing Process Approach*, **pp. 1956–1957.**

Esophageal Tumor

OVERVIEW

- *Benign* tumors of the esophagus, usually in the form of leiomyomas, are uncommon and usually asymptomatic.
- *Malignant* cancerous tumors may develop at any point along the esophagus, evolve as part of a slow process that begins with benign tissue changes, and produce widespread disabling effects.
- The two types of malignant tumors are
  1. Squamous epidermoid tumors, which account for the majority of esophageal cancers and usually develop in the middle third of the esophagus
  2. Adenocarcinomas, which develop in the lower third of the esophagus and are believed to evolve from Barrett's epithelium, possibly created by the presence of chronic reflux.
- Esophageal tumors exhibit rapid local growth and metastatic spread via the lymph nodes.

COLLABORATIVE MANAGEMENT
Assessment
- The nurse records the client's
  1. Alcohol consumption
  2. Tobacco use
  3. History of esophageal disease or problems
  4. Weight loss related to anorexia, dysphagia, or discomfort
- The nurse assesses for
  1. General physical appearance
  2. Persistent and progressive dysphagia
  3. Odynophagia (painful swallowing), reported as a steady, dull, substernal pain, which may radiate
  4. Regurgitation and/or vomiting
  5. Foul breath
  6. Chronic hiccups
  7. Hoarseness from laryngeal spread

Planning and Implementation
NDx: ALTERED NUTRITION: LESS THAN BODY REQUIREMENTS
Nonsurgical Management
- Radiation therapy reduces the tumor's size and offers consistent short-term relief of symptoms.

- Esophageal dilation achieves temporary symptomatic relief of symptoms and is used to reduce tumor obstruction and treat strictures that may occur following radiation therapy.

- A prosthesis may be inserted to bypass disabling dysphagia and maintain an open esophagus, which preserves the client's ability to take oral nutrition.

- Chemotherapy has not proved to be an effective treatment modality and may worsen the client's nutritional status.

- The nurse
  1. Administers antacids and analgesia to provide relief of symptoms
  2. Provides soft or semiliquid foods enriched with skim milk powder or commercial protein supplements to maintain adequate nutritional intake
  3. Provides small, frequent meals, which are better tolerated
  4. Provides care for feeding tubes or hyperalimentation lines that may be required for severe dysphagia

Surgical Management

- Radical surgery is the only definitive treatment for esophageal cancer and the preferred intervention in healthy clients.

- *Subtotal or total esophagogastrectomy* is usually required because tumors are quite large and involve distant lymph nodes.

- The preferred surgical intervention, *esophagogastrostomy*, involves removing the diseased portion of the esophagus and anastamosing the cervical portion to the stomach, which is then brought up into the thorax through the esophageal hiatus, involving both laparotomy and thoracotomy incisions.

- Tumors in the upper esophagus may require *radical neck dissection and laryngectomy* because of spread to the larynx.

- Tumors that spread to the stomach may require *colon interposition*, which requires removal of a section of right or left colon and bringing it up into the thorax to substitute for the esophagus.

- Preoperative care includes provision of nutritional support from 5 days to 2 to 3 weeks prior to surgery by oral supplements, tube feedings, or hyperalimentation.

- The nurse provides preoperative care
  1. Monitors the client's weight, intake and output, and fluid and electrolyte balance

2. Performs meticulous oral care
3. Provides routine preoperative care
4. Teaches the client about the incisions, wound drainage tubes, chest tubes, nasogastric (NG) tube, and intravenous (IV) lines

- The nurse provides postoperative care

    1. Assesses the client's respiratory status
    2. Provides chest physiotherapy, as ordered
    3. Maintains the client in a semi-Fowler's position to support ventilation and prevent reflux
    4. Administers antibiotics, as ordered
    5. Administers supplemental oxygen, as ordered
    6. Ensures patency of the chest tube water seal drainage system
    7. Provides support of the multiple surgical incisions during turning and activity
    8. Assesses for fever, fluid accumulation, general signs of inflammation, and symptoms of early shock
    9. Avoids manipulation and irrigation of the surgically placed NG tube
    10. Provides meticulous mouth care while the NG tube is in place
    11. Maintains nothing by mouth status until gastrointestinal motility is established
    12. Administers IV fluids and hyperalimentation, as ordered
    13. Administers 3 to 5 mL of water every 15 to 30 minutes and assesses client tolerance
    14. Slowly progresses the client's diet to puréed and semisolid foods
    15. Stresses the importance of eating small meals and maintaining an upright position during eating

Discharge Planning

- The nurse provides written postoperative instructions

    1. Respiratory care instructions to ambulate, splint incisions, and provide chest physiotherapy and to report symptoms of respiratory infection to the physician immediately
    2. Inspection of the incision for redness, tenderness, swelling, and drainage

- The nurse reinforces dietary instructions

    1. Increase dietary intake to include high-calorie, high-protein meals that contain soft and easily swallowed foods; meals should be small and frequent
    2. Care for tube feedings and hyperalimentation,

which may be necessary; requires intensive teaching for the client and family caring for the client at home

3. Maintain an upright position after eating and elevate the head of the bed

For more information on esophageal tumors, see *Medical-Surgical Nursing: A Nursing Process Approach*, **pp. 1288–1294.**

External Otitis

OVERVIEW

• External otitis is an infective, inflammatory, or allergic response involving structures of the external auditory canal or the auricle.

• Necrotizing external otitis is the most virulent form and has a 60% to 80% mortality rate, secondary to complications such as meningitis.

• The disease spreads beyond the external auditory canal into the adjacent structures of the ear and skull.

COLLABORATIVE MANAGEMENT

Assessment

• The nurse records the client's

1. Present illness, its course and severity, and possible etiologies
2. Use of earphones, recent changes in hair or other cosmetic products, or changes in soap or laundry detergents
3. History of recent trauma or injury to the ear or external canal
4. Complaints of itching and pain with movement of the pinna or tragus

5. Complaints of feeling as if the ear is plugged and hearing is changed
- The nurse assesses for
    1. Redness and swelling of the external structures of the ear
    2. Greenish-white discharge
    3. Hearing loss
    4. Tender and palpable preauricular or postauricular lymph nodes

Planning and Implementation

NDx: PAIN
- The nurse
    1. Teaches the client to apply heat locally for 20 minutes three times per day
    2. Recommends bed rest because head movements are limited, which thereby reduces pain
    3. Applies topical antibiotic therapy, as ordered
- An earwick (impregnated on the end with medication) is inserted by the physician past the blockage if edema has caused an obstruction of the external canal.
- Systemic oral or intravenous antibiotics such as penicillin (Pen-Vee-K), ampicillin (Polycillin), and cephalothin (Keflin) are used for severe infections.
- Analgesics such as acetylsalicylic acid (aspirin), acetaminophen (Tylenol), or narcotics may be given

NDx: SENSORY/PERCEPTUAL ALTERATION (AUDITORY)
- See Hearing Loss.
- The nurse
    1. Maintains a quiet environment, free from excessive noise, so that the client is able to rest
    2. Approaches the client on the side of the unaffected ear
    3. Speaks in a normal tone of voice

Discharge Planning
- The nurse
    1. Provides drug information
        a. Using all medication in the correct dosage and at the right time
        b. Correct procedure for insertion of eardrops
        c. What to do if a dose is missed or if complications or side effects occur
    2. Stresses the importance of avoiding the use of

items that caused the problem (e.g., earphones, cosmetics)

For more information on external otitis, see *Medical-Surgical Nursing: A Nursing Process Approach,* **pp. 1101–1107.**

Eye Laceration

- The most common areas involved in lacerations of the eye are the eyelids and cornea.
- *Eye lacerations*
  1. Bleed heavily and look more severe than they actually are
  2. Are treated by closing the eye and applying a small ice pack, checking visual acuity, and cleaning and suturing the eyelid
- *Corneal lacerations*
  1. The ocular contents may prolapse through the laceration.
  2. The laceration is manifested by severe eye pain, photophobia, tearing, and decreased visual acuity.
  3. NEVER remove a penetrating object from the eye; it may be holding ocular structures in place.
  4. Treatment includes surgical repair under general anesthesia and antibiotic ointment. An *enucleation* may need to be performed if the ocular contents have protruded through the laceration.
  5. Complications include scarring, which may alter vision.

For more information on eye lacerations, see *Medical-Surgical Nursing: A Nursing Process Approach,* **pp. 1066–1067.**

Fatty Liver

- Fatty liver is caused by the accumulation of triglycerides and other fats in the hepatic cells.
- The most common cause is chronic alcoholism.
- Other causes include malnutrition, diabetes mellitus, obesity, pregnancy, prolonged intravenous hyperalimentation, and exposure to toxic drugs.
- The client is usually asymptomatic; the typical finding is hepatomegaly (an enlarged liver).
- The nurse assesses for
  1. Right upper abdominal pain
  2. Ascites
  3. Edema
  4. Jaundice
  5. Fever
  6. Signs of cirrhosis (see Cirrhosis)
- Liver biopsy confirms the diagnosis.
- Interventions are aimed at removing the underlying cause of the infiltration and dietary restrictions.

For more information on fatty liver, see *Medical-Surgical Nursing: A Nursing Process Approach*, **p. 1505.**

Fibrocystic Breast Disease

- Fibrocystic breast disease (FBD), also called cystic disease or dysplasia, is the most common breast problem in women in their 20s.
- The *first stage* is characterized by premenstrual

bilateral fullness and tenderness, especially in the outer upper quadrant; symptoms resolve after menstruation and recur before the next menstrual cycle.

- In the *second stage*, which occurs in the late 20s and throughout the 30s, bilateral, multicentric nodular areas appear that feel like small marbles, with fullness and soreness.

- The *third stage* occurs between the ages of 35 and 55, when microscopic or macroscopic cysts develop.

- The cysts, which occur suddenly and are associated with pain, tenderness, or burning, are usually three-dimensional, smooth, mobile, and well delineated.

- The cause of FBD is unknown but appears to be related to normal fluctuations in progesterone and estrogen levels during the menstrual cycle.

- Management is symptomatic
    1. Hormonal manipulation is the primary means of intervention and includes oral contraceptives to suppress oversecretion of estrogen.
    2. Other interventions include
        a. Administration of vitamins E and B complex
        b. Administration of diuretics to prevent premenstrual breast engorgement
        c. Avoidance of caffeine
        d. Avoidance of excess salt intake before menses
        e. Administration of mild analgesics
        f. Practice of regular breast self-examination

For more information on fibrocystic breast disease, see *Medical-Surgical Nursing: A Nursing Process Approach*, **pp. 1665–1666.**

Flail Chest

- Flail chest is associated with high-speed motor vehicle accidents.

- Blunt chest trauma results in hemothorax and rib fractures, causing a loose segment of the chest wall to become paradoxical to the expansion and contraction of the rest of the chest wall.

- Paradoxical respiration is the inward movement of the thorax during inspiration with outward movement during expiration; gas exchange and secretion removal are impaired.
- The chest is assessed for paradoxical chest movement, dyspnea, cyanosis, tachycardia, hypotension, pain, and anxiety.
- Interventions include
    1. Humidified oxygen
    2. Pain management
    3. Deep breathing and positioning
    4. Coughing and tracheal aspiration
    5. Psychosocial support
    6. Intubation with mechanical ventilation with positive end-expiratory pressure for severe flail chest associated with respiratory failure and shock

For more information on flail chest, see *Medical-Surgical Nursing: A Nursing Process Approach*, **pp. 2055–2056.**

Food Poisoning

- Food poisoning is caused by ingestion of infectious organisms in food.
- There are two typical types of food poisoning
    1. Staphylococcal food poisoning
        a. *Staphylococcus* grows in meats and dairy products.
        b. Symptoms of staphylococcal infection include abrupt onset of vomiting, with some diarrhea.
        c. The diagnosis is made when stool culture

yields 100,000 enterotoxin-producing staphylococci.

   d. Treatment includes oral or intravenous (IV) fluids.

2. *Botulism*

   a. Botulism is a severe, life-threatening food poisoning with a high mortality rate, commonly acquired from improperly processed canned foods.

   b. *Clostridium botulinum* enters the bloodstream from the intestines and causes symptoms of diplopia, dysphagia, dysphonia, respiratory muscle paralysis, nausea, vomiting, and diarrhea or constipation.

   c. The diagnosis is made by history and stool culture revealing *C. botulinum*.
The serum may be positive for toxins.

   d. Treatment of botulism includes trivalent botulism antitoxin (ABE), stomach lavage, IV fluids, and tracheostomy with mechanical ventilation if respiratory paralysis occurs.

For more information on food poisoning, see *Medical-Surgical Nursing: A Nursing Process Approach*, **pp. 1408–1409.**

Foreign Body, Ocular

• If nothing is seen on the cornea or conjunctiva, the eyelids are everted to examine the palpebral and bulbar conjunctivae for the foreign body.

• The problem is manifested by client complaint of feeling something in the eye, blurry vision, pain, photophobia, or tearing.

- Treatment includes evaluating vision, ophthalmologic irrigation, wearing an eyepatch, and client education on ways to avoid further injury and symptoms of infection.

For more information on ocular foreign bodies, see *Medical-Surgical Nursing: A Nursing Process Approach,* **pp. 1065–1066.**

F

Fracture

OVERVIEW

- A fracture is a break or disruption in the continuity of a bone.
- Fractures can be classified as complete or incomplete
  1. *Complete* fracture: The break is across the entire width of the bone such that the bone is divided into two distinct sections.
  2. *Incomplete* fracture: The fracture does not divide the bone into two distinct sections.
- Fractures can also be grouped according to the extent of the soft tissue damage accompanying the fracture
  1. *Open* or *compound* fracture: The skin surface over the broken bone is disrupted, causing an external wound.
  2. *Closed* or *simple* fracture: does not extend through the skin
- Fractures can also be classified based on cause
  1. *Pathologic* (spontaneous) fracture: occurs after minimal trauma to a bone that has been weakened by disease
  2. *Fatigue* fracture: results from excessive strain and stress on bone

COLLABORATIVE MANAGEMENT

Assessment

- The nurse records
    1. Events leading to the fracture and immediate postinjury care
    2. Previous medical history
    3. Current medication, including over-the-counter and illegal drugs, and alcohol use
    4. Nutritional history
- The nurse assesses for
    1. Trauma to other body systems
    2. Change in bone alignment
    3. Shortening and/or change in bone shape
    4. Neurovascular changes
        a. Skin color
        b. Skin temperature
        c. Movement (if pain is elicited, stop immediately)
        d. Sensation
        e. Pulses distal to injury
        f. Pain: location, nature, frequency
    5. Changes in skin integrity such as ecchymosis, subcutaneous emphysema, or swelling
    6. Capillary refill (if an extremity is involved)
    7. Hemorrhage (open fracture)
    8. Muscle spasm
    9. Respiratory compromise

Planning and Implementation

NDx: PAIN

Nonsurgical Management

- *Closed reduction* involves manipulating the bone ends so that they realign while applying a manual pull, or traction, on the bone.

- *Bandages* and *splints* are used to immobilize areas such as the scapula and clavicle.

- *Casts* are used to hold bone fragments in place after reduction; they allow early mobility, correct and prevent deformity, and reduce pain.

    1. Several cast materials may be used
        a. *Plaster of Paris* requires application of a well-fitted stockinet and web padding prior to the application of wet plaster rolls. The cast takes 24 to 48 hours to dry, and ice may be applied for the first 24 to 48 hours to reduce swelling. The client is warned that heat will be felt immediately after the cast is applied. To facilitate drying, the cast is not covered, and

the client is turned every 1 to 2 hours. The nurse handles the cast with the palms of the hands to prevent indentations and resulting areas of pressure on skin.

    b. *Fiber glass* and *polyester-cotton knit* are lighter weight and take less time to dry.

2. Types of casts

    a. *Arm cast*: When in bed, a sling is used to elevate the arm above the client's head to reduce edema; when out of bed, the arm is supported by a sling placed around the neck.

    b. *Leg cast*: When in bed, the leg is elevated on several pillows.

    c. A *body cast* encircles the body; a *spica cast* encircles a portion of the trunk and one or two extremities. The client is at risk for skin breakdown, pneumonia or atelectasis, joint contracture, or paralytic ileus. *Cast syndrome*, similar to a claustrophobic reaction, may occur.

3. The nurse provides cast care

    a. Petals or finishes the cast if the underlying stockinet does not cover the edges of the cast by placing tape over the rough edges (to prevent skin irritation from rough and crumbling edges)

    b. Recognizes that a window may be cut in the cast by the physician so that the wound can be observed and cared for

    c. Ensures that the cast is not too tight; should be able to insert a finger between the cast and the skin; if it is too tight, the physician may cut it to relieve pressure

    d. Recognizes that the physician may bivalve the cast or cut it lengthwise into two equal pieces; either half can be removed for inspection or provision of care; the two pieces are reunited by an elastic bandage wrap

    e. Encases a long leg or body cast in a protective covering around the perineum to prevent contamination by urine or feces; uses a fracture bedpan

    f. Monitors neurovascular status frequently

    g. Inspects the cast daily for drainage, cracking, crumbling, alignment, and fit once the cast is dry

    h. Circles, dates, and monitors areas of drainage on the cast for change; not unusual for bloody drainage to seep through the cast from an open fracture site

       i. Reports a sudden increase in the amount of drainage or a change in the integrity of the cast to the physician immediately

       j. Cleans a soiled cast with mild detergent and a damp cloth

      k. Does not use lotion or powder on skin around the cast

       l. Teaches the client not to place foreign objects beneath the cast

     m. Smells the cast for foul odor and palpates for hot areas every shift

     n. Has a cast cutter available at all times

4. The nurse observes for and reports complications from casting

    a. Infection
    b. Circulation impairment
    c. Peripheral nerve damage
    d. Pressure necrosis
    e. Contracture of joint
    f. Degenerative arthritis
    g. Muscle atrophy
    h. Thromboembolism

• *Traction* is the application of a pulling force to a part of the body to provide reduction, alignment, and rest; it may also decrease muscle spasm and prevent or correct deformity.

1. Traction types include

    a. *Running,* in which the pulling force is in one direction and the client's body acts as countertraction; moving the bed or body can alter the countertraction force

    b. *Balanced suspension,* which provides the countertraction such that the pulling force of the traction is not altered

2. Classification

    a. *Skin*: the use of a Velcro boot (*Buck's traction*), belt, or halter that is attached to the skin and soft tissues; the purpose is to decrease painful muscle spasms, and weight is limited to 5 to 10 lb

    b. *Skeletal*: pins (Steinmann), wires (Kirschner), tongs (Crutchfield), or screws are surgically inserted directly into bone and therefore allow the use of a longer traction time and heavier weights, usually from 15 to 30 lb.

    c. *Plaster* traction: a combination or skeletal traction and a plaster cast

    d. *Brace* devices: exert a pull to correct alignment deformities

3. The nurse provides care for the client in traction
   a. Maintains correct balance between traction pull and countertraction force
   b. Does not remove weights without a physician's order
   c. Allows the weights to hang freely at all times
   d. Inspects ropes, knots, and pulleys every 8 hours for loosening, fraying, and positioning
   e. Checks the weight for consistency with the physician's order every 8 hours; if not correct, notifies the physician
   f. Notes that if the client complains of severe pain from muscle spasms, the weights may be too heavy or the client may need realignment
   g. Inspects the skin every 8 hours for signs of irritation and inflammation, especially at points of entry of wires, screws, or pins
   h. Performs pin care as required by hospital policy
   i. Performs a neurovascular assessment at least every 8 hours, or more often if clinically indicated

- Large doses of narcotic analgesics, anti-inflammatory drugs, and muscle relaxants may be used.
- Mild tranquilizers such as diazepam (Valium) may be given to relax the client, and to minimize muscle spasm.
- The nurse
  1. Applies ice or heat
  2. Elevates the involved part, when possible
  3. Provides massage or back rubs
  4. Provides distraction, imagery, or music therapy
  5. Teaches progressive relaxation techniques

Surgical Management

- *Open reduction with internal fixation* (ORIF) allows direct visualization of the fracture site and permits early mobilization.
- *External fixation* involves fracture reduction and the insertion of pins into the bone through small percutaneous incisions; the pins are held in place by a large, external metal frame to prevent bone movement.
- The nurse provides preoperative care
  1. Provides routine preoperative care
  2. Recognizes that the client may be placed in traction for a few days prior to surgery
- The nurse provides postoperative care
  1. Provides routine postoperative care
  2. Monitors neurovascular status at least every hour

for the first 24 hours after injury, every 2 hours for the next 12 to 24 hours, and every 4 hours for the next few days
3. Monitors the complete blood count for signs of anemia resulting from blood loss
4. Observes for and reports complications as described below

NDx: Altered (Peripheral) Tissue Perfusion

• The nurse initiates measures to prevent and report complications

1. Compartment syndrome
   a. Characterized by an increase in pressure—external (tight, bulky dressings) or internal (bleeding or fluid accumulation)— within one or more muscle compartments of the extremities, which causes massive compromise of circulation to the area
   b. Is manifested by edema, pain, pallor, unequal or diminished pulses, tense muscle swelling, paresthesia, paresis
   c. Complications include infection, persistent motor weakness, contracture, and myoglobinuric renal failure.
   d. Called *crush syndrome* when multiple compartments are affected; can lead to acidosis, hyperkalemia, shock, myoglobulinuria, and renal failure; death may result

2. Hypovolemic shock (see Shock)
3. Fat embolism syndrome
   a. Clients at risk include those with elevated serum glucose or cholesterol levels, increased capillary fragility, inability to cope with stress, and long-bone or multiple fractures.
   b. Is manifested by respiratory distress, tachycardia, hypertension, tachypnea, fever, petechiae, increased erythrocyte sedimentation rate, and decreased red blood cell and platelet count
   c. Treatment includes bed rest, oxygen, hydration, and possibly steroid therapy.

4. Pulmonary embolism
   a. An obstruction of a pulmonary artery by blood clot(s)
   b. Assessment findings are the same as for a fat embolism except no petechiae.
   c. Treatment consists of preventive measures such as antiembolism stockings and leg exercises, bed rest, oxygen, possibly

228

mechanical ventilation, heparin therapy,
thrombolytics, and possibly surgery (ligation
of vena cava, vena cava umbrella).

5. Infection

   a. May be caused by the wound or the indwelling
      hardware (pins, screws, wires, plates, rods)
   b. Clostridial infections can result in gas
      gangrene or tetanus.
   c. Bone infection can result in osteomyelitis.

6. Avascular necrosis

   a. Can be referred to as aseptic or ischemic
      necrosis
   b. Frequently seen in hip fractures

7. Delayed union, nonunion, and malunion

   a. *Delayed union*, a fracture that does not heal
      within 6 months of injury, is most commonly
      seen in tibial fractures and results in pain and
      immobility; *nonunion* is a fracture that never
      heals; *malunion* is an incorrect union.
   b. Treatments include
      (1) Ilizarov technique, using a circular
          external fixation device that lengthens the
          bone by stimulating bone growth
      (2) Electrical bone stimulation, developed as a
          result of research showing that bone had
          inherent electrical properties that are used
          in healing. Electrodes are placed internally
          or externally at the fracture site to induce
          weak electrical currents in bones called
          pulsing electromagnetic fields.
      (3) Bone grafting, in which chips of bone are
          taken from the client's iliac crest or other
          site and are packed or wired between bone
          ends to facilitate union.

8. Reflex sympathetic dystrophy

   a. A complex syndrome of pain, trophic changes,
      and vasomotor instability
   b. Treatment consists of physical therapy,
      diuretics, pain management, and edema
      control.
   c. If conservative measures fail, sympathetic
      anesthetic blockade or surgical
      sympathectomy is performed.

NDx: POTENTIAL FOR INFECTION
- The nurse
  1. Uses strict aseptic technique for dressing changes,
     wound irrigations, and pin care

2. Monitors for signs of infection, such as swelling, drainage, and fever

NDx: Impaired Physical Mobility

- The nurse employs measures to prevent complications of immobility
  1. Thromboembolic disease
     a. Applies thigh-high antiembolism stockings or sequential compression devices (e.g., Venodyne)
     b. Performs active and/or passive range-of-motion exercises and isometric and isotonic exercises
     c. Administers anticoagulation therapy such as low-dose aspirin, subcutaneous heparin sodium, or warfarin (Coumadin), as ordered
     d. Assesses for the presence of deep-vein thrombosis
  2. Respiratory complications
     a. Encourages the client to turn, cough, and deep breathe every 2 hours and use an incentive spirometer
     b. Assesses for atelectasis or pneumonia
     c. Assists the client to get out of bed as soon as possible
  3. Skin impairment
     a. Inspects the skin for signs of redness or irritation, with particular attention to bony prominences
     b. Uses heel or elbow protectors as needed
  4. Alterations in elimination
     a. Records intake and output, encourages fluids
     b. Provides a diet high in fiber, including raw fruits and vegetables, bran, or prunes
     c. Administers stool softeners and bulk laxatives as needed
  5. Cerebral dysfunction
     a. Recognizes that elderly clients may become disoriented
     b. Keeps a large clock and calendar in the client's view and asks family to bring in personal items and pictures
     c. Keeps side rails up at all times unless they present an accidental hazard (client consistently crawls over them)
     d. Assesses all clients for sensory deprivation
- The nurse collaborates with the physical therapist to promote client mobility.

- *Crutches* require strong upper extremities, balance, and coordination.
    1. To prevent pressure on the axillary nerve, there should be two to three finger widths between the axilla and the top of the crutch when the crutch tip is at least 6 inches diagonally in front of the foot.
    2. The crutch is adjusted so that the elbow is flexed no more than 30 degrees.
- A *walker* is most often used by the elderly client who needs additional support for balance.
- A *cane* is used if minimal support is needed
    1. Is placed on the unaffected side
    2. Should create no greater than 30 degrees flexion of the elbow
    3. Top of cane should be parallel to the greater trochanter of the femur

NDx: ALTERED NUTRITION: LESS THAN BODY REQUIREMENTS
- The nurse
    1. Assesses the client's food likes and dislikes
    2. Collaborates with the dietitian to plan meals that are both appealing and nutritional (high protein, high calorie)
    3. Administers supplements of vitamins B and C, as ordered
    4. Teaches the client to increase his or her dietary intake of milk and milk products, because the client is predisposed to hypocalcemia
    5. Encourages consumption of foods high in iron, because anemia may develop; iron supplement may be ordered

NDx: ANXIETY
- The nurse
    1. Assesses the cause of anxiety
    2. Refers to the appropriate person(s) who can help resolve problems (financial counselor, employer, social worker)
    3. Encourages the client to ventilate his or her feelings

Discharge Planning
- The nurse
    1. Identifies and suggests corrections for hazards in the home prior to discharge
    2. Ensures that the client can use all assistive-adaptive devices ordered for home use prior to discharge

3. Provides verbal and written instructions for the care of casts, splints, braces, or external fixator
4. Provides verbal and written instructions on wound care, as needed
5. Teaches the client/family how to recognize complications such as infection, as well as when and where to contact professional health care should complications arise
6. Provides a detailed plan of care at the time of discharge for clients to be transferred to a long-term-care or rehabilitation facility, if needed
7. Emphasizes the importance of follow-up visits with the physician(s) and other therapists

FRACTURES OF SPECIFIC SITES

• *Clavicular*: self-healing. A splint or bandage is used for immobilization.

• *Scapular*: immobilized with a sling until healing occurs

• *Humeral shaft*: corrected by open reduction and the application of a hanging arm cast or splint. An impacted injury is treated conservatively with a sling. A displaced fracture may require ORIF with pins or a prosthetic device.

• *Olecranon*: treated by closed reduction and application of a cast. Healing may take 2 months. Several additional months may be needed before full use of the elbow returns. For displaced fractures, ORIF is performed, and a splint is worn.

• *Radius* and *ulna*: treated with closed reduction and casting. If displaced, ORIF with intramedullary rods or plates and screws is done.

• *Wrist* and *hand*: treated with closed reduction and casting

• *Hip*: classified as intracapsular (within the joint capsule) or extracapsular (outside the joint capsule). Treatment involves ORIF. Nursing interventions are directed toward management of the following nursing diagnoses:
1. Potential for injury related to subluxation or dislocation
2. Pain related to surgical incision
3. Potential for infection related to impaired skin integrity
4. Impaired physical mobility related to hip precautions and surgical pain

• *Femur*: seldom immobilized by casting; skeletal

traction followed by a cast brace or hip spica cast. ORIF may be needed.

- *Patella*: Repair consists of closed reduction and casting or internal fixation with screws.
- *Tibia* and *fibula*: treated with closed reduction with casting for 8 to 10 weeks; internal fixation and long leg cast for 4 to 6 weeks; or external fixation, used when the fractures cause extensive skin and soft tissue damage.
- *Ankle*: generally create spiral, transverse, or oblique breaks that are difficult to treat and present problems in healing. Treatment consists of a combination of closed and open techniques, depending on the severity and extent of the fracture.
- Fractures of the *foot* or *phalanges* are very painful and are treated with either open or closed techniques.
- *Ribs* and *sternum*: may be treated with an elastic bandage or chest strap, although this is less common. The major complication is puncture of the lungs, heart, or arteries by bone fragments or ends.
- *Pelvic*: the second most common cause of death from trauma after head injuries. When a non–weight-bearing part of the pelvis is fractured, treatment involves bed rest. A weight-bearing fracture may require the use of a pelvic sling, skeletal traction, double hip spica cast, or external fixator.

For more information on fractures, see *Medical-Surgical Nursing: A Nursing Process Approach,* **pp. 780–807.**

Frostbite

- Frostbite is a cold injury of the skin dependent on temperature, duration of exposure, and tissue hypoxia at exposure.
- Cell death is due to microvascular vasoconstriction, with subsequent interference of blood flow and stasis.

- Continued exposure to cold causes vascular necrosis and gangrene.
- Increased risk factors include age, immobility, alcohol use, vascular disease, and psychiatric disorders.
- Treatment includes rapid and continuous rewarming of the tissue in a warm bath for 15 to 20 minutes or until skin flushing occurs; thawing can be painful.
- After thawing, the tissue is exposed so tissue changes can be monitored.
- Frostbite blisters are left intact.
- Over time, the degree of actual tissue destruction is evident, and local care to eschar is indicated.
- Long-term complications of cold injury include amputation, scarring, depigmentation, and thickened nail plates.

For more information on frostbite, see *Medical-Surgical Nursing: A Nursing Process Approach*, **pp. 1210–1211.**

Furuncle, Ear

- A furuncle of the ear is a bacterial infection of a hair follicle located on the outer half of the external ear canal.
- It is manifested by intense pain on light touch.
- The area is swollen and pink, and there may or may not be evidence of a purulent head.
- No drainage is present unless the furuncle has ruptured
- Hearing is impaired if the lesion is large enough to obstruct the canal.

- Treatment consists of local and systemic antibiotics and localized heat; incision and drainage of the lesion may be necessary.

For more information on ear furuncle, see *Medical-Surgical Nursing: A Nursing Process Approach,* **p. 1107.**

F

G

Ganglion

- A ganglion is a round, cystlike lesion often overlying a wrist or joint tendon.
- It is painless on palpation but can cause joint discomfort after prolonged use or minor trauma.
- The fluid within the lesion can be aspirated; total excision is preferred.
- The postoperative care is the same as for other hand surgeries.

For more information on ganglion, see *Medical-Surgical Nursing: A Nursing Process Approach,* **p. 772.**

Gastric Carcinoma

OVERVIEW

- Malignant neoplasms and tumors found in the stomach develop from the mucous membrane.
- In advanced disease, there is invasion to the muscularis or beyond.
- The majority of gastric cancers develop in the pylorus and antrum.
- Methods of extension include spread within the gastric wall into the regional lymphatics and direct organ invasion.
- Adenocarcinomas are the most common type, followed by malignant lymphoma.

COLLABORATIVE MANAGEMENT

Assessment

- The nurse records the client's
  1. Risk factors, including a history of gastric polyps, benign tumors, chronic gastritis, pernicious anemia, gastric surgery, male sex, and age of 50 or older
  2. Diet history, including intake of nitrates, salty foods or salted meats, pickled foods, or starch
  3. Change in appetite or eating habits with or without weight loss
  4. Smoking history
  5. Pain, including onset, duration, frequency, location, and aggravating or alleviating factors.
- The nurse assesses for the late symptoms of disease
  1. Vomiting
  2. Epigastric mass
  3. Hepatomegaly
  4. Ascites
  5. Enlarged lymph nodes

Planning and Implementation

NDx: POTENTIAL FOR INJURY

- Combination drug chemotherapy including fluorouracil, doxorubicin, and mitomycin C has proved more effective than single-agent chemotherapy.
- Radiation therapy is used in conjunction with surgery.
- Surgical management is usually curative in early

disease and involves distal subtotal gastric resection, combined with lymph node dissection.

• Palliative surgical resection in late disease may improve the client's quality of life.

• The nurse provides preoperative care

1. Provides the opportunity for the client and family members to discuss feelings and concerns about the diagnosis, treatment, and expected outcomes
2. Provide specific information about preparatory procedures such as laboratory tests, nothing-by-mouth status, and intravenous catheters
3. Reviews information about informed consent, such as information on the type and length of surgery
4. Discusses expected recovery course, including altered level of functioning, anticipated problems, and potential complications
5. Provides routine preoperative care

• The nurse provides routine postoperative care for the client undergoing general anesthesia (see Intraoperative Care) and care of the nasogastric tube.

NDx: PAIN

• The nurse

1. Administers nonnarcotic agents and narcotics; narcotics may be administered by patient-controlled analgesia pump
2. Provides and teaches relaxation techniques, cutaneous stimulation, and visual imagery

NDx: ALTERED NUTRITION: LESS THAN BODY REQUIREMENTS

• Total parenteral nutrition (TPN) may be required immediately following surgery and in the later recovery period if oral intake is poorly tolerated.

• Postoperative oral intake progresses from oral liquids to small, frequent, solid food feedings; milk and dairy products are often eliminated due to lactose intolerance.

Discharge Planning

• The nurse provides verbal and written postoperative instructions

1. Dietary restrictions individualized to the client
2. Pain management techniques, including medications
3. Inspection of incision for redness, tenderness, swelling, and drainage

4. Dressing change procedures, if necessary
5. Side effects of chemotherapy or radiation treatments

For more information on gastric carcinoma, see *Medical-Surgical Nursing: A Nursing Process Approach*, **pp. 1329–1335.**

Gastritis

OVERVIEW

- Gastritis is defined as the inflammation of the gastric mucosa.
- Mucosal injury occurs and is worsened by histamine release and cholinergic nerve stimulation.
- Hydrochloric acid diffuses into the mucosa and injures small vessels, resulting in edema, hemorrhage, and erosion of the gastric lining.
- Gastritis can be classified as acute or chronic.
  1. *Acute* gastritis, the inflammation of gastric mucosa or submucosa after exposure to local irritants such as alcohol or aspirin, occurs in varying degrees of mucosal necrosis and inflammation, with complete regeneration and healing usually occuring within a few days and complete recovery with no residual damage usually ensuing.
  2. *Chronic* gastritis, a diffuse chronic inflammatory process involving the mucosal lining of the stomach, which usually heals without scarring but can progress to hemorrhage and ulcer formation.
- The three subtypes of chronic gastritis include
  1. Superficial gastritis, in which there is an inflamed, edematous mucosa with hemorrhages and small erosions that are localized in the outer area of the mucosa

2. Atrophic gastritis, in which there is a thickened muscularis with inflammation, and occurs in all areas of the stomach, with decreased fundal, parietal, and chief cells (associated with gastric ulcers and cancer)
3. Gastric atrophy, in which there is total loss of fundal glands with minimal inflammation and thinning of the gastric mucosa

COLLABORATIVE MANAGEMENT

Assessment

- The nurse records the client's
  1. Cigarette use
  2. Dietary intake, including alcohol, caffeine, other irritants, and patterns of eating
  3. Life-style, including perceived stress
  4. Used over-the-counter drugs, such as corticosteroids and anti-inflammatory drugs
  5. Symptoms, including epigastric discomfort, abdominal tenderness, cramps, indigestion, nausea or vomiting, and their onset, duration, location, and frequency, as well as aggravating and alleviating factors
- The nurse assesses for
  1. General appearance, including facial grimacing, restlessness, or moaning
  2. Tenderness in the epigastric area, guarding, and distention
  3. Increased bowel sounds or visual peristaltic waves
  4. Dyspepsia or heartburn
  5. Hematemesis

Planning and Implementation

NDx: Pain

- The nurse
  1. Administers H$_2$ antagonists, as ordered, such as cimetidine (Tagamet), ranitidine (Zantac), famotidine (Pepcid), and nizatidine, to block gastric acid secretions
  2. Administers antacids, as ordered, as buffering agents
  3. Administers vitamin B$_{12}$, as ordered, for clients with pernicious anemia
  4. Avoids drugs associated with gastric irritation, including steroids, aspirin, chemotherapeutic agents, and nonsteroidal anti-inflammatory agents
  5. Avoids foods and spices that contribute to distress, including tea, coffee, cola, chocolate,

mustard, paprika, cloves, pepper, and Tabasco
sauce
6. Teaches the client to avoid large, heavy meals
7. Provides a soft, bland diet
8. Teaches techniques to reduce discomfort, such as
progressive relaxation, cutaneous stimulation,
guided imagery, and distraction
● Surgery is indicated when conservative measures
have failed to control bleeding (See "Surgical
Management" under Peptic Ulcer Disease.)

Discharge Planning
● The nurse teaches the client
1. To stop smoking
2. To reduce caffeine intake
3. To avoid foods and drugs that may be causative
agents

For more information on gastritis, see *Medical-
Surgical Nursing: A Nursing Process Approach*,
pp. 1303–1308.

Gastroenteritis

OVERVIEW
● Gastroenteritis is described as an inflammation of
the mucous membranes of the stomach and intestines,
primarily affecting the small bowel.
● The disease may be viral or bacterial in origin,
causing an inflammatory response in one of three ways
1. Release of enterotoxin, causing local
inflammation and diarrhea
2. Organism penetration of the intestine, causing
cellular destruction, necrosis, and ulceration
(diarrhea occurs with white blood cells or red
blood cells)

3. Organism attachment to mucosal epithelium, destroying cells of the intestinal villi with resultant malabsorption

COLLABORATIVE MANAGEMENT

Assessment

- The nurse records the client's
  1. Onset of diarrhea with accompanying abdominal cramping or pain
  2. Nausea and vomiting
  3. Recent travel experience
- The nurse assesses for
  1. Bloody, mucousy, or watery foul-smelling stool
  2. Fever; temperature may be normal or elevated from 101° to 103° F (38.2° to 39.2° C)
  3. Dehydration exhibited by poor skin turgor, dry mucous membranes, orthostatic blood pressure changes, hypotension, and oliguria
  4. Viral symptoms, such as myalgia, headache, or malaise

Planning and Implementation

NDx: FLUID VOLUME DEFICIT

- The nurse
  1. Administers hypotonic intravenous fluids, as ordered, for severe dehydration
  2. Adds potassium supplements to intravenous fluid, as ordered, if the client is hypokalemic
  3. Advises the client to take small volumes of clear liquids with electrolytes (like ginger ale) and then progress with the diet as tolerated

NDx: DIARRHEA

- The nurse
  1. Provides clear liquid fluids in small amounts as tolerated
  2. Progresses the diet as tolerated, avoiding milk and milk products for 1 week
  3. Avoids intestinal motility suppressants such as antiemetics or anticholinergics for bacterial or viral gastroenteritis
  4. Administers anti-infective agents such as sulfamethoxazole with trimethoprim (Septra, Bactrim) if shigellosis is present
  5. Applies repellent cream, such as zinc oxide, petroleum jelly, Desitin ointment, or Sween products, to protect the skin and anal area

Discharge Planning

- The nurse teaches the client
  1. To minimize the risk of disease transmission by washing his or her hands after bowel movements
  2. To avoid sharing eating utensils, glasses, and dishes and to maintain strict personal hygiene
  3. To follow written instructions for medication dosage, schedule of administration, and side effects, if ordered
  4. To maintain adequate oral fluid intake
  5. To report returning diarrhea or dizziness to the physician

For more information on gastroenteritis, see *Medical-Surgical Nursing: A Nursing Process Approach*, **pp. 1338–1343.**

Gastroesophageal Reflux Disease

OVERVIEW

- Esophageal reflux involves the backward flow of gastrointestinal (GI) contents into the esophagus, exposing the esophageal mucosa to the irritating effects of gastric and/or duodenal contents.
- Gastroesophageal reflux disease (GERD) develops when an inflammatory response is initiated.
- The degree of inflammation is related to the acid concentration of the refluxed material, the number of reflux episodes, and the length of time the esophagus is exposed to the irritant.

COLLABORATIVE MANAGEMENT
Assessment

- The nurse records the client's
  1. Symptoms, including onset, frequency, and

severity, and the environmental factors associated with them
2. Ingestion of corrosive substances
3. Previous radiation treatment to the head and neck
4. Infections involving structures of the mouth
5. Current medical treatment and over-the-counter medications
6. Work and leisure-time activities
- The nurse assesses for
    1. Physical appearance and nutritional status
    2. Pain location
    3. Swallowing and smoothness of laryngeal movement
    4. Heartburn or pyrosis, the primary symptom, described as a burning sensation; severe heartburn may radiate to the neck or jaw or may be referred to the back
    5. Pain aggravated by bending over, straining, or lying in a recumbent position
    6. Pain occurring after each meal and persists from 20 minutes to 2 hours
    7. Regurgitation not associated with belching or nausea; warm fluid traveling up the throat, resulting in a sour or bitter taste in the mouth
    8. Waterbrash (reflex salivary hypersecretion)
    9. Dysphagia (difficulty in swallowing)
    10. Chest pain from esophageal spasm
    11. Belching and a feeling of flatulence or bloating after eating

Planning and Implementation

NDx: PAIN

Nonsurgical Management
- The nurse
    1. Teaches the client to avoid fatty foods, coffee, tea, cola, chocolate, spicy foods, acidic foods, and alcohol
    2. Provides four to six small meals a day
    3. Teaches the client to avoid evening snacking and no eating 3 hours prior to bedtime
    4. Instructs the client to eat slowly and chew food thoroughly
    5. Encourages weight reduction if the client is obese
    6. Elevates the head of the bed by 6 to 12 inches to prevent nighttime reflux
    7. Administers antacids, as ordered, for acid-neutralizing effects
    8. Administers histamine receptor antagonists, such as cimetidine (Tagamet) or ranitidine

(Zantac), as ordered, which reduce gastric acid production, provide symptom improvement, and support healing of the inflamed esophageal tissue
9. Administers bethanecol (Urecholine), as ordered, to increase lower esophageal pressure and increase the rate of esophageal clearance
10. Administers metoclopramide (Reglan), as ordered, to increase the rate of gastric emptying
11. Avoids drugs that decrease lower esophageal sphincter (LES) pressure or delay gastric emptying, such as anticholinergics, calcium channel blockers, theophylline (Theo-Dur), and diazepam (Valium)

Surgical Management

• Antireflux surgery is performed only in healthy clients who have not responded to aggressive medical management.

• The three major surgical procedures are *Nissen fundoplication*, *Belsey's repair*, and *Hill's repair*.

• These procedures involve wrapping and suturing the gastric fundus around the esophagus, which anchors the LES area below the diaphragm and reinforces the high-pressure area.

• The nurse provides routine preoperative care.

• Following wrapping procedures, the nurse provides postoperative care

1. Provides routine postoperative care
2. Avoids repositioning or replacing the nasogastric tube, which was inserted during surgery
3. Avoids performing endotracheal suctioning on a client with esophageal anastamosis or repair
4. Assesses the cutaneous suture line for redness, drainage, and other signs of infection
5. Observes the surgical dressing for bleeding
6. Cleanses the suture line once each shift with half-strength peroxide, as ordered, and applies antibacterial ointment, as ordered
7. Elevates the head of the bed 30 degrees at rest and 90 degrees when feeding is instituted
8. Encourages the client to continue to follow the basic antireflux regime

• Synthetic *Angelchik prosthesis* placement is an alternate minor surgical procedure used for clients unable or unwilling to face major surgery.

• A laparotomy is performed, and a C-shaped silicone prosthesis filled with gel is tied around the distal esophagus, anchoring the LES in the abdomen and reinforcing sphincter pressure.

- Prior to the Angelchik procedure, the nurse provides routine preoperative care.
- Postoperative care closely parallels that used for laparotomy procedure.
- The nurse additionally
  1. Pays special attention to respiratory care because the surgery is performed close to the diaphragm
  2. Provides adequate analgesia so the client can cough effectively and clear the airway
  3. Teaches the client that mild dysphagia is common but resolves in time
  4. Encourages the client to eat smaller meals to avoid overdistention of the stomach

Discharge Planning

- The nurse
  1. Provides written instructions concerning diet modifications, side effects of medications, and life-style modifications.
  2. Stresses the importance of follow-up visits with the physician(s) and reporting increased or returned symptoms.

For more information on gastroesophageal reflux disease, see *Medical-Surgical Nursing: A Nursing Process Approach*, **pp. 1271–1281.**

Genital Herpes Simplex

OVERVIEW

- Genital herpes simplex is a sexually transmitted disease of the herpes simplex virus (HSV).
- The two types of herpes simplex are
  1. *Type 1* HSV, which causes most nongenital lesions, including cold sores

2. *Type 2* HSV, which causes genital lesions
- The incubation period is 2 to 20 days, with the average being 1 week.

COLLABORATIVE MANAGEMENT

- Clinical manifestations include
    1. Tingling sensation on the skin
    2. Appearance of vesicles (blisters) in a characteristic cluster on the penis, scrotum, vulva, perineum, vagina, cervix, and/or perianal region
    3. Headaches
    4. Fever
    5. Generalized malaise
    6. Painful urination
- After lesions heal, the virus remains in a dormant state in the nerve ganglia.
- Periodically, the virus may activate, and episodes of infection recur.
- Activation may be stimulated by factors that include stress, fever, sunburn, menses, and sexual activity.
- Viral shedding occurs, and the client is infectious.
- Management is focused on decreasing pain, promoting healing without secondary infection, decreasing viral excretion, and preventing transmission of the infection.
- Treatment includes measures
    1. To decrease pain and promote comfort, such as
        a. Oral analgesics
        b. Topical steroids
        c. Local anesthetic sprays or ointments
        d. Ice or warm compresses to lesions
        e. Sitz baths
    2. To prevent dysuria or to relieve retention of urine
        a. Encouraging increased fluid intake
        b. Encouraging frequent voiding
        c. Pouring water over genitalia while voiding or encourage voiding while sitting in a tub of water or standing in a shower
        d. Catheterizing the client, if needed
    3. To prevent infection
        a. Encouraging genital hygiene and keeping the skin clean and dry
        b. Wearing gloves while applying ointments
        c. Avoiding sexual activity when lesions are present
        d. Using condoms during all sexual activity

- Acyclovir, an antiviral drug, partially controls signs and symptoms and accelerates healing.

For more information on genital herpes simplex, see *Medical-Surgical Nursing: A Nursing Process Approach,* **pp. 1777–1781.**

Glaucoma

OVERVIEW

- Glaucoma is a group of ocular diseases characterized by increased ocular pressure.
- Left untreated, glaucoma can result in blindness.
- Types of glaucoma include
    1. *Primary,* in which the structures that are involved in circulation and/or reabsorption of the aqueous humor undergo direct pathologic change
        a. Open angle, or chronic
        b. Angle closure, also known as closed angle, narrow angle, or acute
    2. *Secondary,* which results from ocular diseases that cause a narrowed angle or an increased volume of fluid within the eye
    3. *Congenital,* which results from the failure of mesodermal tissue to create a functioning trabecular meshwork

COLLABORATIVE MANAGEMENT
Assessment
- The nurse assesses for
    1. Previous or existing eye-related problems
    2. Family history of glaucoma
    3. Increased intraocular pressure

4. Diminished accommodation
5. Visual field losses
6. Decreased visual acuity not correctable with glasses
7. Appearance of halos around lights
8. Headache or eye pain (pain is sudden and excruciating in acute glaucoma)
9. Anxiety and fear

Planning and Implementation

NDx: SENSORY PERCEPTUAL ALTERATION (VISUAL)
Nonsurgical Management

- The nurse administers drug therapy, as ordered
    1. Miotics to constrict the pupil and contract the ciliary muscle, such as pilocarpine hydrochloride (Pilocar, Isopto-Carpine), carbachol (Isopto Carbachol), and echothiophate iodide (Phospholine Iodide), which may cause blurred vision for 1 to 2 hours after use and adaptation to dark environments may be difficult
    2. Agents to inhibit formation of aqueous humor, which include timolol (Timoptic), betaxotol (Betoptic), and levobunolol (Betagan)
    3. Carbonic anhydrase inhibitors, such as acetazolamide (Diamox) and methazolamide (Neptazane), to reduce production of aqueous humor, with side effects that include numbness and tingling of the hands and feet, nausea, or malaise
    4. Systemic osmotic agents given to clients with acute glaucoma to reduce ocular pressure, including oral glycerin (Osmoglyn)

Surgical Management

- *Laser trabeculoplasty* is performed under local anesthesia for open-angle glaucoma to produce scars in the trabecular meshwork, causing them to tighten and thereby increase the outflow of aqueous humor.

- For angle-closure glaucoma, the laser is used to create a hole in the periphery of the iris, which allows aqueous humor to flow from the posterior chamber to the anterior chamber and then into the trabecular meshwork.

- A postoperative ocular steroid ointment may be prescribed following laser surgery.

- Complications of laser surgery are indicated by a headache that is unrelieved by acetaminophen and/or that is accompanied by nausea, brow pain, and/or a change in visual acuity.

- Other surgical procedures include filtering procedures, fistulizing sclerectomy, peripheral iridectomy, and cyclodialysis.
- The nurse provides preoperative care
    1. Provides routine preoperative care
    2. Administers medications to lower intraocular pressure, given topically or intravenously, as ordered
    3. Instills topical antibiotics, as ordered
- The nurse provides postoperative care
    1. Provides routine postoperative care
    2. Provides the antibiotic that is administered subconjunctivally by the ophthalmologist
    3. Adjusts the head of the bed to the position of comfort
    4. Assists the client with ambulating and eating as needed as soon as the effects of anesthesia are worn off
    5. Reports any drainage to the physician immediately but does not remove the original dressing unless specific orders are written to do so
    6. Instructs the client not to lie on the operative side
    7. Instructs the client to report symptoms of brow pain, severe eye pain, or nausea
    8. Observes for and reports complications of glaucoma surgery
        a. Increased intraocular pressure, manifested by ocular pain, pain above the eyebrow, and nausea; the client is instructed to avoid bending from the waist, lifting heavy objects, straining while having a bowel movement, coughing, and vomiting
        b. Hypotony—decreased intraocular pressure, which can lead to choroidal hemorrhage, or choroidal detachment, manifested by pain deep in the eye, with a definite onset, diaphoresis, or change in vital signs
        c. Infection
        d. Scar tissue

Discharge Planning

- The nurse
    1. Assists with the identification and correction of hazards in the home prior to discharge
    2. Refers the client/family to a home health service and/or Meals on Wheels, as needed
    3. Teaches the administration of eyedrops
    4. Provides drug information, as needed
    5. Stresses the importance of wearing protective eyewear during the day and the eye shield at night

6. Emphasizes the importance of follow-up visits with the physician(s)

For more information on glaucoma, see *Medical-Surgical Nursing: A Nursing Process Approach,* **pp. 1046–1052.**

Glomerulonephritis, Acute

OVERVIEW

- Acute glomerulonephritis is an inflammatory process of the glomeruli initiated by activation of immunologic responses.
- Two mechanisms of antigen-antibody reaction cause glomerular injury
  1. Antigen-antibody complexes that circulate and are deposited in glomerular tissue
  2. Immune complexes that form directly in the glomerular tissue as a result of local interaction
- Immune complexes are deposited in the mesangium and in the subendothelium and subepithelium of the walls of the glomerular capillary membrane.
- Activation of complement and release of vasoactive substances cause additional glomerular membrane injury.
- Red blood cells and protein molecules move into Bowman's capsule.
- *Primary* causes from the immune response to pathogens include
  1. Group A beta-hemolytic streptococcus
  2. Staphylococcal or pneumococcal bacteremia
  3. Syphilis
  4. Visceral abscesses
  5. Bacterial endocarditis
  6. Hepatitis B
  7. Infectious mononucleosis
  8. Measles

9. Mumps
10. Cytomegaloviral infections
11. Parasitic, fungal, or viral infections
- *Secondary* causes related to systemic disease include
    1. Systemic lupus erythematosus
    2. Progressive systemic sclerosis
    3. Thrombocytopenia purpura
    4. Postpartum renal failure
    5. Henoch-Schönlein purpura
    6. Goodpasture's syndrome
    7. Wegener's granulomatosis
    8. Polyarteritis nodosa
    9. Hemolytic-uremic syndrome

COLLABORATIVE MANAGEMENT
Assessment

G

- The nurse records the client's
    1. History of recent infections
    2. Recent travel
    3. Activities with exposure to viruses, bacteria, fungi, or parasites
    4. Recent illnesses
    5. Recent surgeries or invasive procedures
    6. Known systemic diseases
- The nurse assesses for
    1. Skin lesions or incisions
    2. Edema of the face, eyelids, hands, and peripheral tissue
    3. Hypertension
    4. Changes in patterns of urination
    5. Smoky, reddish-brown, or cola-colored urine
    6. Dysuria
    7. Decreased amount of urine output
    8. Difficulty breathing
    9. Orthopnea
    10. Nocturnal or exertional dyspnea
    11. Changes in weight
    12. Rales in lung fields
    13. S_3 heart sound
    14. Neck vein engorgement
    15. Fatigue and malaise
    16. Anorexia, nausea, and/or vomiting

Planning and Implementation
NDx: ALTERED NUTRITION: LESS THAN BODY REQUIREMENTS
- For the client with normal urine output, no diet modifications are necessary; the nurse encourages foods from all food groups.

- For the client with oliguria, fluid intake is restricted to the amount of urine in 24 hours plus 500 cc for insensible losses; sodium, protein, and potassium intake is restricted.
- The nurse provides frequent mouth care for the client with uremic symptoms.

NDx: Fluid Volume Excess
- Refer to "Collaborative Management" under Renal Failure, Chronic.

Discharge Planning
- The nurse
   1. Reviews prescribed medication instructions, including purpose, timing, frequency, duration, and side effects
   2. Discusses dietary and fluid intake modifications
   3. Advises the client to measure weight and blood pressure daily
   4. Teaches the importance of regular exercise with rest schedules
   5. Instructs the client about peritoneal or vascular access care if short-term dialysis is required to control fluid volume excess or uremic symptoms
   6. Reviews dialysis schedules and routines

For more information on acute glomerulonephritis, see *Medical-Surgical Nursing: A Nursing Process Approach*, **pp. 1850–1853.**

Glomerulonephritis, Chronic

OVERVIEW
- Chronic glomerulonephritis, or chronic nephritic syndrome, is the diagnostic name given to known and unknown causes of renal deterioration or renal failure.
- The exact pathogenesis is unknown; changes are

believed to be due to effects of hypertension, intermittent or recurrent infections and inflammation, and altered metabolism and hemodynamics.

- Kidney tissue atrophies, and the functional mass of nephrons decreases, which alters glomerular filtration.
- Glomerular injury results in proteinuria due to increased permeability of the glomerular basement membrane.
- The process eventually results in end-stage renal disease (ESRD) and uremia, requiring dialysis and/or transplantation.

COLLABORATIVE MANAGEMENT

- The nurse records the client's
  1. Health problems, including systemic disease
  2. Renal or urologic problems
  3. Childhood infectious diseases, such as *streptococcus*
  4. Recent exposure to infections
  5. Overall assessment of health status
  6. Changes in urinary status, including frequency of voiding and changes in urine color, clarity, and odor
  7. Changes in activity tolerance
  8. Presence of edema
  9. Changes in mental concentration or memory
- The nurse
  1. Inspects the skin for yellow color, ecchymosis, and rashes
  2. Inspects for evidence of edema in tissues
  3. Measures blood pressure and weight
  4. Auscultates the heart for an S_3 sound
  5. Auscultates the lungs for the presence of rales or crackles
  6. Observes the rate and depth of breathing pattern
  7. Inspects neck veins for engorgement
  8. Inspects and analyzes urine
- Management of chronic glomerulonephritis is similar to conservative management for ESRD.

For more information on chronic glomerulonephritis, see *Medical-Surgical Nursing: A Nursing Process Approach*, **pp. 1854–1855**.

Gonorrhea

- Gonorrhea is a sexually transmitted disease (STD) caused by *Neisseria gonorrhoeae*, a gram-negative diplococcus.
- The disease is transmitted by direct sexual contact and through an infected birth canal to the neonate.
- Initial symptoms occur 3 to 10 days after sexual contact with an infected person, or the client may be asymptomatic.
- Clinical manifestations include
    1. Male
        a. Dysuria
        b. Penile discharge that is either profuse yellowish-green fluid or clear, scant fluid
        c. Anal itching and irritation
        d. Rectal bleeding
        e. Painful defecation
        f. Pharyngitis
    2. Female
        a. Change in vaginal discharge
        b. Urinary frequency
        c. Dysuria
        d. Anal itching and irritation
        e. Rectal bleeding
        f. Painful defecation
        g. Pharyngitis
- In men, the urethra is the site most commonly affected but can spread to prostate, seminal vesicles, and epididymis.
- In women, the cervix and urethra are the most common sites, but upward spread can cause pelvic inflammatory disease, endometritis, salpingitis, and pelvic peritonitis.
- Assessment includes
    1. Sexual history
        a. Types and frequency of sexual activity
        b. Number of sexual contacts
        c. Past history of sexually transmitted disease
        d. Potential sites of infection
        e. Sexual preference
    2. Chief complaint
    3. Inspection for lesions, rashes, and discharges from the urethra, vagina, and/or rectum
    4. Gram stain smears for gram-negative diplococci

- Culture results provide a definitive diagnosis.
- Treatment includes antibiotics.
- Client education includes information about
  1. Transmission and treatment
  2. Prevention of reinfection
  3. Avoidance of sexual activity until the infection is cured
  4. Use of condoms if sexually active
  5. Need to report the disease

For more information on gonorrhea, see *Medical-Surgical Nursing: A Nursing Process Approach*, **pp. 1783–1785.**

Gout

OVERVIEW

- Gout is a systemic disease in which urate crystals deposit in joints and other body tissues.
- Two major types are
  1. *Primary* gout, which results from one of several inborn errors of purine metabolism. Uric acid production exceeds the kidney's excretion capability, and sodium urate deposits in synovium and other tissues, resulting in inflammation.
  2. *Secondary* gout, which involves excessive uric acid in the blood that is caused by another disease
- Four phases of the disease process include
  1. Asymptomatic hyperuricemia, in which there are no symptoms but serum uric acid is elevated
  2. *Acute* gout, which is characterized by excruciating pain and inflammation of one or more small joints, especially the great toe

3. *Intercritical,* or *intercurrent,* gout, which is asymptomatic, with no abnormalities found on examination (period between acute attacks)
4. *Chronic* gout, in which repeated episodes of acute gout result in the deposit of urate crystals under the skin and within major organs, especially the renal system

COLLABORATIVE MANAGEMENT
Assessment
- The nurse assesses for
  1. Family history of the disease
  2. Joint inflammation
  3. Excruciating pain in the involved joint(s)
  4. Tophi, hard, fairly large, and irregular-shaped deposits in the skin that may break open, with a yellow, gritty substance discharged (seen in chronic gout)
  5. Renal stones or dysfunction

Planning and Implementation
NDx: PAIN
- The nurse administers drug therapy, as ordered
  1. For *acute* gout only, colchicine and nonsteroidal anti-inflammatory drugs (NSAID) until the inflammation subsides, usually for 4 to 7 days or until severe diarrhea occurs
  2. For *chronic* gout, allopurinol (Zyloprim) or probenecid (Benemid), with serum uric acid levels monitored to determine the effectiveness of the drug
- Dietary restrictions are controversial but may include a strict low-purine diet with avoidance of organ meats, shellfish, and oily fish with bones.
- Excessive alcohol intake and fad "starvation" diets can cause a gout attack.
- The nurse instructs the client to avoid
  1. Aspirin in any form and diuretics
  2. Excessive physical or emotional stress

NDx: POTENTIAL FOR ALTERED PATTERNS OF URINARY ELIMINATION
- The nurse teaches the client
  1. To force fluids
  2. To increase urinary pH by eating alkaline ash foods, such as citrus fruits and juices, milk, and other dairy products

Discharge Planning

• The nurse teaches the client to follow the prescribed medication regimen even when there are no symptoms.

For more information on gout, see *Medical-Surgical Nursing: A Nursing Process Approach,* **pp. 706–708.**

G

Guillain-Barré Syndrome

OVERVIEW

• Guillain-Barré syndrome (GB), also called acute idiopathic polyneuritis, infectious polyneuritis, or Landry's paralysis, is an acute inflammation and demyelinization of the peripheral nervous system.

• Three stages include

1. *Initial* period, which begins with the onset of the first definitive symptoms and ends when no further deterioration is noted (usually 1 to 3 weeks)
2. *Plateau* period, which is a time of little change and lasts several days to 2 weeks
3. *Recovery* period, which is thought to coincide with remyelination and axonal regeneration and lasts 4 to 6 months

• Three types of GB include

1. *Ascending,* the most common clinical pattern, with weakness beginning in the lower extremities and progressing upward to include the trunk and arms; sometimes affecting the cranial nerves and sometimes with respiratory compromise
2. *Descending,* in which there is weakness of the face or bulbar muscles of the jaw, the sternocleidomastoid muscles, and muscles of the tongue, pharynx and larynx, and progressing downward to involve the limbs; respiratory compromise can occur quickly

3. *Miller-Fisher* variant, which consists of a triad of ophthalmoplegia, areflexia, and severe ataxia, with normal motor strength and intact sensory function

COLLABORATIVE MANAGEMENT
Assessment
- The nurse records the client's
  1. Past medical and surgical history
     a. Occurrence of antecedent illness 3 to 4 weeks prior to the onset of GB
     b. Description of symptoms (in chronological order)
- The nurse assesses for
  1. Paresthesia (numbness or tingling)
  2. Pain, resembling that of a charley horse
  3. Cranial nerve dysfunction: facial weakness, dysphagia, diplopia
  4. Difficulty walking
  5. Muscle weakness or flaccid paralysis without muscle wasting
  6. Respiratory compromise or failure: dyspnea, decreased breath sounds, decreased tidal volume and/or vital capacity
  7. Bowel and bladder incontinence
  8. Autonomic dysfunction evidenced by orthostatic hypotension and/or tachycardia
  9. Decreased or absent deep-tendon reflexes
  10. Ophthalmoplegia (level of consciousness, cerebral functioning, and/or pupillary signs are not affected)
  11. Ability to cope with illness
  12. Anxiety, fear, and panic
  13. Anger and depression

Planning and Implementation
NDx: INEFFECTIVE BREATHING PATTERN; INEFFECTIVE AIRWAY CLEARANCE; IMPAIRED GAS EXCHANGE
- The nurse
  1. Performs a respiratory assessment
     a. Assesses every 4 hours
     b. Observes for dyspnea, air hunger, and/or subjective complaints of shortness of breath
     c. Measures vital capacity every 2 to 4 hours
     d. Obtains arterial blood gases as indicated by the client's clinical status
     e. Keeps equipment for intubation and a ventilator available

2. Performs chest physiotherapy; encourages the client to cough and deep breathe
3. Changes the client's position frequently

NDx: IMPAIRED PHYSICAL MOBILITY

- A grading system is used for muscle testing
  - 0: no contraction
  - 1: flicker or trace contraction
  - 2: active movement with gravity eliminated
  - 3: active movement against gravity
  - 4: active movement against gravity and resistance
  - 5: normal power
- The nurse
  1. Applies thigh-high antiembolism stockings
  2. Administers subcutaneous heparin, as ordered, every 12 hours
  3. Performs range-of-motion (ROM) exercises

- Plasmapheresis may be performed in which the client's plasma is separated from whole blood, and its abnormal constituents are removed or the plasma is exchanged with normal plasma or a colloidal substitute. It has led to reductions in the length of hospital stay and in the amount of time for the client to resume walking.

- The nurse monitors vital and neurologic signs routinely throughout the plasmapheresis procedure.

- Complications of plasmapheresis include hypovolemia, hypokalemia, hypocalcemia, temporary circumoral and distal extremity paresthesia, muscle twitching, nausea, and vomiting.

- The nurse
  1. Administers adrenocorticotropic hormone (ACTH) (Acthar), as ordered, to shorten the duration of the disease
  2. Administers cyclophosphamide (Cytoxan) and azathioprine (Imuran), as ordered, which have met with variable success

NDx: IMPAIRED SKIN INTEGRITY

- The nurse
  1. Assesses skin integrity every 4 hours, especially the tips of the ears, heels, and bony prominences
  2. Positions the client frequently
  3. Massages the skin and bony prominences with lotion
  4. Keeps the skin clean and dry; uses commercial skin wash and ointment after incontinence
  5. Uses pressure-prevention devices
     a. Cushions, flotation devices

259

b. Eggcrate or alternating-pressure mattresses
c. Air-fluidized beds
6. Monitors nutritional intake

NDx: POWERLESSNESS

- The nurse
    1. Encourages the client to verbalize feelings concerning the illness and its effects
    2. Provides information regarding the disease process
    3. Allows the client to participate in his or her care and make choices as much as possible
    4. Provides encouragement and positive reinforcement
    5. Identifies factors that increase coping abilities through asking the client/family to describe situations that they have successfully coped with in the past
    6. Keeps necessary items (call light, radio or TV control) within the client's reach
    7. Uses a communication board if the client is unable to speak

NDx: ANXIETY; ANTICIPATORY GRIEVING

- The nurse
    1. Assesses the client/family for verbal and nonverbal behaviors indicative of anxiety, fear, and grieving
    2. Establishes a trusting, therapeutic nurse-client relationship
    3. Encourages the client/family to discuss their fears and concerns
    4. Allows the family to participate in care (if willing and able), such as ROM exercises and massages

NDx: TOTAL SELF-CARE DEFICIT

- The nurse
    1. Assesses the client's ability to perform activities of daily living; provides assistance based on the level of the client's ability
    2. Monitors response or tolerance of activity
    3. Provides adequate rest periods between activities and therapy sessions
    4. Collaborates with physical, occupational, and speech therapy to identify and obtain needed assistive-adaptive devices

Discharge Planning

- The nurse
    1. Identifies and suggests corrections of hazards in the home prior to discharge

2. Ensures the client can correctly use all adaptive-assistive devices ordered for home use

3. Provides a detailed plan of care at the time of discharge for clients to be transferred to a long-term-care or rehabilitation facility (Rehabilitation may be lengthy. See Rehabilitation.)

4. Assesses the client's and family's knowledge and understanding of the disease

5. Provides oral and written information
   a. Techniques to facilitate mobility
   b. Prevention of skin breakdown
   c. ROM exercises

6. Reinforces the teaching provided by other health care disciplines

7. Refers the client to local or community agencies for assistance in the home setting

For more information on Guillain-Barré syndrome, see *Medical-Surgical Nursing: A Nursing Process Approach,* **pp. 960–968.**

Gynecomastia

• Gynecomastia is a benign condition of breast enlargement, usually bilateral, in males.

• The condition is caused by proliferation of the glandular tissue, including mammary ducts and ductal stroma.

• Etiologic factors include drugs, aging, and obesity; underlying diseases causing estrogen excess, such as malnutrition, liver disease, and/or hyperthyroidism; and androgen deficiency states, such as aging and/or chronic renal failure.

- The client with gynecomastia is evaluated for breast cancer.

For more information on gynecomastia, see *Medical-Surgical Nursing: A Nursing Process Approach*, **pp. 1666–1667.**

Hallux Valgus

- Hallux valgus, also referred to as a bunion, is a foot problem in which the great toe deviates laterally at the metatarsophalangeal (MTP) joint.
- As the deviation worsens, the bony prominence enlarges and causes pain, particularly when wearing shoes.
- The treatment consists of a *bunionectomy*, which involves removing the bony overgrowth and bursa.
- When other toe deformities accompany the condition or if the bony overgrowth is large, several *osteotomies*, or bone resections, may be performed.
- Kirschner wires are inserted vertically through the toes for about 3 weeks postoperatively.

For more information on hallux valgus, see *Medical-Surgical Nursing: A Nursing Process Approach*, **p. 772.**

Hammertoe

- A hammertoe is the dorsiflexion of any metatarsophalangeal joint with plantar flexion of the adjacent proximal interphalangeal joint; the second toe is most often affected.
- As the deformity worsens, corns may develop on the dorsal side of the toe.
- As a result, clients are uncomfortable when walking or wearing shoes.
- Surgical treatment consists of *osteotomies* and the insertion of Kirschner wires for fixation.
- The client uses crutches until full weight bearing is allowed, in 3 to 4 weeks.

H

For more information on hammertoe, see *Medical-Surgical Nursing: A Nursing Process Approach,* **pp. 772–773.**

Headache, Cluster and Migraine

OVERVIEW

- A *migraine* headache is a severe unilateral headache often accompanied by nausea, vomiting, and sensitivity to light.
- *Cluster* headaches, also known as migrainous neuralgia, Horton's syndrome, histamine cephalalgia, or paroxysmal nocturnal cephalalgia, occur at about the same time(s) every day (often at night) and are characterized by excruciating pain lasting for 30 to 60 minutes.

- Two forms of headaches are
  1. *Episodic*, which occur most often, with the headache pattern continuing for 6 to 8 weeks and followed by a period of remission that may last for months or years
  2. *Chronic*, in which there has been no remission for more than a year

COLLABORATIVE MANAGEMENT

Assessment

- The nurse records the client's
  1. Onset of menses, use of contraceptive hormones
  2. Age at onset of first headache, precipitating factors
  3. Description of the characteristics of the headache
  4. Alcohol intake, foods that precipitate an attack
  5. Current medications, including prescribed and over the counter
  6. Typical work and leisure activities

- The nurse records additional information about *migraine* headache
  1. Presence of aura, time between aura and onset of headache, length of the attack
  2. Occurrence of nausea and/or vomiting
  3. Treatment: prescribed and over-the-counter medication, lying down in a darkened room, ice bag to forehead
  4. Family history of migraine headache

- The nurse records additional information about *cluster* headaches—sequence of events for headaches, including duration, frequency in 24 hours, and number of weeks before remission.

- The nurse assesses the client during a *migraine* headache for
  1. Presence of aura, precipitating factors such as strong sensory stimuli (light, smells, noises)
  2. Visual changes, numbness and/or tingling of the lips and/or tongue
  3. Slowness of thought or confusion, drowsiness, vertigo
  4. Nausea and/or vomiting
  5. Location and intensity of the pain, time headache begins and ends
  6. Mood change (irritability, euphoria, depression) or no prodromal sign

- The nurse assesses the client during a *cluster* headache for
  1. Behavior during the headache, such as an

inability to sit still or lie down, pacing, rocking while sitting
2. Presence of lacrimation, rhinorrhea, and/or congestion
3. Facial flushing or pallor
4. Ptosis and miosis on the side of the headache
5. Presence of bradycardia
6. Distension and tenderness of the temporal artery on the affected side
7. Ability to handle stress, usual coping mechanisms, and means of relaxation
8. Degree to which attack is incapacitating

Planning and Implementation

NDx: PAIN

- The nurse administers drug therapy, as ordered
  1. For *migraine* headache
     a. Beta-blockers such as propranolol (Inderal), ergot derivatives such as methysergide (Sansert), and antidepressants such as imipramine hydrochloride (Tofranil)
     b. Ergotamine tartrate (Ergomar, Gynergen), indomethacin (Indocin) and/or naproxen (Naprosyn)
  2. For *cluster* headache
     a. Ergotamine (Gynergen) administered 2 hours before the attack is expected or immediately at the onset
     b. Prednisone (Deltasone) or lithium citrate (Cibalith-S) given prophylactically
- Antiemetics are used to control nausea and vomiting.
- Bed rest in a darkened room with uninterrupted sleep often reduces the pain.

Discharge Planning

- The nurse
  1. Obtains a dietary consultation to help the client select personal food preferences that reduce the risk of precipitating a headache
  2. Teaches the client to follow the prescribed rest and recreation program
  3. Reinforces stress-reduction techniques
  4. Provides drug information
     a. Taking all medications in the correct dosage, at the right time, and by the right route
     b. What to do if a dosage is missed or if complications or side effects occur

265

5. Reviews measures to prevent future attacks

For more information on headache, see *Medical-Surgical Nursing: A Nursing Process Approach,* **pp. 864–877.**

Head Trauma

OVERVIEW

• Head trauma is a traumatic insult to the brain caused by an external force that may produce a diminished or altered state of consciousness and changes in cognitive abilities, physical functioning, and/or behavioral and emotional functioning.

• The damage most frequently occurs to the frontal and temporal lobes.

• An *open* head injury occurs when the skull is fractured or penetrated by an object, violating the integrity of brain and dura and exposing them to environmental contaminants.

• Types of cranial fractures include
  1. *Linear*, a simple, clean break
  2. *Depressed*, in which bone is pressed inward into brain tissue to at least the thickness of the skull
  3. *Open*, in which the scalp is lacerated, creating a direct opening to the brain tissue
  4. *Basilar*, which occurs at the base of the skull, usually along the paranasal sinus, and results in a cerebrospinal fluid (CSF) leak from the nose or ear, possibly resulting in damage to cranial nerves I, II, VII, and VIII and infection

• *Closed* head injuries are caused by blunt trauma and lead to concussions, contusions, and lacerations of the brain.

  1. A *concussion* is characterized by a brief loss of consciousness.

2. A *contusion* causes bruising of the brain tissue.
3. A *laceration* causes actual tearing of the cortical surface vessels and may lead to secondary hemorrhage.

• Secondary responses include any neurologic damage that occurs after the initial injury and may result in increased morbidity and mortality, including

1. Increased intracranial pressure (ICP)
2. Edema: vasogenic, interstitial
3. Hemorrhage: epidural, subdural, intracranial
4. Impaired cerebral autoregulation
5. Hydrocephalus

COLLABORATIVE MANAGEMENT

Assessment

• The nurse records the events surrounding the injury

1. When, where, and how the injury occurred
2. The client's level of consciousness immediately after the injury and upon admission to the hospital/unit and if there have been any changes or fluctuations
3. Presence of seizure activity

• The nurse records the client's

1. Age, sex, and race
2. Past medical and social history
3. Hand dominance
4. Allergies to medications and foods, especially seafood (clients allergic to seafood are often allergic to the medium use in diagnostic testing)
5. Alcohol and illegal drug consumption

• The nurse assesses for

1. Impaired airway or breathing pattern
2. Signs and symptoms of hypovolemic shock or hemorrhage, which may indicate abdominal bleeding or bleeding into soft tissue around major fractures
3. Indications of spinal cord injury
4. Cardiac arrhythmias from chest trauma, bruising of the heart, and/or interference with the autonomic system
5. Impaired cerebral autoregulation manifested by changes in vital signs
6. Changes in neurologic status/indications of increased ICP

   a. Decreased level of consciousness (stuporous, coma)
   b. Pupils that are large (or pinpoint) and nonreactive to light

H

    c. Decreased or absent motor strength in the extremities, hemiparesis or hemiplegia
    d. Inability to follow commands, confused
    e. Behavioral changes
    f. Cranial nerve dysfunction, especially I, III, VI, VII, and IX
    g. Ataxia, changes in muscle tone
    h. Aphasia
    i. Complaint of severe headache, nausea, or vomiting
    j. Seizure activity
    k. Drainage of CSF from the ear or nose

7. Indication of posttraumatic sequelae in the client who experienced a minor head injury; symptoms may persist for weeks or months

    a. Persistent headache
    b. Weakness
    c. Dizziness

8. Personality and behavior changes
9. Loss of memory
10. Problems with perception, reasoning abilities, and concept formation
11. Changes in personality and behavior, such as temper outbursts, risk-taking behavior, depression, and denial of disability
12. Loss of short-term memory and recent memory
13. Ability to learn new information, to concentrate, and to plan

NDx: Altered Cerebral Tissue Perfusion
Nonsurgical Management

- The nurse performs a neurologic assessment every hour
    1. Verbal response, orientation
    2. Eye opening, pupil size, and reaction to light
    3. Motor response
    4. Vital signs
- The nurse
    1. Elevates the head of the bed 30 to 45 degrees (unless contraindicated, e.g., spinal cord injury)
    2. Avoids activities that may increase ICP
        a. Positions the client to avoid extreme hip or neck flexion
        b. Avoids clustering nursing procedures
        c. Provides a quiet environment
- The client on a respirator may be hyperventilated to maintain an arterial carbon dioxide (PCO_2) level of 25 to 30 mmHg and an arterial oxygen maintained at 80 to 100 mmHg.

- The client may be placed in barbiturate coma using pentobarbital or thiopental to decrease the metabolic demands of the brain. This requires sophisticated hemodynamic monitoring techniques, mechanical ventilation, and ICP monitoring. Complications include cardiac dysrhythmias, hypotension, and fluid and electrolyte disturbances. Some facilities use narcotic sedation rather than barbiturates.
- The nurse administers drug therapy, as ordered
  1. Glucocorticoid (dexamethasone, methylprednisolone) to reduce edema (although the effectiveness is being questioned)
  2. Osmotic diuretics (mannitol) given through or drawn up through a needle with a filter to eliminate microscopic crystals
  3. Loop diuretics (e.g., furosemide) to treat increased ICP
  4. Paralytic agents (pancuronium), used if the client is mechanically ventilated to control restlessness and agitation in those at risk for increased ICP
- The client with head trauma is at risk for hyperglycemia, diabetes insipidus, syndrome of inappropriate antidiuretic hormone, fluid overload, and/or dehydration.
- The nurse
  1. Monitors electrolytes and serum and urine osmolarity
  2. Measures intake and output every hour
  3. Measures urine specific gravity every hour

Surgical Management

- A *craniotomy* may be indicated to
  1. Evacuate a subdural or epidural hematoma
  2. Treat uncontrolled increased ICP; ischemic tissue or tips of temporal lobe removed
  3. Treat hydrocephalus
- Surgical insertion of an intracranial pressure-monitoring device is often performed. Types of devices include
  1. Intraventricular
  2. Epidural monitor
  3. Subdural bolt or screw

NDx: SENSORY/PERCEPTUAL ALTERATION

- The nurse
  1. Provides a hazard-free environment
  2. Checks the temperature of food and beverages on the tray before serving
  3. Keeps the side rails up while the client is in bed and the seat belt on while the client is in a chair

269

4. Initiates a sensory stimulation program
5. Orients the client to environment, time, place, and the reason for hospitalization
6. Reassures the client that family/significant others know where he or she is and explains when they will visit
7. Maintains a normal sleep-wake cycle
8. Has the family bring in familiar objects, such as pictures
9. Monitors the client's reaction to television or radio; often, the client is unable to differentiate these programs from what is happening within her or his own environment

NDx: IMPAIRED PHYSICAL MOBILITY

- The nurse
  1. Performs active and passive range-of-motion exercises at least once per shift
  2. Positions the client carefully and uses splints and braces correctly
  3. Applies high-top tennis shoes if the client's feet are flaccid; uses them with clients who are spastic only after consultation with physical therapy
  4. Applies thigh-high antiembolism stockings to prevent pulmonary embolism

NDx: POTENTIAL FOR INJURY

- The nurse
  1. Maintains seizure precautions
  2. Keeps the bed in a low position and the side rails up
  3. Restrains the client's extremities only if necessary; uses a chest restraint or hand mittens

NDx: IMPAIRED GAS EXCHANGE

- The nurse
  1. Performs chest physiotherapy and encourages the client to breathe deeply
  2. Turns and repositions the client at least once every 2 hours
  3. Suctions the client as needed

NDx: BODY IMAGE DISTURBANCE; ALTERED ROLE PERFORMANCE

- The nurse
  1. Establishes a trusting relationship with the client
  2. Allows the client to direct and participate in his or her care and decision making regarding treatment as much as possible
  3. Encourages the client to verbalize feelings, anxieties, and fears

4. Emphasizes the client's abilities while assisting the client to adapt to disabilities

NDx: ALTERED NUTRITION: LESS THAN BODY REQUIREMENTS

- The nurse
  1. Begins nutritional support as soon as possible via hyperalimentation, tube feedings (nasal or gastrostomy), or oral feedings
  2. Checks for a positive gag reflex and evaluates swallowing abilities before beginning oral feedings; clients often have subtle dysfunction, which places them at risk for silent aspiration

Discharge Planning

- The nurse
  1. Provides a detailed plan of care at the time of discharge for clients to be transferred to a rehabilitation or long-term-care facility (rehabilitation may be a lengthy process; see Rehabilitation)
  2. Refers the client to the local head injury support group
  3. Teaches the client/family measures to treat sensory dysfunctions
     a. The home should have functioning smoke detectors (the client may have loss of sense of smell).
     b. Keeping objects and furniture in the same place is important.
     c. The measures described under "Sensory/ Perceptual Alteration" are relevant here also.
     d. The nurse helps the family and client to develop a home routine that is structured, repetitious, and consistent.

- For minor head injury, the nurse discusses symptoms of posttraumatic syndrome, informs the client this is "normal," and refers to a support group if symptoms persist.

For more information on head injury, see *Medical-Surgical Nursing: A Nursing Process Approach,* **pp. 923–937.**

Hearing Loss

OVERVIEW

- Hearing loss is generally thought of as conductive, sensorineural, or a combination of the two.
    1. *Conductive* hearing loss occurs when sound waves are blocked from coming to the inner-ear nerve fibers because of external-ear or middle-ear disorders, such as an inflammatory process or an obstruction.
    2. *Sensorineural* hearing loss is caused by a pathologic process of the inner ear or of the sensory fibers that lead to the cerebral cortex (VIII cranial nerve).
    3. *Mixed conductive-sensorineural* hearing loss is a combination of the two.
- The etiology of hearing loss determines the degree to which the hearing loss can be corrected and the amount of normal hearing that will return.

COLLABORATIVE MANAGEMENT

Assessment

- The nurse assesses for *early* warning signs of a hearing loss: the client
    1. Frequently asks people to repeat statements
    2. Understands words better in small groups
    3. Strains to hear
    4. Turns the head to favor one ear or leans forward
    5. Complains of ringing in the ears
    6. Fails to respond when not looking in the direction of the sound
    7. Exhibits irritability
    8. Answers questions incorrectly
    9. Raises the volume of television or radio
    10. Avoids large groups
- The nurse assesses for (for *conductive* hearing loss)
    1. Causes of the hearing loss, such as obstruction or inflammation caused by cerumen, a foreign body, edema, infection, tumor, or otosclerosis
    2. Abnormality of the tympanic membrane
    3. Client's speaking softly
    4. Client's hearing best in a noisy environment
    5. Abnormal Rinne's test: air conduction is greater than bone conduction
    6. Abnormal Weber's test: lateralization to the affected ear

- The nurse assesses for (for *sensorineural* hearing loss)
  1. Causes of hearing loss that include prolonged exposure to loud noise, ototoxic drugs, presbycusis, Meniere's syndrome, acoustic neuroma, diabetes mellitus, labyrinthitis, infection, and/or myxedema
  2. High-pitched, continuous tinnitus
  3. Occasional dizziness
  4. Client's speaking loudly
  5. Client's hearing poorly in a loud environment; high-frequency soft-discriminating consonants are lost first, especially sounds such as *s*, *sh*, *f*, *th*, and *ch*
  6. Abnormal Rinne's test: air conduction is less than bone conduction
  7. Abnormal Weber's test: lateralization to the unaffected ear

Planning and Implementation

NDx: SENSORY PERCEPTUAL ALTERATION (AUDITORY)

- The nurse
  1. Uses the written word if the client is able to see, read, and write
  2. Uses pictures of familiar phrases and objects
  3. Eliminates distracting noises when talking to the client
  4. Ensures that there is adequate lighting in the room, especially if the client can read lips, when appropriate
  5. Does not shout
  6. Keeps her or his hands and other objects away from the mouth when talking to the client
  7. Moves close to the client (positions self in front of the client) and speaks slowly and clearly
  8. Uses lower tones when communicating with a client with a high-frequency hearing loss
  9. Validates with the client the understanding of statements made by asking the client to repeat what was said

- Cochlear implant is a new and experimental means to treat a sensorineural hearing loss.

- Hearing with a hearing aid can be much different from normal hearing. The nurse
  1. Encourages the client to start using the aid slowly to develop an appreciation for the device
  2. Reminds the client that background noises will be amplified as well
  3. Reminds the client to remove the hearing aid when he or she is fatigued

- The nurse
  1. Assesses the client for depression, fear, and despair
  2. Uses techniques described under "NDx: Sensory Perceptual Alteration (Auditory)"
  3. Collaborates with the client's family and friends to identify activities the client enjoys and assist the client to identify ways these activities can be enjoyed again
  4. Refers the client to the American Speech-Language-Hearing Association, National Association of Hearing and Speech Agencies, and Self-Help for Hard-of-Hearing People (Shhh)

Discharge Planning

- The nurse
  1. Informs the client that telephone amplifiers increase the volume of sound carried by the telephone
  2. Informs the client that flashing lights are available that are activated by the ringing of the telephone or doorbell to alert the client visually
  3. Refers the client for use of a Hearing Aid dog, which alerts the client to the telephone, doorbell, cries of other people, and potential dangers, if appropriate
  4. Refers the client and family to classes for sign language and lip reading

For more information on hearing loss, see *Medical-Surgical Nursing: A Nursing Process Approach,* **pp. 1096–1100.**

Heart Failure

OVERVIEW

• *Heart failure* is the term describing the state in which the heart can no longer pump an adequate supply of blood or cardiac output to meet the demands of the body.

• Heart failure results in inadequate tissue perfusion and pulmonary and systemic congestion.

• Basic cardiac physiologic mechanisms, such as stroke volume, heart rate, cardiac output, and contractility, are altered in heart failure.

• Compensatory mechanisms to maintain normal cardiac function are

   1. Increased sympathetic nervous system response, causing increased heart rate, increased myocardial contractility, and venous and arterial vasoconstriction
   2. The Frank-Starling response (the cardiac muscles contract more forcibly the more they are stretched) increases preload, which sustains cardiac output.
   3. Myocardial hypertrophy provides more muscle mass, resulting in more effective cardiac contractility, and further increasing cardiac output.

• Compensatory mechanisms may eventually cause deleterious effects on pump function, contributing to increased myocardial oxygen consumption, causing the signs and symptoms of heart failure.

• The classifications of heart failure include

   1. *Backward versus forward failure*

      a. Backward failure results when the ventricle is unable to pump out its volume of blood, causing blood to accumulate and raising the pressure within the ventricles, the atria, and the venous system.
      b. Forward failure results when the heart is unable to maintain cardiac output, diminishing perfusion.

   2. *Left versus right ventricular failure*

      a. Left ventricular (LV) failure is caused by hypertensive disease, coronary artery disease (CAD), and/or valvular insufficiency, involving the mitral or aortic valves;

H

pulmonary congestion and edema usually signal the onset of LV failure.
- b. Right ventricular (RV) failure is most often caused by LV failure.
- c. Sustained pulmonary hypertension also develops into RV failure, leading to systemic venous congestion and peripheral edema.
3. *Low- versus high-cardiac output syndrome*
   - a. Low-output syndrome occurs when the heart fails as a pump, resulting in impaired peripheral circulation and vasoconstriction.
   - b. High-output syndrome results when cardiac output remains normal or above normal but the metabolic needs of the body are not met; causes include increased metabolic needs as seen in hyperthyroidism, fever, and pregnancy.
4. *Acute versus chronic failure*
   - a. Acute heart failure results from a marked decrease in LV failure due to myocardial infarction (MI), acute valvular dysfunction, or hypertensive crisis.
   - b. Chronic heart failure develops over time and is the end result of an increasing inability of the compensatory mechanisms to be effective; it occurs in hypertension, valvular disease, or chronic obstructive pulmonary disease.

COLLABORATIVE MANAGEMENT

Assessment

- The nurse records the client's
  1. Past medical history
     - a. Hypertension
     - b. Angina
     - c. MI
     - d. Rheumatic heart disease
     - e. Valvular disorders
     - f. Endocarditis
     - g. Pericarditis
  2. Perception of breathing pattern
  3. Fluid retention
  4. Response to activity
  5. Complaint of exertional or paroxysmal noctural dyspnea
  6. Cough
  7. Changes in mental status
  8. Irregular heartbeat
  9. Peripheral edema
  10. Weight gain

11. Gastrointestinal complaints
12. Nutritional history

- The nurse assesses for
  1. Breathlessness
  2. Weakness
  3. Fatigue
  4. Dizziness
  5. Confusion
  6. Pulmonary congestion
  7. Hypotension
  8. Increased heart size by palpating the precordium
  9. Tachycardia
  10. S_3 or S_4 heart sounds
  11. Crackles and wheezes
  12. Jugular venous distention
  13. Hepatomegaly
  14. Dependent edema
  15. Ascites

Planning and Implementation

NDx: DECREASED CARDIAC OUTPUT
Nonsurgical Management

- The nurse administers drug therapy
  1. Inotropic agents, such as digoxin (Lanoxin, Lanoxicaps) to improve pump performance and enhance contractility, as ordered
  2. Sympathomimetic agents, such as dopamine (Intropin) and dobutamine (Dobutrex), to clients whose condition is severely compromised by heart failure, as ordered
  3. Diuretics, as ordered, to enhance renal excretion of sodium and water, reducing circulating blood volume, decreasing preload, and reducing systemic and pulmonary congestion
  4. Vasodilators, as ordered, to increase cardiac output by dilating peripheral vascular vessels and reducing impedence or resistance to LV outflow

- Oxygen therapy, is administered, as ordered.

- The nurse
  1. Provides a low-sodium diet to control water retention
  2. Introduces a weight-reduction program, if needed, in consultation with the dietitian
  3. Provides physical and emotional rest
  4. Places the client in a semi- or high Fowler's position
  5. Obtains and records daily weights
  6. Maintains accurate intake and output measurements
  7. Implements fluid restriction

H

Surgical Management

• Heart transplantation may be required for end-stage heart failure or cardiomyopathy. This major surgery, performed at special centers, consists of removal of the diseased heart, leaving the posterior walls of the client's atria, followed by the anastamosis of the atria, aorta, and pulmonary arteries.

• Immunosuppressant drugs are administered to prevent rejection. (For more information on immunosuppression, see Cancer, General.)

Discharge Planning

• The nurse
  1. Assists the client in identifying factors that might precipitate symptoms
  2. Instructs the client to watch for and report to the physician: a weight gain of 2 to 3 lb, swelling ankles and feet, persistent cough, or frequent urination at night
  3. Provides oral and written instructions concerning medications, such as digoxin administration, including the importance of monitoring heart rate and rhythm, and side effects
  4. Reviews the signs and symptoms of hypokalemia for clients on diuretics and provides information on foods high in potassium
  5. Recommends the client restrict dietary sodium and provides written instructions on low-salt diets and identifying food flavorings to use as a substitute for salt, such as lemon, garlic, and herbs
  6. Stresses the importance of follow-up visits with the physician(s)

For more information on heart failure, see *Medical-Surgical Nursing: A Nursing Process Approach*, **pp. 2163–2171.**

Hemangioma

- Hemangiomas are benign vascular neoplasms occurring shortly after birth.
- They may regress in size or expand with growth.
- The *nevus flammeus* is a congenital vascular neoplasm involving mature capillaries.
- The lesions favor the face and upper body and occur as well-demarcated macular patches ranging in color from pink to bluish-purple.
- The *port-wine stain* grows proportionately with the child and remains unchanged in adult life.
- It usually occurs as a solitary lesion.
- Treatment is cosmetic and depends on the size and location of the lesion; it includes laser therapy, surgical excision with or without skin graft, or covering with opaque make-up.

For more information on hemangioma, see *Medical-Surgical Nursing: A Nursing Process Approach*, **p. 1208.**

Hemolytic Blood Transfusion Reaction

- A hemolytic blood transfusion reaction occurs when a recipient is given ABO-incompatible blood.
- The most common causes are a mistake in the labeling of blood and transfusion of blood to the wrong individual.

- Symptoms usually occur within 15 minutes of the start of the transfusion and include
  1. Burning along the vein
  2. Facial flushing
  3. Headache
  4. Chest pain
  5. Low back pain
  6. Fever, chills, and labored respirations
- Treatment includes
  1. Immediately stopping the blood transfusion
  2. Continuing infusion of normal saline
  3. Notifying the physician
  4. Monitoring vital signs and output frequently
  5. Treating shock with epinephrine, fluids, and oxygen
  6. Sending a sample of the client's blood to the laboratory
  7. Sending a urine sample to the laboratory for determination of hemoglobin
  8. Administering mannitol (Osmitrol) for renal involvement

For more information on hemolytic blood transfusion reaction, see *Medical-Surgical Nursing: A Nursing Process Approach,* **pp. 664–665.**

Hemophilia

- Hemophilia is a group of several hereditary bleeding disorders resulting from deficiencies of specific clotting factors that impair the hemostatic response and the capacity to form a stable fibrin clot.
- *Hemophilia A* (classic hemophilia) is a deficiency of factor VIII and accounts for 80% of all cases.
- *Hemophilia B* (Christmas disease) is a deficiency of factor IX and accounts for 20% of all cases.

- Abnormal bleeding occurs, which may be mild, moderate, or severe, depending on the degree of factor deficiency in response to any trauma.
- The nurse assesses for
  1. Excessive hemorrhage from minor cuts or abrasions
  2. Joint and muscle hemorrhages (degenerative)
  3. Tendency to bruise easily
  4. Prolonged postoperative hemorrhage
  5. Laboratory tests: prolonged partial thromboplastin time, normal bleeding time, and prothrombin time
- Management includes administration of factor VIII cryoprecipitate.

H

For more information on hemophilia, see *Medical-Surgical Nursing: A Nursing Process Approach*, **pp. 2276–2277.**

Hemorrhoid

OVERVIEW

- Hemorrhoids are unnaturally swollen or distended veins in the anorectal region that are common and not significant unless they cause pain and/or bleeding.
- Increased intra-abdominal pressure causes elevated systemic and portal venous pressure, which is transmitted to the anorectal veins.
- *Internal* hemorrhoids cannot be seen on inspection of the perianal area and lie above the anal sphincter.
- *External* hemorrhoids can be seen on inspection and lie below the anal sphincter.
- *Prolapsed* hemorrhoids can become thrombosed or inflamed.

- Common causes of repeated increased abdominal pressure are straining at stool, pregnancy, and portal hypertension.

COLLABORATIVE MANAGEMENT

- Common symptoms are bleeding, which is characteristically bright red and found on toilet tissue or outside the stool, pain associated with thrombosis, itching, and mucous discharge.
- Diagnosis is made by inspection, digital examination, and proctoscopy.
- Conservative treatment is aimed at reducing symptoms, including application of cold packs to the anorectal area followed by hot sitz baths; witch hazel soaks and topical anesthetics such as lidocaine (Xylocaine); over-the-counter remedies such as Nupercainal ointment; and high-fiber diets and fluids to promote regular bowel movements without straining and stool softeners.
- Surgical methods are indicated for recurring symptoms, including sclerotherapy, rubber band ligation, cryosurgery, and hemorrhoidectomy.
- The nurse teaches clients with hemorrhoids
    1. To adhere to a high-fiber, high-fluid diet to promote regular bowel patterns
    2. To utilize the local treatments for symptom relief
- Postoperative care includes
    1. Assisting the client to a side-lying position
    2. Keeping ice packs over the dressing, if ordered, until the packing is removed by the physician
    3. Utilizing moist heat (e.g., sitz baths) three to four times a day
    4. Administering stool softeners, such as docusate sodium (Colace), as ordered
    5. Assisting the client with the first defecation
    6. Adminstering narcotic analgesia prior to the first defecation
    7. Monitoring for urinary retention

For more information on hemorrhoids, see *Medical-Surgical Nursing: A Nursing Process Approach*, **pp. 1403–1404.**

Hemothorax

- Hemothorax is a common problem following blunt chest trauma.
- Simple hemothorax is a blood loss of less than 2000 mL into the thoracic cavity.
- The bleeding is caused by injuries to the lung parenchyma associated with rib and sternal fractures.
- Massive intrathoracic bleeding stems from injury to the heart, great vessels, or major systemic arteries.
- Physical assessment findings depend on the size of the hemothorax
  1. Asymptomatic for small hemothorax
  2. Respiratory distress for large hemothorax with diminished breath sounds and a dull percussion note on the affected side
- Interventions are aimed at blood evacuation to normalize pulmonary function and prevent infection and include anterior and posterolateral chest tube insertion.

For more information on hemothorax, see *Medical-Surgical Nursing: A Nursing Process Approach*, **p. 2056.**

Hepatic Abscess

- Hepatic (liver) abscesses occur when the liver is invaded by bacteria or protozoa.
- Liver tissue is destroyed.
- The resulting necrotic cavity becomes filled with infected, liquefied liver cells and tissue and leukocytes.

- Liver abscess has an uncommon occurrence with a high mortality rate.

- Pyrogenic abscesses are caused by bacteria such as *Escherichia coli*, *Klebsiella*, *Enterobacter*, *Salmonella*, *Staphylococcus*, and *Enterococcus*.

- Abscesses can result following cholangitis, liver trauma, peritonitis, sepsis, or infection extension and occur as multiple abscesses.

- Amebic hepatic abscesses occur following amebic dysentery as a single abscess in the liver's right upper quadrant.

- The nurse assesses for
  1. Right upper quadrant abdominal pain
  2. Tender, palpable liver
  3. Anorexia
  4. Weight loss
  5. Nausea and vomiting
  6. Fever and chills
  7. Shoulder pain
  8. Dyspnea

- Hepatic abscesses are usually diagnosed by liver scan.

- Surgical drainage is indicated only for a single, pyrogenic abscess or for an amebic abscess that fails to respond to long-term antibiotics.

For more information on hepatic abscess, see *Medical-Surgical Nursing: A Nursing Process Approach*, **p. 1505.**

Hepatitis

OVERVIEW

- Hepatitis is the widespread inflammation of liver cells, resulting in enlargement of the liver and congestion with inflammatory cells.

- *Viral hepatitis* is the most prevalent type, caused by one of four viruses

1. *Hepatitis A (HAV)*
   a. HAV, spread by the fecal-oral route, is characterized by a mild course and often goes unrecognized.
   b. Sources of infection include contaminated water, shellfish caught in contaminated water, and food contaminated by food handlers infected with the HAV.
   c. The incubation period is usually between 2 and 6 weeks, with an average of 4 weeks.
2. *Hepatitis B (HBV)*
   a. Formerly known as serum hepatitis, HBV is transmitted via the percutaneous route by contamination with blood and blood products.
   b. It is also spread via the mucous membranes by contact with infected body fluids, direct contamination of open wounds, handling infected equipment or items, and through sexual contact.
   c. The clinical course is varied, with an insidious onset and mild symptoms to serious sequelae, such as fulminant hepatitis, chronic active or persistent hepatitis, cirrhosis, or hepatocellular carcinoma.
   d. The incubation period is generally between 40 and 180 days.
3. *Hepatitis C (non-A, non-B)*
   a. The causative virus is similar to HBV.
   b. It is transmitted through blood and blood products and sexual contact.
   c. Symptoms develop 40 to 100 days after exposure to the virus.
4. *Delta hepatitis (Hepatitis D)*
   a. Hepatitis D is caused by infection with the hepatitis D virus.
   b. It is transmitted by nonpercutaneous routes, particularly close personal contact.

- HDV coinfects with HBV, and the duration of the HDV is dependent on the HBV infection.

- *Toxic* and *drug-induced hepatitis* result from exposure to hepatotoxins such as industrial toxins, alcohol, and/or medication.

COLLABORATIVE MANAGEMENT

Assessment

- The nurse records the client's
  1. Known exposure to HAV or HBV
  2. Recent blood transfusions

3. History of hemodialysis
4. Sexual preferences, including homosexual or bisexual
5. Intravenous drug use
6. Ear piercing
7. Tattooing
8. Living accommodations, including crowded facilities
9. Health care employment history
10. Recent travel to foreign countries
11. Recent ingestion of shellfish or contaminated water

- The nurse assesses for
  1. Weakness and fatigue
  2. Loss of appetite
  3. General malaise
  4. Myalgias
  5. Arthritislike joint pain
  6. Dull headaches
  7. Irritability
  8. Depression
  9. Nausea and vomiting
  10. Liver tenderness in the right upper quadrant
  11. Jaundice of the skin, mucous membranes, and sclera
  12. Dark urine
  13. Clay-colored stools
  14. Rashes
  15. Fever

Planning and Implementation

NDx: ACTIVITY INTOLERANCE

- The nurse
  1. Maintains physical rest alternating with periods of activity to promote liver cell regeneration by reducing the liver's metabolic needs
  2. Promotes emotional and psychologic rest

NDx: POTENTIAL FOR INFECTION

- The nurse
  1. Adheres to blood and body fluid precautions in the hospital setting and at home
  2. Wears gloves when in contact with the hepatitis A client's feces

NDx: ALTERED NUTRITION: LESS THAN BODY REQUIREMENTS

- A special diet is not required, although increased carbohydrates and calories with moderate fat and protein may be given.

- The nurse
  1. Determines food preferences
  2. Consults with the dietitian
  3. Gives supplemental vitamins, as ordered
  4. Administers antiemetics, as ordered, to relieve nausea

Discharge Planning
- The nurse provides client/family education
  1. Modes of transmission of hepatitis
  2. Observation of measures to prevent infection transmission
  3. Avoiding alcohol and nonprescription hepatotoxic drugs
  4. Determination of activity tolerance, rest
  5. Eating small, frequent meals of high-carbohydrate and low-fat foods
  6. Avoiding sexual activity until hepatitis B surface antigen (HBsAg) testing results are negative
  7. Importance of follow-up visits with the physician(s)

H

For more information on hepatitis, see *Medical-Surgical Nursing: A Nursing Process Approach*, **pp. 1497–1505.**

Hernia

OVERVIEW
- A hernia is a weakness in the abdominal muscle wall through which a segment of bowel or other structure protrudes, resulting from a defect in the integrity of the muscular wall and increased intra-abdominal pressure.
- Common types of hernias include
  1. *Indirect inguinal* hernias, which occur through the inguinal ring and follow the spermatic cord through the inguinal canal

2. *Direct inguinal* hernias, which pass through the abdominal wall in an area of muscle weakness
3. *Femoral* hernias, which occur through the femoral ring as a plug of fat in the femoral canal, which enlarges and pulls the peritoneum and the bladder into the sac
4. *Umbilical* hernias, classified as incisional or ventral and occurring at a surgical incision.

• *Reducible* hernias allow the contents of the hernial sac to be reduced or placed back into the abdominal cavity.

• *Irreducible*, or incarcerated, hernias cannot be reduced or placed back into the abdominal cavity.

• *Strangulated* hernias result when the blood supply to the herniated segment of the bowel is cut off by pressure from the hernial ring, causing ischemia and obstruction of the bowel loop.

COLLABORATIVE MANAGEMENT
Assessment
• The nurse records the client's
   1. Weight, height, and body build
   2. Concurrent medical conditions
   3. Lifting history
   4. Previous history of hernia
   5. Report of "feeling something pop" when straining or lifting
• The nurse assesses for
   1. Presence of the hernia on abdominal inspection
   2. Presence of bowel sounds (absence may indicate obstruction)
   3. Palpable hernia and its location

Planning and Implementation
NDx: POTENTIAL FOR INJURY

• *Herniorrhaphy*, the surgical treatment of choice, involves replacing the contents of the hernial sac into the abdominal cavity and closing the opening.

• *Hernioplasty* may be required to reinforce the weakened muscular wall with mesh, fascia, or wire.

• The nurse provides routine preoperative care.

• The nurse gives the client postoperative instructions
   1. Avoid coughing
   2. Deep breathe and turn frequently to promote lung expansion
   3. For indirect inguinal hernia repair, wear a scrotal support and apply an ice bag to the scrotum to prevent swelling

4. Elevate the scrotum with a soft pillow
5. Encourage early ambulation, if the client is able
6. Use specified techniques to stimulate voiding
7. Ensure an intake of at least 1500 to 2400 mL of fluids per day

Discharge Planning

- The nurse teaches the client
    1. How to care for the incision
    2. To limit activity, including avoiding lifting and straining, for 2 weeks after surgery
    3. To inspect the incision for redness, tenderness, swelling, and drainage and report the findings to the physician.
    4. How to take and monitor pain medication

For more information on hernia, see *Medical-Surgical Nursing: A Nursing Process Approach*, **pp. 1368–1371.**

Hiatal Hernia

OVERVIEW

- Esophageal or diaphragmatic hiatal hernias occur when the lower portion of the esophagus, or a portion of the stomach, or both, move into the thorax through the esophageal hiatus.
- There are two major types of hiatal hernia
    1. *Sliding* hernias, which occur when the esophagogastric junction and a portion of the fundus of the stomach are displaced through the hiatus into the thorax, with the hernia moving freely and sliding into and out of the thorax when there are changes in position or intra-abdominal pressure increases
    2. *Paraesophageal* or rolling hernias, which occur when the gastroesophageal junction stays below

the diaphragm but the fundus and portions of the greater curvature of the stomach roll into the thorax beside the esophagus

COLLABORATIVE MANAGEMENT
Assessment
- The nurse records the client's
    1. Weight and body build
    2. Daily work and leisure activities
    3. Usual diet pattern
    4. Occurrence of reactive symptoms, if any, to specific foods or activities
- The nurse assesses for
    1. General appearance and nutritional status
    2. Heartburn
    3. Regurgitation
    4. Chest pain that may mimic angina
    5. Dysphagia
    6. Belching
    7. Feeling of fullness after eating
    8. Feeling of breathlessness or suffocation
    9. Increased symptoms when in a recumbent position

Planning and Implementation
NDx: PAIN

Nonsurgical Management
- The nurse
    1. Administers antacids, histamine receptor antagonists, and cholinergic drugs, as ordered, in an attempt to control esophageal reflux and its symptoms
    2. Teaches the client to avoid fatty foods, coffee, tea, cola, chocolate, and alcohol, as well as spicy and acidic foods, such as orange juice
    3. Encourages the client to eat four to six small meals per day
    4. Teaches the client to avoid nighttime snacking to ensure that the stomach is empty
    5. Encourages weight reduction since obesity increases intra-abdominal pressure
    6. Elevates the head of the bed 6 to 12 in to reduce the incidence of esophageal reflux
    7. Instructs the client to avoid lying down several hours after eating

Surgical Management
- Surgery is indicated when the risk of complications such as aspiration are high and damage from chronic reflux is severe.

• Current surgical approaches for sliding hernias involve reinforcement of the lower esophageal sphincter (LES) to restore sphincter competence and prevent reflux, through some degree of *fundoplication*, or the wrapping of a portion of the stomach fundus around the distal esophagus to anchor it and reinforce the LES.

• Refer to Esophageal Tumor for preoperative and postoperative care.

Discharge Planning

• The nurse teaches the client

1. Activity restriction following hiatal hernia repair, including avoidance of straining and lifting and restriction on climbing stairs
2. Inspection of the surgical wound daily and reporting the incidence of swelling, redness, tenderness, or discharge to the physician
3. The importance of reporting fever to the physician
4. Avoidance of prolonged coughing episodes to prevent dehiscence of the fundoplication
5. Smoking cessation
6. Diet restrictions, including modifying the size and timing of meals, avoiding irritating foods or liquids, and reporting recurrence of reflux symptoms to the physician

H

For more information on hiatal hernia, see *Medical-Surgical Nursing: A Nursing Process Approach*, **pp. 1281–1285.**

Hodgkin's Disease

OVERVIEW

• Hodgkin's disease is a neoplastic disorder originating in a single lymph node or a single chain of nodes, which metastasizes to other lymphoid structures and eventually invades nonlymphoid tissues.

- This malignancy occurs primarily in young adults.
- Factors implicated as causes include viral infections and exposure to alkylating chemical agents.

COLLABORATIVE MANAGEMENT

- The nurse assesses for staging of Hodgkin's disease
  1. Stage Ia, confined to a single lymph node region or only one extranodal site
  2. Stage Ib, confined to a single lymph node region or only one extranodal site, and with the client experiencing symptoms of persistent fever, night sweats, and weight loss
  3. Stage IIa, confined to either two or more lymph node regions on the same side or contiguous extranodal sites on the same side of the diaphragm
  4. Stage IIb, confined to either two or more lymph node regions on the same side or contiguous extranodal sites on the same side of diaphragm, and with the client experiencing systemic symptoms
  5. Stage IIIa, extending to lymph node regions on both sides of diaphragm
  6. Stage IIIb, extending to lymph node regions on both sides of the diaphragm, and with the client experiencing systemic symptoms
  7. Stage IIIs, extending to lymph node regions on both sides of the diaphragm, with the client experiencing systemic symptoms and involvement of the spleen
  8. Stage IV, with widely disseminated foci of involvement
- The nurse assesses for
  1. Greatly enlarged, painless lymph nodes
  2. Persistent fever
  3. Malaise
  4. Night sweats
  5. Weight loss
- Treatment includes extensive external radiation of involved lymph node regions for stages I and II without mediastinal node involvement; more extensive disease requires radiation coupled with aggressive multiagent chemotherapy.
- The nurse monitors for side effects of radiation or drug therapy
  1. Prevention of infection

2. Nausea and vomiting
3. Skin irritation and breakdown

For more information on Hodgkin's disease, see
*Medical-Surgical Nursing: A Nursing Process
Approach*, **pp. 2271–2272.**

Huntington's Chorea

● Huntington's chorea is a hereditary disorder
transmitted as an autosomal dominant trait at the time
of conception.

● The two main symptoms of the disease are
progressive mental status changes, leading to dementia,
and choreiform movements.

● Other clinical manifestations of Huntington's chorea
include poor balance, hesitant or explosive speech,
dysphagia, impaired respirations, and bowel and
bladder incontinence.

● There is no known cure or treatment of the disease.

● The only way to prevent transmission of the gene is
for those affected to refrain from having children.

● Management of the disease is symptomatic.

● Nursing interventions are directed toward treating
nursing diagnoses

1. Impaired physical mobility
2. Altered nutrition: less than body requirements
3. Total incontinence
4. Total self-care deficit
5. Body image disturbance and altered role
   performance
6. Potential for injury
7. Ineffective airway clearance, ineffective breathing
   pattern, and impaired gas exchange

293

- As the symptoms progress, the client's status deteriorates, and death occurs from complications of immobility, such as pneumonia or sepsis.

For more information on Huntington's chorea, see *Medical-Surgical Nursing: A Nursing Process Approach,* **pp. 921–922.**

Hydrocele

- A hydrocele is a cystic mass, usually filled with straw-colored fluid, that forms around the testis.
- A hydrocele is the result of a disorder in the lymphatic drainage of the scrotum, causing a swelling of the tunica vaginalis, which surrounds the testes.
- A hydrocele may be aspirated via needle and syringe or surgically removed.
- Postoperatively the client wears a scrotal support to keep the scrotal dressing in place and keeps the scrotum elevated to prevent edema.

For more information on hydrocele, see *Medical-Surgical Nursing: A Nursing Process Approach,* **p. 1766.**

Hydronephrosis/ Hydroureter/Urethral Stricture

OVERVIEW

- Several disorders are associated with obstruction of the outflow of urine.
- In *hydronephrosis*, the kidney becomes enlarged as urine accumulates in the renal pelvis and the calyces; obstruction within the pelvis or ureteropelvic junction results in renal pelvic distention, and extensive damage to the vasculature and renal tubules can result.
- *Hydroureter* is the obstruction of the ureter at the point of the iliac vessel crossing or the ureterovesical entry; dilation of the ureter occurs at the point proximal to the obstruction as urine accumulates.
- A *urethral stricture* is the most distal point of obstruction, with bladder distention occurring before hydroureter and hydronephrosis.
- Urinary tract obstruction results in direct pressure buildup on the tissue, causing structural damage.
- Within the nephron, the tubular filtrate pressure increases as drainage through the collecting system is impaired, resulting in decreased glomerular filtration and renal failure.
- Causes of hydronephrosis and hydroureter include tumors, stones, trauma, congenital structural defects, and retroperitoneal fibrosis; pregnancy may cause ureteral dilation.
- Urethral stricture occurs from chronic inflammation.

COLLABORATIVE MANAGEMENT

- The nurse records the client's
  1. History of known renal or urologic disorders
  2. Childhood urinary tract problems
  3. Pattern of urination, including amount and frequency
  4. Description of urine, including color, clarity, and odor
  5. Report of symptoms, including flank and/or abdominal pain, chills, fever, and malaise
- The nurse assesses for
  1. Flank asymmetry and pain
  2. Abdominal tenderness or pain

3. Bladder distention
4. Urine leakage with abdominal pressure

• Urinary retention and potential for infection are primary problems.

• Treatment measures are aimed at correcting the obstruction. (See specific etiologies elsewhere in the book.)

For more information on urinary obstructions, see *Medical-Surgical Nursing: A Nursing Process Approach*, **pp. 1863–1865.**

Hyperaldosteronism

OVERVIEW

• Hyperaldosteronism is defined as an increased secretion of aldosterone by the adrenal glands, resulting in a state of mineralocorticoid excess.

• Primary hyperaldosteronism (Conn's syndrome), due to excessive secretion of aldosterone, is usually caused by the presence of an adenoma.

• Secondary hyperaldosteronism, the continuous excessive secretion of aldosterone resulting from higher levels of angiotensin II, is usually caused by poor renal perfusion, mechanical obstruction of the renal vessels, and/or the use of thiazide diuretics.

• Hyperaldosteronism is manifested by hypernatremia, hypokalemia, alkalosis, and hypertension.

COLLABORATIVE MANAGEMENT

• *Adrenalectomy* is the surgery of choice in most cases.
• The nurse
  1. Provides a low-sodium diet preoperatively as ordered but no restrictions postoperatively

2. Administers temporary glucocorticoid replacement if a unilateral adrenalectomy is performed or permanent replacement if a bilateral adrenalectomy is performed, as ordered
3. Administers spironolactone (Aldactone) therapy as ordered, if surgery is inadvisable
4. Instructs the client about side effects of spironolactone
   a. Hyperkalemia (in the client with impaired renal function or excessive potassium intake)
   b. Hyponatremia
   c. Gynecomastia
   d. Diarrhea
   e. Urticaria, rash
   f. Inability to maintain an erection, hirsutism, and amenorrhea

H

For more information on hyperaldosteronism, see *Medical-Surgical Nursing: A Nursing Process Approach,* **p. 1555.**

Hypercalcemia

OVERVIEW

- Hypercalcemia is defined as a serum calcium level greater than 10.5 mg/dL or 5.5 mEq/L.
- Small increases in serum calcium can have profound effects on physiological function.
- Common causes of hypercalcemia include
  1. Increased absorption of calcium
     a. Excessive oral intake of calcium
     b. Excessive oral intake of vitamin D
  2. Decreased excretion of calcium
     a. Renal failure
     b. Use of thiazide diuretics

3. Increased bone resorption of calcium
   a. Hyperparathyroidism
   b. Malignancy
      (1) Direct invasion (cancers of breast, lung, prostate, and osteoclastic bone and multiple myeloma)
      (2) Indirect resorption (liver cancer, small cell lung cancer, cancer of the adrenal gland)
   c. Hyperthyroidism
   d. Immobility
   e. Use of glucocorticoids
4. Hemoconcentration
   a. Dehydration
   b. Use of lithium
   c. Adrenal insufficiency

COLLABORATIVE MANAGEMENT

Assessment

- The nurse records the client's
  1. Age
  2. Use of prescribed and over-the-counter medications
     a. Antacids
     b. Thiazide diuretics
     c. Glucocorticoids
     d. Thyroid replacement drugs
     e. Calcium supplements
     f. Vitamin D supplements
  3. Current and past medical and surgical history
     a. Malignancy
     b. Chronic conditions
     c. Heart disease
     d. Parathyroid or other endocrine problems
  4. Activity level, especially the amount of weight-bearing activities
  5. Diet history: excessive ingestion of foods high in calcium, such as dairy products, legumes, broccoli, salmon, sardines, and tofu
- The nurse assesses for
  1. Cardiovascular changes, the most serious and life-threatening manifestations
     a. Increased heart rate
     b. Increased blood pressure
     c. Bounding, full peripheral pulses
     d. Electrocardiogram (ECG) abnormalities
        (1) Shortened ST segment
        (2) Widened T wave

e. Potentiation of digitalis-associated toxicities
   f. Decreased clotting time
   g. Late phase
      (1) Bradycardia
      (2) Cardiac arrest, sinus arrest

2. Neuromuscular changes
   a. Disorientation, lethargy, coma
   b. Profound muscle weakness
   c. Diminished or absent deep-tendon reflexes

3. Gastrointestinal changes
   a. Decreased motility
   b. Hypoactive bowel sounds
   c. Anorexia, nausea
   d. Abdominal distention
   e. Constipation

4. Respiratory changes (ineffective respiratory movement related to profound skeletal muscle weakness)

5. Renal changes
   a. Increased urinary output
   b. Dehydration
   c. Formation of renal calculi

6. Psychosocial changes
   a. Behavioral changes
   b. Mood changes
   c. Impaired short- and long-term memory
   d. Disordered thought processes

Planning and Implementation
NDx: Decreased Cardiac Output

- The nurse administers drug therapy, as ordered
   1. Immediately stops all intravenous (IV) infusions and oral medications containing calcium
   2. Administers IV infusion of normal saline if the client's renal status is normal and cardiopulmonary status can handle the extra fluid
   3. Stops thiazide diuretics; furosemide (Lasix) may be administered to increase the excretion of calcium
   4. May administer calcium chelators or binders
      a. Mithramycin (Plicamycin)
      b. Penicillamine (Cupramine)
   5. May administer drugs that inhibit calcium resorption from the bone
      a. Phosphorus
      b. Calcitonin (Calcimar)
      c. Prostaglandin synthesis inhibitors (aspirin, nonsteroidal anti-inflammatory drugs)

6. Should not administer multiple vitamins, calcium supplements, and antacids

- The nurse recognizes that diet therapy has a minimal beneficial effect.

- Peritoneal dialysis, hemodialysis, and/or blood ultrafiltration may be used to treat the client with life-threatening hypercalcemia. The dialyzing fluid should contain little calcium.

- The nurse institutes cardiac monitoring, as ordered
    1. Compares recent ECG tracings with the client's baseline tracings or tracings obtained when the client's serum calcium was normal
    2. Examines the ECG for changes in T waves and the QT interval, as well as for changes in rate and rhythm

NDx: CONSTIPATION

- The nurse
    1. Assesses bowel activity before giving oral food or liquids
    2. Assesses for paralytic ileus, decreased bowel sounds
    3. Administers drug therapy, as ordered, such as stool softeners and laxatives
    4. Encourages fluids as tolerated

NDx: POTENTIAL ALTERED TISSUE PERFUSION

- The nurse administers drugs to increase clotting time, as ordered (unless contraindicated)
    1. Aspirin
    2. Heparin
    3. Warfarin (Coumadin)
    4. Does not use aspirin and heparin together

- The nurse teaches the client that foods high in vitamin K such as green leafy vegetables should be restricted.

- The nurse promotes venous return
    1. Assesses the client for venous stasis
    2. Removes or loosens restrictive clothing
    3. Uses antiembolism stockings
        a. Carefully measures the client's legs to ensure that the correct size is ordered
        b. Orders two pair and applies a fresh pair daily
        c. Assesses fit (neither too tight nor too loose)
    4. Instructs the client in the correct performance of isometric exercises, especially of the legs
    5. Teaches the client how to perform active and passive range-of-motion exercises
    6. Encourages the client to keep leg joints straight when in bed

7. Ensures that the knee gatch of the bed is not elevated and that the bed is not bent at the client's hips
8. Encourages the client to ambulate and to avoid standing or keeping the legs in a static dependent position
9. Encourages the client to lie in the side-lying position especially if his or her abdomen is large
10. Encourages deep breathing exercises for 5 minutes every hour while awake
11. Assesses for indications of thrombus formation

NDx: POTENTIAL FOR INJURY (FRACTURE)

- The nurse
1. Provides a hazard-free environment to prevent falls
2. Ambulates the client with assistance
3. Provides the client with nonskid shoes when ambulating or getting out of bed
4. Keeps the side rails up and the bed in a low position
5. Places the call light within easy reach
6. Avoids excessive pressure or pulling or pushing movements when positioning the client

Discharge Planning

- The nurse
1. Teaches the client how to determine the electrolyte content of prepared foods and medications by carefully reading labels
2. Obtains a dietary consultation for assistance in providing information on the planning and preparation of palatable meals whenever a specific electrolyte restriction is necessary
3. Teaches the client about specific food or fluid restrictions
4. Reviews the signs and symptoms of the specific imbalance for which the client is at risk, as well as what specific information should be reported immediately to the primary health care provider
5. Provides drug information, as needed

For more information on hypercalcemia, see *Medical-Surgical Nursing: A Nursing Process Approach,* **pp. 301–309.**

Hyperglycemic Hyperosmolar Nonketotic Syndrome

OVERVIEW

- Hyperglycemic hyperosmolar nonketotic syndrome (HHNKS) occurs as an emergency in diabetes care by much the same process as diabetic ketoacidosis (DKA), except there is not excessive formation of ketones.

- People experiencing HHNKS do not usually manifest Kussmaul's respirations or elevated levels of serum or urinary ketones.

- The hyperosmolar state leads to serious fluid volume depletion and shock.

- Features of the disease include
  1. Gradual onset
  2. Precipitated by infection, other stressors, poor fluid intake
  3. Clinical manifestations

     a. Polyuria
     b. Fatigue
     c. Decreased temperature
     d. Lethargy
     e. Confusion
     f. Coma
     g. Seizures
     h. Hemiplegia
     i. Rapid pulse
     j. Dehydration

  4. Laboratory findings

     a. Serum glucose: greater than 800 mg/dL
     b. Osmolarity: greater than 350 mOsm/L
     c. Serum acetone: nondetectable or small
     d. Serum HCO_3: 17 mEq/L
     e. Arterial pH: about 7.26
     f. Serum Na: normal to high
     g. Serum K: low
     h. Serum P: not known
     i. Anion gap: normal
     j. Blood urea nitrogen: high

- Treatment measures for HHNKS are similar to DKA, except there is increased need for fluid replacement and assessment of fluid overload and less need for regular insulin.

For more information on hyperglycemic hyperosmolar nonketotic syndrome, see *Medical-Surgical Nursing: A Nursing Process Approach*, **pp. 1594–1595.**

Hyperkalemia

OVERVIEW

- Hyperkalemia is defined as a serum potassium level of greater than 5.0 mEq/L.
- The consequences can be life threatening, and the imbalance is generally not seen in healthy individuals.
- Causes include
    1. Excessive potassium intake
        a. Potassium-containing foods or medications
        b. Salt substitutes
        c. Potassium chloride (KCl) administration
        d. Rapid infusion of potassium-containing intravenous (IV) solution
    2. Decreased potassium excretion, which may be seen in Addison's disease and renal failure
    3. Movement of potassium from intracellular fluid to extracellular fluid
        a. Tissue damage
        b. Acidosis
        c. Hyperuricemia

COLLABORATIVE MANAGEMENT
Assessment
- The nurse records the client's
    1. Age

2. Past medical and surgical history
3. Medication use, particularly diuretics containing potassium
4. Urinary output and frequency
5. Diet history, including the use of salt substitutes and methods of preparing food (steaming, baking)

- The nurse assesses for
    1. Cardiovascular changes (the most common cause of death)
        a. Irregular heart rate, usually slow
        b. Decreased blood pressure
        c. Electrocardiogram (ECG) abnormalities
            (1) Tall T waves
            (2) Widened QRS complexes
            (3) Prolonged PR intervals
            (4) Flat P waves
        d. Ectopic beats
        e. Late changes: dysrhythmias, ventricular fibrillation, cardiac arrest in diastole
    2. Neuromuscular changes
        a. Early phase or mild hyperkalemia
            (1) Muscle twitches, cramps
            (2) Paresthesia
        b. Late phase or severe
            (1) Profound weakness
            (2) Ascending flaccid paralysis in distal to proximal direction involving arms or legs
    3. Gastrointestinal changes
        a. Increased motility
        b. Hyperactive bowel sounds
        c. Diarrhea
    4. Respiratory changes (unaffected until late, when profound weakness of skeletal muscles causes respiratory failure)

Planning and Implementation

NDx: Decreased Cardiac Output

- The nurse
    1. Immediately stops infusions of IVs containing potassium; leaves the IV line open
    2. Administers IVs containing substantial amounts of glucose and insulin, as ordered (250 mL of 10% to 20% glucose with 10 to 20 units of insulin)
    3. Withholds oral potassium supplements
    4. Administers transfusions of whole blood or packed red blood cells, which should be given only if absolutely necessary
    5. Maintains a potassium-restricted diet

6. Gives sodium bicarbonate, as ordered, if hyperkalemia is accompanied by or caused by metabolic acidosis
7. Monitors the client closely for hypokalemia or hypoglycemia
8. Administers oral or rectal cation exchange resins such as sodium polystyrene sulfonate (Kayexalate), as ordered

- Dialysis may be necessary when potassium levels reach lethal levels.
- The nurse
  1. Compares ECG tracings to baseline (notes changes in rate, rhythm, and waveform)
  2. Marks chest lead placement with a nonerasable pen since changes in tracing patterns are more reliable when chest leads are consistently placed
  3. Obtains a dietary consultation when hyperkalemia is chronic or when it is related to inappropriate renal handling of potassium; when severe or sudden onset of hyperkalemia occurs, diet therapy is of little value

H

NDx: Diarrhea

- The nurse
  1. Uses caution regarding the amount and frequency of any antidiarrheal medications
  2. Recognizes that overmedication can result in paralytic ileus or constipation
  3. Has the client avoid high-fiber and high-residue foods
  4. Encourages fluids, as tolerated (however, excessive fluid intake could increase peristalsis and diarrhea)

Discharge Planning

- The nurse reviews diet therapy with the client/family, as needed
  1. Teaches the client how to determine the electrolyte content of food and medications
  2. Obtains a dietary consultation for assistance in providing information on the planning and preparation of meals
  3. Teaches the client to adhere to specific food or fluid restriction

For more information on hyperkalemia, see *Medical-Surgical Nursing: A Nursing Process Approach,* **pp. 274–279.**

Hypermagnesemia

- Hypermagnesemia exists when the serum magnesium level is greater than 2.5 mEq/L.
- Common causes of hypermagnesemia include
    1. Excessive ingestion of antacids with a high concentration of magnesium (Maalox, milk of magnesia, magnesium sulfate)
    2. Renal insufficiency
- Clinical manifestations include
    1. Bradycardia
    2. Peripheral vasodilation
    3. Hypotension
    4. Electrocardiogram changes
        a. Prolonged PR interval
        b. Widened QRS complex
    5. Drowsy and lethargic, progressing to coma
    6. Diminished or absent deep-tendon reflexes
    7. Respiratory insufficiency
- Management of hypermagnesemia include
    1. Intravenous fluids
    2. Loop diuretics
    3. Calcium for severe cardiac manifestations
    4. Dietary restrictions of meat, nuts, legumes, fish, vegetables, and whole-grain cereal products

For more information on hypermagnesemia, see *Medical-Surgical Nursing: A Nursing Process Approach,* **pp. 313–314.**

Hypernatremia

OVERVIEW

- Hypernatremia is defined as a serum sodium level above 145 mEq/L. Common causes include
    1. Decreased sodium excretion
        a. Hyperaldosteronism
        b. Renal failure
        c. Corticosteroids
        d. Cushing's syndrome
    2. Increased sodium intake
        a. Excessive oral sodium ingestion
        b. Excessive administration of sodium-containing intravenous (IV) fluids
    3. Decreased water intake, nothing by mouth
    4. Increased water loss
        a. Increased rate of metabolism
        b. Fever
        c. Hyperventilation
        d. Infection
        e. Excessive diaphoresis
        f. Watery diarrhea
        g. Dehydration

COLLABORATIVE MANAGEMENT

Assessment

- The nurse records the client's
    1. Age
    2. Medications, including prescription and over-the-counter; use of antacids
    3. Past medical and surgical history
    4. Current medical history, including presence of chronic diseases
    5. Actual fluid intake in the previous 24 hours, types of fluids ingested
    6. Recent changes in weight
    7. Diet history
        a. Consumption of high-sodium foods, such as canned foods, processed and packaged foods, snack foods, crackers, cheese, and smoked meats
        b. Use of sodium-containing condiments, such as soy sauce, ketchup, steak sauces, meat tenderizers
    8. Amount of strenuous physical exercise and

H

environmental temperature and humidity present
during the activity
- The nurse assesses for
    1. Neuromuscular changes
        a. Hypernatremia with normovolemia or
           hypovolemia (agitation, confusion, seizures)
        b. Hypernatremia with hypervolemia (lethargy,
           stupor, coma)
        c. Mild or early changes
            (1) Spontaneous muscle twitches
            (2) Irregular contractions
        d. Severe or late changes
            (1) Skeletal muscle weakness
            (2) Deep-tendon reflexes diminished or absent
    2. Cardiovascular changes
        a. Decreased myocardial contractility
        b. Diminished cardiac output
        c. Heart rate and blood pressure responsive to
           vascular volume
    3. Respiratory changes (problems associated with
       pulmonary edema when hypernatremia is
       accompanied by hypervolemia)
    4. Renal changes
        a. Decreased urinary output
        b. Increased specific gravity
    5. Integumentary changes
        a. Dry, flaky skin
        b. Presence or absence of edema related to
           accompanying fluid volume changes
    6. Psychosocial changes (agitation or manic
       behavior)

Planning and Implementation

NDx: ALTERED NUTRITION: GREATER THAN BODY REQUIREMENTS FOR SODIUM

- The nurse restores fluid balance, as ordered, when
caused by fluid loss
    1. IV infusions of D_5W
    2. IV infusion of isotonic D_5W sodium chloride
       solutions if hypernatremia is caused by fluid and
       sodium loss

- The nurse administers natriuretic (enhance sodium
loss) diuretics, generally loop diuretics, if the condition
is caused by inadequate renal excretion of sodium
    1. Furosemide (Lasix, Furoside, Novosemide,
       Uritol)
    2. Bumetanide (Bumex)

3. Ethacrynic acid (Edecrin)

- The nurse assesses the client frequently for symptoms that indicate excessive loss of fluids, sodium, or potassium.
- Dietary restriction of sodium is prescribed.
- Fluid restriction may be needed.

NDx: Altered Oral Mucous Membrane

- Drug therapy for decreasing oral mucosal dryness is available but of dubious effectiveness.
- The nurse
  1. Moistens the client's lips with a petroleum-based lubricant
  2. Provides frequent mouth care, including brushing and flossing the teeth
  3. Rinses the client's mouth frequently
     a. Does not use commercial mouthwashes that contain alcohol or glycerin washes and swabs because these products tend to dry the oral mucosa further and may increase the discomfort by stinging or burning open fissures in the mucosa
     b. Rinses the mouth no more than two to three times per day with dilute hydrogen peroxide
     c. Uses lukewarm saline or tap water rinses
  4. Assists the client with oral hygiene before meals or snacks
- When mouth dryness is present, the client should avoid foods that are highly spiced or mechanically hard; bland, soft, cool foods are most easily tolerated.

NDx: Anxiety

- Medications used to decrease nerve and muscle responsiveness to stimuli are given
  1. Diazepam (Valium, Neo-Calme, E-Pam)
  2. Chlordiazepoxide (Librium, Solium)
  3. Lorazepam (Ativan)
  4. Methocarbamol (Robaxin, Delaxin)
  5. Orphenadrine (Banflex, Myolin, Norflex)

Discharge Planning

- The nurse reviews diet therapy with the client/family
  1. Teaches the client how to determine the electrolyte content of prepared foods and medications by carefully reading labels
  2. Obtains a dietary consultation for assistance in providing information on the planning and preparation of palatable meals whenever a specific electrolyte restriction is necessary

3. Teaches the client to adhere to specific food or fluid restrictions
- The nurse reviews signs and symptoms of the specific imbalance for which the client is at risk, as well as what specific information should be reported immediately to the primary health care provider.
- The nurse provides drug information, as needed.

For more information on hypernatremia, see *Medical-Surgical Nursing: A Nursing Process Approach,* **pp. 287–294.**

Hyperparathyroidism

OVERVIEW

- Primary hyperparathyroidism results when one or more hyperfunctioning glands is unresponsive to the normal feedback of serum calcium.
- Secondary hyperparathyroidism is a response to the hypocalcemia in chronic renal disease and in vitamin D deficiency.

COLLABORATIVE MANAGEMENT

Assessment

- The nurse records the client's
  1. Family history of disease
  2. Mothers whose newborns developed tetany (prime suspects for primary hyperparathyroidism)
  3. Use of over-the-counter medications and prescription medications
  4. Previous medical history
     a. Bone fractures, pathological fractures
     b. Radiation treatment

- The nurse assesses for
    1. Headache
    2. Drowsiness, fatigue
    3. Epigastric pain
    4. Muscle weakness
    5. Gastrointestinal disturbances, such as anorexia, nausea, and vomiting
    6. Depression
    7. Weight loss
    8. Waxy pallor of the skin
    9. Bone deformities in the extremities and back
    10. Renal calculi
    11. Decreased deep-tendon reflexes

Planning and Implementation
NDx: Potential for Decreased Cardiac Output

Nonsurgical Management
- Hydration (usually with intravenous normal saline) and the administration of furosemide (Lasix) are used to reduce serum calcium levels.
- The nurse
    1. Records strict intake and output measurements
    2. Observes for changes in blood pressure, rate or rhythm of pulses, and increasing confusion, lethargy, or irritation
    3. Assesses the need for cardiac monitoring
    4. Monitors for congestive heart failure secondary to fluid overload
    5. Monitors serum calcium levels frequently
    6. Instructs the client to report any nausea, vomiting, palpitations, tingling sensations, or numbness
    7. Administers drug therapy, as ordered

        a. Phosphates to inhibit bone resorption and interfere with calcium absorption (used only when calcium levels must be lowered rapidly)
        b. Calcitonin to decrease skeletal calcium release and increase the renal clearance of calcium (must be given in conjunction with glucocorticoids)
        c. Mithramycin, a cytotoxic antibiotic, the most effective agent to lower calcium levels (monitor closely for thrombocytopenia and renal and hepatic toxicity)

Surgical Management
- The surgery of choice is the removal of the parathyroid glands.

- The nurse provides preoperative care
  1. Stabilizes calcium levels per the physician's order
  2. Monitors bleeding times and coagulation studies
  3. Monitors complete blood count
  4. Provides routine preoperative care
- The nurse provides postoperative care
  1. Monitors serum calcium levels every 4 hours
  2. Monitors vital signs frequently per protocol
  3. Checks neck dressing for abnormal amounts of drainage or bleeding
  4. Observes for respiratory distress
  5. Has emergency equipment such as a tracheostomy tray and oxygen at the bedside
  6. Monitors for signs of hypocalcemia, such as tingling and twitching of the extremities and face
  7. Checks for Trousseau's and Chvostek's signs
  8. Administers calcium and vitamin D, as ordered

Discharge Planning

- The nurse teaches the client
  1. The importance of follow-up calcium levels
  2. The importance of follow-up visits with the physician(s)
  3. Actions and side effects of medication, if ordered

For more information on hyperparathyroidism, see *Medical-Surgical Nursing: A Nursing Process Approach,* **pp. 1575–1580.**

Hyperphosphatemia

- Hyperphosphatemia exists with a serum phosphate level greater than 4.5 mg/dL.
- Elevations of phosphate are well tolerated.
- Problems are associated with the hypocalcemia induced as a result of the increase in serum phosphorus levels.

- Common causes include
    1. Renal insufficiency
    2. Aggressive treatment of neoplasms
    3. Increased intake of phosphorus
    4. Hypoparathyroidism
- Management of hyperphosphatemia includes management of the underlying hypocalcemia.

For more information on hyperphosphatemia, see *Medical-Surgical Nursing: A Nursing Process Approach,* **pp. 311–312.**

H

Hyperpituitarism

OVERVIEW

- Hyperpituitarism is a pathologic state that occurs as a result of a hormone-secreting adenoma (pituitary tumor) and also as a result of hypothalamic dysfunction.
- Common secretory tumors include the prolactinoma (lactotrophic [PRL] secreting tumor), causing decreased reproductive functioning, and the growth hormone (GH) somatotrophic-producing adenoma, causing gigantism or acromegaly
    1. *Gigantism*, characterized by rapid proportional growth in the length of all bones
    2. *Acromegaly*, characterized by increased skeletal thickness, hypertrophy of the skin, and enlargement of visceral organs.
- Hypersecretion of adrenocorticotropic hormone results in overstimulation of the adrenal cortex and may lead to the development of Cushing's disease.

COLLABORATIVE MANAGEMENT
Assessment
- The nurse records the client's
    1. Age, sex, and family history

2. Complaints of change in hat, glove, ring, or shoe size
3. Visual difficulties
4. Sexual history/functioning
   a. Female clients
      (1) Amenorrhea
      (2) Irregular menses
      (3) Difficulty becoming pregnant
      (4) Decreased libido
      (5) Painful intercourse
   b. Male clients
      (1) Decreased libido
      (2) Impotence
- The nurse assesses for
  1. Changes in facial features
     a. Increase in lip and nose size
     b. Prominent supraorbital ridge
  2. Enlarging head, hand, and foot size
  3. Prominent jaw
  4. Dysphagia, difficulty chewing, and/or dentures that do not fit
  5. Arthritic changes causing pain and decreased mobility
  6. Arrowhead or tufted characteristics on x-ray films and a thickened appearance of the distal phalanges
  7. Increased perspiration and oil secretion on the client's skin
  8. Increased metabolism and strength (initially with acromegaly and gigantism)
  9. Lethargy and weakness (in later stages of gigantism and acromegaly)
  10. Visual changes
  11. Organomegaly (cardiac or hepatic)
  12. Hypertension
  13. Deepening of the voice because of hypertrophy of the larynx
  14. Hyperprolactinemia (observed with hypogonadism and galactorrhea)
  15. Changes in body image
  16. Depression and emotional distress

Planning and Implementation
NDx: BODY IMAGE DISTURBANCE
Nonsurgical Management
- The nurse
  1. Encourages the client to verbalize concerns and fears related to his or her altered physical appearance

2. Helps the client to identify his or her strengths and positive characteristics
3. Administers bromocriptine mesylate (Parlodel), as ordered, to treat hyperprolactinemia or acromegaly by reducing GH levels and decreasing tumor size
4. Instructs the client regarding drug side effects, which include postural hypotension, gastric irritation, nausea, headaches, abdominal cramps, and constipation
5. Teaches the client to take the drug with meals or a snack
6. Instructs the client to stop the drug immediately if she becomes pregnant

• Proton beam or alpha particle radiation therapy is usually effective but slow. Side effects include hypopituitarism, optic nerve damage, oculomotor dysfunction, and/or visual field defects.

Surgical Management

• Surgical removal of the tumor or pituitary gland (*hypophysectomy*) is performed, usually via the transsphenoidal approach
1. The client is placed in a semisitting position, and an initial incision is made at the inner aspect of the upper lip.
2. The sella turcica is entered through the sphenoid sinus, and the gland or tumor is removed.
3. A muscle graft is taken, often from the anterior thigh, to pack the dura and prevent leakage of cerebrospinal fluid (CSF).
4. Nasal packing is inserted and a dressing applied under the nose to prevent the packing from dislodging.

• A transfrontal craniotomy is performed if the tumor is inaccessible through the transsphenoidal route.
• The nurse
1. Provides routine preoperative care
2. Explains to the client that nasal packing will remain in place for 2 to 3 days, which necessitates mouth breathing
3. Explains that toothbrushing, coughing, sneezing, nose blowing, and bending must be avoided postoperatively
4. Provides routine postoperative care
   a. Monitors for changes in neurologic status
   b. Carefully measures intake and output
   c. Observes and reports signs of diabetes insipidus, such as low urine specific gravity, and polyuria

d. Instructs the client to report postnasal drip
e. Records the amount and color of nasal drainage (clear drainage is tested for glucose, whose presence indicates that the fluid is CSF)
f. Elevates the head of the bed at all times
g. Reports severe persistent headache to the physician immediately (may indicate that CSF has leaked into the sinus area)
h. Observes the client for indications of meningitis, such as headache, fever, and nuchal rigidity

NDx: SEXUAL DYSFUNCTION

- The nurse
  1. Identifies the specific problem(s) and encourages the client to discuss any effect that sexual dysfunction has had on the relationship with his or her sexual partner
  2. Instructs the client that medication may be helpful
  3. Informs the client that sexual dysfunction may occur after a hypophysectomy

Discharge Planning

- The nurse identifies the need for adaptive-assistive equipment in the home.
- The nurse teaches the client
  1. To avoid bending over to pick things up or tie shoes
  2. To avoid straining during a bowel movement
  3. To rinse the mouth and use dental floss until brushing of teeth can be resumed after the incision has healed
  4. To expect a decreased sense of smell for 3 to 4 months

For more information on hyperpituitarism, see *Medical-Surgical Nursing: A Nursing Process Approach,* **pp. 1533–1538.**

Hypertension

OVERVIEW

- Hypertension is defined as systolic blood pressure greater than or equal to 140 mmHg and/or diastolic blood pressure greater than or equal to 90 mmHg occurring in a client on at least three separate occasions.
- Hypertension is the major risk factor for coronary, cerebral, renal, and peripheral vascular disease.
- Systemic arterial pressure is a product of cardiac output and total peripheral resistance.
- Four control systems play a major role in maintaining blood pressure: arterial baroreceptors, body fluid volume, renin-angiotensin system, and vascular autoregulation.
- There are two major classifications of hypertension
  1. *Essential*, primary or idiopathic
  2. *Secondary*, from known causes, such as estrogen-containing oral contraceptives, renal vascular and renal parenchymal disease, dysfunction of adrenal medulla or adrenal cortex, coarctation of the aorta, neurogenic disorders such as brain tumors and encephalitis, and psychiatric disorders.

COLLABORATIVE MANAGEMENT

Assessment

- The nurse records the client's
  1. Age
  2. Race
  3. Family history of hypertension
  4. Alcohol intake
  5. Salt intake
  6. Smoking history
  7. Exercise habits
  8. Past and present history of renal or cardiovascular disease
  9. Medication use (prescribed and over the counter)
  10. Sexual history
- The nurse assesses for
  1. Symptoms of hypertension
     a. Headache
     b. Edema
     c. Nocturia

317

    d. Lethargy
    e. Nosebleeds
    f. Vision changes
2. Blood pressure readings in both arms
3. Blood pressure readings in supine and erect positions
4. Peripheral pulse rate, rhythm, and force
5. Bruits over the carotid and abdominal arteries
6. Psychosocial stressors

Planning and Implementation

NDx: KNOWLEDGE DEFICIT

- The nurse
  1. Advises the client to avoid adding table salt to food, cooking with salt, adding seasonings that contain sodium, and limit eating canned, frozen, and other processed foods
  2. Teaches the client to use salt substitutes
  3. Monitors the client's weight
  4. Advises the client to restrict alcohol intake
  5. Implements a regular exercise program
  6. Teaches or refers the client to stress management programs
  7. Administers drug therapy, as ordered
     a. *Diuretics*
        (1) *Thiazide* diuretics prevent sodium and water reabsorption in the kidney's distal tubules, while promoting potassium excretion (e.g., hydrochlorothiazide [HydroDIURIL]).
        (2) *Loop* diuretics depress sodium reabsorption in the ascending loop of Henle and promote potassium excretion (e.g., furosemide [Lasix]).
        (3) *Potassium-sparing* diuretics act on the kidney's distal tubule to inhibit reabsorption of sodium in exchange for potassium ions, thereby retaining potassium (e.g., spironolactone [Aldactone]).
     b. *Beta-blocking* agents lower blood pressure by blocking beta receptors in the heart and peripheral vessels, reducing cardiac rate and output (e.g., propranolol [Inderal]).
     c. *Calcium channel blockers* lower blood pressure by interfering with transmembrane influx of calcium ions, resulting in vasoconstriction (e.g., nifedipine [Procardia]).

d. *Angiotensin-converting-enzyme inhibitors* convert angiotensin I to angiotensin II (e.g., Captopril [Capoten]).

e. *Adrenergic inhibitors* stimulate alpha receptors in the brain to lower blood pressure, which inhibits the sympathetic nervous system vasomotor center and sympathetic outflow (e.g., clonidine hydrochloride [Catapres]).

f. *Vasodilators* relax vascular smooth muscle tone, reducing peripheral resistance (e.g., minoxidil [Loniten]).

NDx: Potential for Noncompliance

- The nurse
  1. Instructs the client that pharmacologic treatment for essential hypertension usually requires lifetime medication control
  2. Explains the side effects of hypertension
  3. Identifies potential reasons for noncompliance, such as the client's assumption that hypertension is under control when symptoms are gone, adverse side effects, and cost factors

Discharge Planning

- The nurse provides educational information for hypertension control
  1. Salt restriction
  2. Weight maintenance or reduction
  3. Stress reduction
  4. Alcohol restriction
  5. Exercise program

- The nurse gives oral and written information on medication therapy
  1. Indications
  2. Dosage
  3. Times of administration
  4. Side effects
  5. Drug interactions
  6. Importance of renewing prescriptions
  7. Reporting side effects to the physician

- The nurse instructs the client in the technique of blood pressure monitoring if equipment is available for use at home.
- The nurse teaches the client to record blood pressure readings in a log book/diary.

- The nurse emphasizes the importance of follow-up visits with the physician(s).

For more information on hypertension, see *Medical-Surgical Nursing: A Nursing Process Approach*, **pp. 2195–2205.**

Hyperthyroidism

OVERVIEW

- Hyperthyroidism occurs as a result of excessive thyroid hormone secretion.
- The most common cause is Graves' disease (toxic diffuse goiter).
- Thyrotoxicosis refers to the clinical signs and symptoms that appear when body tissues are stimulated by increased thyroid hormones.
- Hyperthyroidism produces a state of hypermetabolism with increased sympathetic nervous system activity; it may be transient or permanent.

EMERGENCY CARE

- Thyroid storm is a life-threatening event.
    1. The nurse assesses for signs and symptoms triggered by a major stressor such as trauma or infection
        a. Fever
        b. Tachycardia, systolic hypertension
        c. Gastrointestinal symptoms: nausea, vomiting, diarrhea
        d. Agitation, tremors, and anxiety
        e. Restlessness, confusion, psychosis
        f. Seizures

2. The nurse provides interventions, as ordered
   a. Maintains a patent airway and adequate ventilation
   b. Administers antithyroid drugs (propylthiouracil [PTU], methimazole [Tapazole])
   c. Administers sodium iodide solution
   d. Administers propranolol (Inderal) if life-threatening arrhythmias are present
   e. Administers glucocorticoids to prevent release of thyroid hormone
   f. Provides comfort measures
   g. Monitors vital signs frequently
   h. Administers nonsalicylate antipyretics to reduce fever

COLLABORATIVE MANAGEMENT

Assessment

- The nurse records the client's
   1. Age and sex
   2. Usual weight (the client may report weight loss and increased appetite)
   3. Heat intolerance, diaphoresis
   4. Palpitations, chest pain
   5. Changes in breathing pattern (dyspnea with or without excretion may occur)
   6. Changes in vision: blurring, double vision, eyes tiring easily
   7. Changes in ability to perform activities of daily living (ADL): fatigue, weakness, insomnia
   8. Changes in menses (amenorrhea, decreased menstrual flow)
   9. Increased libido
   10. Previous medical history
       a. Thyroid surgery
       b. Radiation therapy to the neck (some clients may be resistant to radiation therapy)
       c. Current medications
- The nurse assesses for
   1. Two types of ophthalmopathy
      a. Eyelid retraction and eyelid lag
      b. Globe lag
   2. Exophthalmos (seen in Graves' disease)
      a. Impaired vision
      b. Problems with focusing
      c. Possible corneal ulcerations and infections
   3. Mass or general enlargement of the thyroid gland

Planning and Implementation

NDx: POTENTIAL FOR DECREASED CARDIAC OUTPUT

Nonsurgical Management

- The nurse
    1. Monitors vital signs at least every 4 hours
    2. Instructs the client to report palpitations, dyspnea, vertigo, and/or chest pain immediately
    3. Provides a quiet, restful environment
    4. Administers drug therapy as ordered
        a. Antithyroid drugs
        b. Iodide preparations
        c. Lithium carbonate
        d. Beta-adrenergic blocking agents

- The nurse teaches the client about radioactive iodine therapy
    1. ^{131}I is taken orally (one dose usually on an outpatient basis).
    2. Radiation precautions generally are not required.
    3. Relief of symptoms usually does not occur for 6 to 8 weeks.
    4. Hypothyroidism may occur as a complication.

Surgical Management

- All (total thyroidectomy) or part of the thyroid gland (subtotal thyroidectomy) may be removed.
- The nurse provides preoperative care
    1. Provides routine preoperative care
    2. Administers antithyroid drugs and iodine preparations, as ordered, to place the client in a euthyroid state and to decrease the size and vascularity of the gland
    3. Monitors cardiac status
    4. Monitors nutritional status
- The nurse provides postoperative care
    1. Provides routine postoperative care
    2. Places sandbags or pillows to support the client's head and neck
    3. Maintains the client in a semi-Fowler's position
    4. Administers pain medication as ordered and the client needs it
    5. Provides humidification
    6. Turns, coughs, and deep breathes the client every 1 to 2 hours
    7. Inspects the neck dressing for drainage (a moderate amount of drainage is expected if a drain is left in place)
    8. Keeps equipment for a tracheostomy at the bedside

9. Keeps calcium gluconate or calcium chloride at the bedside
10. Administers fluids as ordered
11. Applies an ice bag to the neck to reduce swelling
12. Observes for complications
   a. Hemorrhage
   b. Respiratory distress
   c. Hypocalcemia and tetany, caused by parathyroid gland injury
      (1) Tingling around the mouth or of the toes and fingers
      (2) Muscular twitching
      (3) Positive Chvostek's and Trousseau's signs
      (4) Damage to laryngeal nerves

NDx: ALTERED NUTRITION: LESS THAN BODY REQUIREMENTS

- The nurse
   1. Obtains a dietary consultation
   2. Weighs the client daily
   3. Provides frequent high-calorie, high-protein, and high-carbohydrate meals

NDx: POTENTIAL FOR SENSORY/PERCEPTUAL ALTERATION (VISUAL)

- The infiltrative ophthalmopathy of Graves' disease is not influenced by medical therapy.
- The nurse
   1. For mild symptoms
      a. Elevates the head of the bed at night
      b. Applies eye lubricant/artificial tears
   2. For severe symptoms
      a. Tapes the eyes closed
      b. Administers short-term steroids as ordered
      c. Administers diuretics as ordered

Discharge Planning

- The nurse teaches the client
   1. Pertinent drug information
   2. The necessity to report any temperature elevation, sore throat, or symptoms of infection
   3. The signs and symptoms of hyperthyroidism or hypothyroidism

4. The importance of follow-up visits with the physician(s)

For more information on hyperthyroidism, see *Medical-Surgical Nursing: A Nursing Process Approach*, **pp. 1559–1569.**

Hyphema

- A hyphema is the presence of blood in the anterior chamber of the eye.
- If the hyphema is large, it may obstruct the pupil and reduce visual acuity.
- Treatment includes
  1. Bed rest in a semi-Fowler's position
  2. Restriction of eye movements for 3 to 5 days
  3. Restriction of reading and television
  4. Cycloplegic eyedrops, such as atropine
  5. An eye shield and patch
- Nursing management includes monitoring visual acuity and adherence to activity restrictions, providing alternative forms of sensory stimulation, and reporting any sudden increase in eye pain immediately.

For more information on hyphema, see *Medical-Surgical Nursing: A Nursing Process Approach*, **pp. 1064–1065.**

Hypocalcemia

OVERVIEW

• Hypocalcemia is defined as a serum calcium level of less than 8 mg/dL or 4.5 mEq/L.

• Relatively small fluctuations in serum calcium levels have profound effects on physiological function.

• Hypocalcemia is usually not a primary disease or condition but a result of other diseases or conditions.

• Common causes of hypocalcemia include

1. Inhibition of calcium absorption from the gastrointestinal (GI) tract
   a. Inadequate oral intake of calcium
   b. Lactose intolerance
   c. Malabsorption syndromes
      (1) Celiac sprue
      (2) Crohn's disease
   d. Inadequate intake of vitamin D

2. Increased calcium excretion
   a. Renal failure
   b. Diarrhea
   c. Steatorrhea
   d. Wound drainage (especially gastrointestinal)

3. Conditions that decrease the ionized fraction of calcium
   a. Alkalosis
   b. Calcium chelators or binders
      (1) Citrate
      (2) Mithramycin
      (3) Penicillamine (Cupramine)
      (4) Cellulose sodium phosphate (Calcibind)
   c. Acute pancreatitis
   d. Hyperphosphatemia
   e. Immobility

4. Endocrine disturbances
   a. Removal or destruction of the parathyroid glands
      (1) Thyroidectomy
      (2) Radiation to the thyroid
      (3) Strangulation
      (4) Neck injuries

H

COLLABORATIVE MANAGEMENT

Assessment

- The nurse records the client's
  1. Age (incidence tends to increase with age)
  2. Sex (more common in females)
  3. Race (50% to 70% of American blacks have some degree of lactose intolerance)
  4. Activity level
  5. Diet history, including the use of a calcium supplement
  6. History of frequent, painful muscle spasms (charley horses) in the calf of the leg during periods of inactivity or sleep
  7. History of orthopedic surgery or bone healing
- The nurse assesses for
  1. Neuromuscular changes (the system most affected)
     a. Anxiety, irritability, psychosis
     b. Paresthesia followed by numbness
     c. Irritable skeletal muscles—twitches, cramps, tetany, seizures
     d. Hyperactive deep-tendon reflexes
     e. Positive Trousseau's sign
        (1) Testing is accomplished by placing a blood pressure cuff around the upper arm, inflating the cuff to greater than systolic pressure, and keeping it there for 1 to 4 minutes.
        (2) The hand and fingers spasm in palmar flexion.
        (3) Spasms continue for 20 to 30 seconds after the cuff has been released.
     f. Positive Chvostek's sign (tapping on the face just below and anterior to the ear—over the facial nerve—triggers facial twitching that includes one side of the mouth, nose, and cheek)
  2. GI changes
     a. Increased gastric motility
     b. Hyperactive bowel sounds
     c. Abdominal cramping
     d. Diarrhea
  3. Cardiovascular changes
     a. Increased heart rate
     b. Decreased myocardial contractility
     c. Diminished peripheral pulses
     d. Hypotension

e. Electrocardiogram abnormalities
   (1) Prolonged ST interval
   (2) Prolonged QT interval
4. Respiratory changes
   a. Not affected directly
   b. Respiratory failure or arrest, which can occur as a result of decreased respiratory movement secondary to muscle tetany or seizure activity
5. Psychosocial changes
   a. Subtle behavior changes
   b. Increasing sensitivity to extraneous environmental noise and activity
   c. Irrational thinking
   d. Frank psychosis

Planning and Implementation

NDx: ALTERED NUTRITION: LESS THAN BODY REQUIREMENTS OF CALCIUM

H

- The nurse administers drug therapy, as ordered
  1. Oral supplements of calcium carbonate, calcium gluconate, and calcium lactate used for mild hypocalcemia (administer 30 minutes before meals)
  2. Parenteral calcium for severe hypocalcemia
     a. Give a slow intravenous (IV) drip, unless life threatening, of calcium chloride or calcium gluconate.
     b. Monitor cardiovascular status; ideally the client should be on a cardiac monitor.
     c. Assess Chvostek's and Trousseau's signs every 15 minutes.
     d. Monitor frequent serum calcium levels (every hour).
     e. Assess the infusion site every 15 minutes.
        (1) Infiltration can cause tissue hypoxia and necrosis.
        (2) Poor blood return, pain at infusion site, edema, or any other indication of infiltration warrants stopping the infusion and changing the IV site.
        (3) Vitamin D enhances the intestinal absorption of calcium.
        (4) Aluminum hydroxide, magnesium chloride, and/or magnesium sulfate increases calcium levels.
- The nurse provides diet therapy, as ordered
  1. High-calcium, low-phosphorus diet for mild cases

and those with chronic pathologic conditions that put them at risk for hypocalcemia
2. Foods high in calcium

    a. Low-fat yogurt
    b. Skim and whole milk
    c. Raw collard greens
    d. Rhubarb
    e. Cheddar and American cheese
    f. Tofu
    g. Broccoli

3. Small, frequent meals for clients who are weak or fatigued
4. Adequate vitamin D intake for dietary calcium to be beneficial

    a. Increased client exposure to sunlight unless contraindicated
    b. Other sources of vitamin D
        (1) Fortified milk
        (2) Liver
        (3) Eggs
        (4) Fatty fish
        (5) Butterfat

NDx: DIARRHEA

- The nurse administers medications to decrease peristalsis and intestinal motility
    1. Exercises caution regarding the amount and frequency of administration of these drugs
    2. Recognizes that overmedication can result in constipation or paralytic ileus

NDx: POTENTIAL FOR INJURY

- The nurse
    1. Administers drugs to decrease the degree of nerve and muscle responsiveness and overstimulation, as ordered

        a. Methocarbamol (Robaxin, Skelaxin, Delaxin)
        b. Orphenadrine (Banflex, Flexoject, Myolin)
        c. Carisoprodol (Soma, Rela)
        d. Diazepam (Valium, Rival, E-Pam)
        e. Magnesium sulfate

    2. Minimizes environmental stimuli
    3. Minimizes activity (stimulation can increase muscular twitching, cramps, and tetany)
    4. Restricts the client to bed rest if Chvostek's or Trousseau's sign is positive and provides total care
    5. Restricts visitors
    6. Implements seizure precautions

7. Keeps emergency equipment readily available in anticipation of complications
   a. Oxygen and suctioning equipment
   b. Tracheostomy tray
   c. Ambu bag

Discharge Planning

- The nurse
  1. Reviews diet therapy with the client/family
     a. Teaches the client to read labels carefully to determine the electrolyte content of prepared foods and medications
     b. Obtains a dietary consultation for assistance in providing information on the planning and preparation of palatable meals whenever a specific electrolyte restriction is necessary
     c. Teaches the client to adhere to specific food or fluid restriction
  2. Reviews signs and symptoms of the specific imbalance for which the client is at risk, as well as what specific information should be reported immediately to the primary health care provider
  3. Provides drug information, as needed

For more information on hypocalcemia, see *Medical-Surgical Nursing: A Nursing Process Approach,* **pp. 294–301.**

Hypoglycemia

- Hypoglycemia is called by a variety of names, including insulin reaction, insulin shock, and low blood sugar.
- Clinical manifestations include
  1. Adrenergic manifestations
     a. Sweating

b. Palpitations
   c. Pallor
   d. Irritability
   e. Angina
   f. Anxiety
   g. Tremulousness
   h. Hunger
   i. Piloerection

2. Neuroglycopenic manifestations

   a. Blurred vision
   b. Diplopia
   c. Headache
   d. Slurred speech
   e. Weakness
   f. Inability to make decisions
   g. Agitation
   h. Seizures
   i. Unconsciousness
   j. Confusion

- Symptoms occur if the blood glucose level falls below normal levels (a plasma glucose level less than 60 mg/dL) or rapidly changes from one level to another.
- Treatment depends on the level of hypoglycemia
   1. Glucose levels of 40 to 60 mg/dL respond to ingestion of food such as milk or crackers.
   2. Glucose levels of 20 to 40 mg/dL respond to simple sugar, such as 15 g of honey, table sugar, or juice, followed by a well-balanced meal.
   3. A 50% dextrose solution by intravenous push is the treatment of choice for the client in seizure or the unconscious person with hypoglycemia.
   4. Glucagon is the drug of choice at home or other nonhospital setting.

For more information on hypoglycemia, see *Medical-Surgical Nursing: A Nursing Process Approach*, **pp. 1596–1597.**

Hypokalemia

OVERVIEW

- Hypokalemia is defined as a serum potassium ion (K^+) level below 3.5 mEq/L.
- Hypokalemia is potentially life threatening because the symptoms affect virtually every body system.
- Common causes include
    1. Inappropriate or excessive use of diuretics, digitalis, or corticosteroids
    2. Increased secretion of aldosterone
    3. Diarrhea, vomiting
    4. Wound drainage, excessive drainage from ostomies
    5. Prolonged nasogastric suction
    6. Heat-induced excessive diaphoresis
    7. Inadequate potassium intake such as occurs when the client has nothing by mouth for several days
    8. Cushing's syndrome
    9. Metabolic acidosis
    10. Presence of excess amounts of insulin in the blood, such as during hyperalimentation infusions and/or during treatment of uncontrolled diabetes

COLLABORATIVE MANAGEMENT

Assessment

- The nurse records the client's
    1. Age
    2. Medication use (prescribed and/or over the counter)
    3. Current medical history, presence of acute and/or chronic diseases
    4. Dietary history
- The nurse assesses for
    1. Cardiovascular changes
        a. Variable pulse rate, more often rapid
        b. Pulse thready and weak
        c. Peripheral pulses difficult to palpate
        d. Postural hypotension
        e. Electrocardiogram abnormalities
            (1) ST depression
            (2) Inverted T wave
            (3) Prominent U wave
            (4) Heart block

H

2. Respiratory changes
    a. Shallow, ineffective respirations
    b. Diminished breath sounds
3. Neuromuscular changes
    a. Anxiety, lethargy, confusion, coma
    b. Loss of tactile discrimination
    c. General skeletal muscle weakness
    d. Deep-tendon hyporeflexia
    e. Eventual flaccid paralysis
4. Gastrointestinal changes
    a. Decreased motility
    b. Hypoactive to absent bowel sounds
    c. Nausea, vomiting
    d. Abdominal distention
    e. Paralytic ileus
    f. Constipation
5. Renal changes
    a. Decreased ability to concentrate urine
    b. Polyuria
    c. Decreased specific gravity

Planning and Implementation
NDx: POTENTIAL FOR INJURY

- The nurse administers drug therapy, as ordered
    1. Parenteral potassium is a tissue irritant and may irritate the veins, causing a chemical phlebitis. It must be diluted well and administered slowly; rapid increases of serum potassium level depress cardiac muscle contractility and can lead to serious arrhythmias and cardiac arrest.
    2. Oral potassium has a strong, unpleasant taste. It must not be given on an empty stomach as it may cause nausea and vomiting.
    3. Diuretics that increase renal excretion of potassium are common causes of hypokalemia; potassium-sparing diuretics may be appropriate, including Spironolactone (Aldactone), Triamterene (Dyrenium), and Amiloride (Midamor).
- The nurse
    1. Provides foods high in potassium, including avocados, bananas, cantaloupe, raisins, and whole-wheat bread
    2. Instructs the client to avoid long cooking of vegetables and fruits in water
    3. Provides frequent rest periods for the client prone to skeletal muscle weakness
    4. Maintains a hazard-free environment

5. Assists the client with ambulation
6. Keeps the side rails up

NDx: CONSTIPATION
- The nurse
    1. Administers laxatives that add bulk or fiber to stimulate peristalsis
    2. Administers drugs such as metoclopramide (Reglan, Maxeran), as ordered
    3. Provides a high-fiber diet and encourages fluids
    4. Encourages physical activity and exercise to promote gastric motility

Discharge Planning
- The nurse
    1. Obtains a dietary consultation to help the client select personal food preferences high in essential nutrients
    2. Provides drug information, as needed
    3. Teaches early recognition of the signs and symptoms of hypokalemia
        a. Slow or irregular heartbeat
        b. Numbness or tingling sensations in the hands and feet, cramping of large leg muscles
        c. Sensations of weakness
        d. Difficulty in maintaining mental concentration, slight confusion or forgetfulness
        e. Constipation, abdominal distention, nausea

For more information on hypokalemia, see *Medical-Surgical Nursing: A Nursing Process Approach,* **pp. 268–274.**

Hypomagnesemia

- Hypomagnesemia exists when the serum magnesium ion level is less than 1.5 mEq/L.
- Common causes include
    1. Malnutrition or starvation

2. Prolonged nasogastric suctioning
3. Diarrhea or steatorrhea
4. Loss or destruction of intestinal mucosa
5. Alcoholism, especially when accompanied by liver disease
6. Increased renal excretion of magnesium
   a. Certain drugs
      (1) Loop diuretics, such as furosemide (Lasix, Uritol)
      (2) Osmotic diuretics, such as mannitol and urea
      (3) Aminoglycosides, such as kanamycin (Kantrex), gentamicin (Garamycin), and tobramycin (Nebcin)
      (4) Some neoplastic agents, such as cisplatin (Platinol)
   b. Hypoparathyroidism
   c. Primary hyperaldosteronism
- Clinical manifestations include
  1. Hyperactive deep-tendon reflexes
  2. Painful paresthesia
  3. Tetanic muscle contractions
  4. Positive Chvostek's and Trousseau's signs
  5. Tetany and seizures
  6. Depression
  7. Frank psychosis
  8. Confusion
- Management of hypomagnesemia includes
  1. Stopping drugs that contribute to the development of hypomagnesemia
  2. Intravenous infusion of magnesium sulfate
  3. Increasing the client's intake of foods high in magnesium, such as meats, nuts, legumes, fish, and vegetables

For more information on hypomagnesemia, see *Medical-Surgical Nursing: A Nursing Process Approach,* **pp. 312–313.**

Hyponatremia

OVERVIEW

- Hyponatremia is defined as a serum sodium level of less than 136 mEq/L.
- The condition is one of the most common electrolyte imbalances that occurs among hospitalized clients.
- Common causes include
  1. Increased sodium excretion
     a. Excessive diaphoresis
     b. Diuretics
     c. Wound drainage (especially gastrointestinal)
     d. Decreased secretion of aldosterone
     e. Hyperlipidemia
     f. Renal disease
  2. Inadequate sodium intake
     a. Nothing by mouth (NPO)
     b. Low-salt diet
  3. Dilution of serum sodium
     a. Excessive ingestion of hypotonic fluids
     b. Psychogenic polydipsia
     c. Freshwater drowning
     d. Renal failure (nephrotic syndrome)
     e. Irrigation with hypotonic fluids
     f. Syndrome of inappropriate antidiuretic hormone (SIADH)
     g. Hyperglycemia
     h. Congestive heart failure

COLLABORATIVE MANAGEMENT

Assessment

- The nurse records the client's
  1. Age (young children and elderly are more prone to electrolyte imbalance)
  2. Height and weight
  3. Past medical and surgical history
  4. Recent history of vomiting, diarrhea, fever, and/or wound drainage
  5. Urinary output, including frequency and amount of voiding
  6. Types of fluids and actual fluid intake in general and specifically during the last 24 hours
  7. Use of over-the-counter and prescribed medications, especially diuretics, morphine, and chemotherapeutic agents

H

8. Diet history
9. Amount of strenuous physical activity, including environmental temperature and humidity
- The nurse assesses for
  1. Neuromuscular changes
     a. Generalized skeletal muscle weakness
     b. Diminished deep-tendon reflexes
     c. Personality changes
     d. Headache
     e. Seizures
  2. Gastrointestinal changes
     a. Increased motility
     b. Nausea
     c. Hyperactive bowel sounds
     d. Diarrhea
     e. Abdominal cramping
  3. Cardiovascular changes
     a. Normovolemic
        (1) Rapid pulse rate
        (2) Normal blood pressure
     b. Hypovolemic
        (1) Rapid pulse rate
        (2) Pulse thready and weak
        (3) Hypotensive
        (4) Central venous pressure normal or low
        (5) Flat neck veins
  4. Respiratory changes (secondary to the influence of low serum sodium on cerebral function and circulatory status); late manifestations related to
     a. Skeletal muscle weakness
     b. Shallow, ineffective respiratory movements
     c. Hypervolemia
     d. Pulmonary edema
        (1) Rapid, shallow respirations
        (2) Moist rales
  5. Renal changes
     a. Increased urinary output
     b. Decreased specific gravity of urine

Planning and Implementation
NDx: ALTERED THOUGHT PROCESSES
- The nurse performs neurologic checks every 4 hours
  1. Level of consciousness
  2. Orientation

3. Recent and past memory
4. Ability to concentrate
5. Cognitive function
6. Muscle strength and tone

- The nurse administers drug therapy, as ordered

    1. Isotonic (0.9%) or hypertonic (3% to 5%) intravenous solutions (rate of infusion should be regulated by the rate of the sodium or fluid loss)
    2. Diuretics, primarily hydrouretic (water excreting), when hyponatremia is accompanied by fluid excess

        a. Osmotic diuretics such as mannitol
        b. Urea or dexamethasone when cerebral edema is profound

    3. Hyponatremia as a result of inappropriate or excessive secretion of antidiuretic hormone (ADH) may be treated with agents such as demeclocycline or lithium that antagonize ADH or agents that block ADH receptors

        a. Antidotes to these agents must be kept on hand during the time the client is receiving them.
        b. The antidote for demeclocycline is amiloride; for lithium, it is acetazolamide.

- The underlying pathology is treated when hyponatremia is not a *direct* disturbance of sodium balance.
- The nurse monitors and maintains diet therapy, as needed

    1. Increases oral sodium and restricts oral intake of fluids to some extent, in consultation with the dietitian; common food sources of sodium are table salt, soy sauce, cured pork, cottage cheese, and American cheese
    2. Accurately measures intake and output
    3. Reinforces the rationale for fluid restriction

- Diet therapy has little effect on severe hyponatremia.
- The nurse maintains a safe environment

    1. Assists the client to process information correctly
    2. Orients the client to time and place at every interaction
    3. Places large clocks and calendars where the client can see them
    4. Is sure that the client wears glasses and hearing aids, if needed, when awake
    5. Reduces extraneous noise and environmental stimuli
    6. Ambulates the client with assistance

7. Keeps the side rails up and the bed in a low position at all times when the client is in bed

• Based on assessment data and facility policy, restraints are used as needed if all other protective measures fail; seizure precautions are implemented.

NDx: PAIN (HEADACHE)

• Headache may be caused by increased intracranial pressure (ICP).

• Drug therapy is aimed at decreasing the frequency and intensity of the Valsalva maneuver, which increases ICP

1. Stool softeners and laxatives
2. Antihistamine or decongestant medications (some of these medications may further increase ICP; the nurse checks actions and side effects before administering)

• The nurse

1. Administers analgesics, as ordered (morphine derivatives should not be used)
2. Positions the client to decrease ICP

    a. Elevates the head of the bed 15 to 30 degrees
    b. Makes sure that venous return from the head is not obstructed by tight collars, dressings on the neck, or poor positioning
    c. Cautions the client to avoid bending, lifting, or straining

3. Reduces environmental stimuli
4. Plans the client's schedule to allow for frequent periods of rest; reschedules activities that are not of an immediate priority

Discharge Planning

• The nurse reviews diet therapy with the client/family

1. Has the client determine the electrolyte content of prepared foods and medications by carefully reading labels
2. Obtains a dietary consultation for assistance in providing information on the planning and preparation of palatable meals whenever a specific electrolyte restriction is necessary
3. Teaches the client to adhere to specific food or fluid restrictions

• The nurse reviews signs and symptoms of the specific imbalance for which the client is at risk, as well as what specific information should be reported immediately to the primary health care provider.

- The nurse provides drug information, as needed.

For more information on hyponatremia, see *Medical-Surgical Nursing: A Nursing Process Approach,* **pp. 279–287.**

Hypophosphatemia

- Hypophosphatemia is a serum phosphate level of less than 2.5 mg/dL.
- Body functions are not significantly impaired as a result of rapid, wide fluctuations in serum levels.
- Alterations in function are more obvious when hypophosphatemia is chronic.
- Common causes include
  1. Malnutrition or starvation
  2. Ingestion of large amounts of antacids containing aluminum hydroxide (Alternagel, Amphojel) and/or magnesium (Bisodol, milk of magnesia)
  3. Diarrhea
  4. Excessive use of laxatives
  5. Loss or destruction of intestinal tissue
  6. Osmotic diuresis
  7. Hyperglycemia
  8. Rapid administration of total parenteral nutrition and/or hyperalimentation fluids
  9. Excessive carbohydrate ingestion
- Clinical manifestations do not appear until the decrease in serum phosphate levels is severe or prolonged and include
  1. Decreased stroke volume
  2. Decreased cardiac output
  3. Peripheral pulses slow, difficult to find, and easy to obliterate
  4. Weak, ineffective myocardial contractions
  5. Generalized skeletal muscle weakness

6. Ineffective respiratory movements, possibly leading to respiratory failure if skeletal muscle weakness is present
7. Infection
8. Prolonged bleeding time in response to relatively slight trauma or tissue injury
9. Easy bruising
10. Increased irritability
11. Seizure activity
12. Coma
13. Decreased bone density, alterations in bone shape, fractures
14. Renal calculi

- Treatment of hypophosphatemia includes
  1. Stopping all drugs such as antacids, osmotic diuretics, and calcium supplements
  2. Administering oral supplements of phosphates and vitamin D, as ordered
  3. Administering parenteral phosphate only when the serum phosphate level is less than 1 mg/dL and the client is experiencing serious signs and symptoms of hypophosphatemia
  4. Encouraging the clients to eat foods high in phosphorus, such as beef, pork, beans, and other legumes

For more information on hypophosphatemia, see *Medical-Surgical Nursing: A Nursing Process Approach,* **pp. 309–311.**

Hypopituitarism

OVERVIEW

- Hypopituitarism is a deficiency of one or more of the anterior pituitary hormones.
- The clinical features and symptoms vary depending on the severity of the disease and the number of deficient hormones.

COLLABORATIVE MANAGEMENT
Assessment
- The nurse records the client's
  1. Loss of secondary sex characteristics
     a. Adult males may report
        (1) Loss of facial and body hair
        (2) Episodes of impotence
        (3) Decreased libido
     b. Adult females may report
        (1) Secondary amenorrhea
        (2) Difficulty becoming pregnant
        (3) Painful intercourse because of decreased vaginal secretions
        (4) Decreased libido
  2. History and/or family history of
     a. Chronic renal failure
     b. Pancreatic, liver, and/or bone disease
     c. Diabetes mellitus
     d. Hypothyroidism
     e. Administration of gonadal hormones
     f. Nutritional deficits, such as an inadequate supply of protein, carbohydrates, fats, vitamin D, calcium, and/or phosphorus
     g. Gastrointestinal malabsorption syndromes
     h. Failure to thrive in infancy and childhood
- The nurse assesses for
  1. Neurologic manifestations
     a. Changes in visual acuity and peripheral vision
     b. Bilateral temporal headaches
     c. Diplopia and ocular muscle paralysis secondary to cranial nerve III, IV, and VI dysfunction
  2. Decrease or loss of facial and/or body hair
  3. Decrease in muscle mass and tone
  4. Testicular atrophy in males
  5. Loss or decreased axillary and pubic hair and atrophy of the breasts in females
  6. Changes in body image and self-worth secondary to changes in physical appearance

Planning and Implementation
NDx: BODY IMAGE DISTURBANCE
- The nurse
  1. Encourages the client to verbalize feelings of concern and/or anxiety about body changes
  2. Stresses the role of hormonal replacement, which usually corrects the loss of secondary sex

characteristics (isolated growth hormone [GH] deficiency may be treated with exogenous GH)

3. Respects the client with GH deficiency and resultant short stature in a manner appropriate for the client's age
4. Teaches the side effects of hormonal replacement
   a. Insulin resistance (for hyperglycemia and glycosuria)
   b. Headache
   c. Localized muscle pain
   d. Weakness
   e. Mild, transient edema
   f. Hypothyroidism (ensure that the client has periodic thyroid function tests)

NDx: SEXUAL DYSFUNCTION

- The nurse
  1. Instructs the client about hormone replacement therapy, which usually corrects the physiologic problems related to sexual activity
  2. Administers androgens (testosterone) intramuscularly for males, as ordered; the nurse
     a. Instructs the client in self-administration
     b. Begins dosage at 50 mg, which is gradually increased to 200 mg, based on age, as ordered
     c. Teaches the client that injections are usually required every 4 to 6 weeks depending on clinical evaluation and recurrence of symptoms
     d. Teaches the side effects of testosterone, which include gynecomastia, baldness, and prostatic hypertrophy
     e. Alerts the client that the maximal effects of treatment include
        (1) Increase in penis size, libido, and muscle mass
        (2) Increased growth of facial, pubic, and axillary hair
        (3) Deepened voice
        (4) Increased bone size and strength
        (5) Increased self-esteem and improved body image
  3. Administers human chorionic gonadotrophin (hCG) therapy for achieving fertility, as ordered
  4. Administers hormone replacement with a combination of estrogen and progesterone administered in a cyclic manner to females, as ordered, and teaches the client about adverse effects of drug therapy, such as hypertension and thrombophlebitis.

- The nurse
  1. Assists the client to identify sources of support
  2. Helps the client identify his or her particular strengths
  3. Encourages the use of support groups, as needed
  4. Encourages psychological counseling, as needed

Discharge Planning

- The client with GH deficiency may need home modifications as a result of short stature.
- The nurse ensures that the client can correctly use all adaptive-assistive devices ordered for home use.
- The nurse teaches the client/family
  1. To take all medication in the correct dosage, at the right time, and by the correct route
  2. To use the proper technique for intramuscular injection
  3. To rotate injection sites correctly
  4. To know what to do if a dose is missed or if complications or side effects occur
- The nurse
  1. Stresses that changes in secondary sex characteristics occur gradually
  2. Emphasizes the importance of follow-up visits with the physician

For more information on hypopituitarism, see *Medical-Surgical Nursing: A Nursing Process Approach,* **pp. 1529–1533.**

Hypothyroidism

OVERVIEW

- Hypothyroidism results from inadequate peripheral tissue thyroid hormone levels.
- The majority of cases occur as a result of thyroid surgery and radioactive iodine treatment of thyrotoxicosis.

- *Primary* hypothyroidism is a result of pathological changes in the thyroid gland itself.
- *Secondary* hypothyroidism may result from inadequate pituitary production of thyroid stimulating hormone.
- Goiter is an enlargement of the thyroid gland due to inadequate production of thyroid hormone.
- Myxedema coma is a rare but serious presentation of hypothyroidism, manifested by coma, hypotension, hyponatremia, respiratory failure, and hypoglycemia.

COLLABORATIVE MANAGEMENT

Assessment

- The nurse records the client's
  1. Change in sleep habits (usually significantly increased)
  2. Generalized weakness, anorexia, muscle aches, paresthesia, and cold intolerance
  3. Change in bowel pattern (usually constipation)
  4. Past medical history, with special attention to use of drugs such as lithium, aminoglutethimide, sodium or potassium perchlorate, thiocyanates, or cobalt
- The nurse assesses for
  1. Integumentary changes
     a. Cool, pale or yellowish, dry, coarse, scaly skin
     b. Thick, brittle nails
     c. Decreased hair growth, loss of eyebrow hair
  2. Pulmonary changes
     a. Hypoventilation
     b. Pleural effusion
  3. Cardiovascular changes
     a. Bradycardia
     b. Other dysrhythmias
     c. Enlarged heart
     d. Decreased exercise or activity tolerance
  4. Gastrointestinal changes
     a. Anorexia
     b. Constipation
     c. Abdominal distension
  5. Neurologic changes
     a. Slowing of intellectual functions
     b. Slowness or slurring of speech
     c. Impaired memory
     d. Inattentiveness

    e. Lethargy
    f. Confusion
    g. Paresthesia
    h. Decreased deep-tendon reflexes
6. Physiologic/emotional changes
    a. Apathy
    b. Agitation
    c. Depression
    d. Paranoia
7. Metabolic changes
    a. Decreased basal metabolic rate
    b. Decreased body temperature
    c. Cold intolerance
8. Reproductive changes
    a. Females: changes in menses, infertility, decreased libido
    b. Males: decreased libido, impotence
9. Other changes
    a. Periorbital edema
    b. Facial puffiness
    c. Nonpitting edema of the hands and feet
    d. Goiter
    e. Anemia
    f. Easy bruising

Planning and Implementation

NDx: Decreased Cardiac Output

- Clients with chronic hypothyroidism may have cardiovascular disease.
- The nurse
  1. Monitors blood pressure, heart rate, and rhythm
  2. Observes closely for signs of hemodynamic compromise
     a. Hypotension
     b. Decreasing urinary output
     c. Mental status changes
- The nurse teaches the client about lifelong replacement of thyroid hormone
  1. Administers synthetic hormone preparations: levothyroxine sodium (Synthroid, Levoid, Levothroid)
  2. Observes closely for chest pain and dyspnea when initiating therapy
  3. Monitors for signs and symptoms of hyperthyroidism that can occur during replacement therapy

NDx: INEFFECTIVE BREATHING PATTERN

- The nurse
    1. Observes and records the rate and depth of respirations
    2. Auscultates lungs and notes abnormalities, such as decreased breath sounds
    3. Recognizes that severe respiratory distress may be associated with myxedema coma
    4. Avoids sedating the client as it may contribute to respiratory distress; if sedation must be used, the usual dosage is decreased because hypothyroidism increases sensitivity to these drugs

NDx: ALTERED THOUGHT PROCESSES

- The nurse
    1. Notes the presence and severity of symptoms, such as lethargy, memory deficit, inattentiveness, and mental slowness
    2. Notes the resolution of symptoms with thyroid hormone replacement therapy

Discharge Planning

- The nurse teaches the client
    1. About the possible need for extra heat or clothing owing to cold intolerance if the symptoms have not cleared before discharge
    2. Drug information
        a. Taking all medication in the correct dosage, at the right time, and by the right route
        b. What to do if a dose is missed or if complications or side effects occur
        c. Contraindications of over-the-counter medications that may interact with the thyroid medication
        d. Importance of wearing a Medic Alert bracelet or necklace because many thyroid medications potentiate and interact with many other drugs.
    3. Diet information to prevent constipation
    4. Importance of follow-up visits with the physician(s)

For more information on hypothyroidism, see *Medical-Surgical Nursing: A Nursing Process Approach*, **pp. 1568–1574.**

Immunodeficiencies

- B cell, or antibody-mediated, immunity normally protects the host from a variety of bacterial infections and some viral infections through the production of specific antibodies; lack of this protection leads to recurrent infections with encapsulated bacteria and/or a history of treatment failure.

- In *antibody-mediated immunodeficiency*, laboratory studies reveal hypogammaglobulinemia—either a selective deficiency or a panhypogammaglobulinemia.

- Types of antibody-mediated immunodeficiency include

  1. Bruton's, or X-linked, agammaglobulinemia
     a. Congenital antibody-mediated immunodeficiency
     b. Overall good prognosis if hormonal replacement begins early in life, except for clients who develop polio, chronic echovirus infection, or a lymphoreticular malignancy
     c. Treatment with intravenous (IV) or intramuscular (IM) immune serum globulin

  2. Common variable immunodeficiency, or acquired hypogammaglobulinemia
     a. Appears in adolescents or young adults
     b. Is characterized by recurrent infections with pyogenic bacteria
     c. Complications include giardiasis, bronchiectasis, gastric carcinoma, lymphoreticular malignancy, and cholelithiasis
     d. Treated by the regular administration of IV or IM immune serum globulin and the use of antibiotics intermittently or chronically

  3. Immunoglobulin A (IgA) deficiency
     a. May be asymptomatic or have chronic recurrent respiratory tract infections, atopic diseases, and/or collagen-vascular diseases; may see malabsorption syndrome
     b. Treatment limited to appropriate and vigorous treatment of infection

- In *cell-mediated immunodeficiencies*, the client lacks cell-mediated immunity with a partial or absolute defect in T cell function and clinically presents with recurrent infections with opportunistic fungi, viruses, and parasites. There is a high incidence of malignancy, growth retardation, wasting, and diarrhea. Treatment is aimed at reconstituting or enhancing T cell immunity. The life span for the client is short.

- *Combined immunodeficiencies* are those states in which both antibody-mediated and cell-mediated immunity are compromised or deficient. Treatment includes

    1. Early identification and prompt treatment of infection
    2. Minimizing the client's exposure to infected persons or contaminated objects
    3. Removing Foley catheters, IV lines, and other invasive tubes as soon as possible.
    4. Irradiation of blood and blood products
    5. Avoidance of live, attenuated vaccines

- Client/family education includes

    1. Signs and symptoms of infection
    2. Diagnostic procedures, pre- and postcare
    3. Medications
    4. General health and hygiene measures
    5. Referral to genetic counseling if appropriate

- *Iatrogenic* immunodeficiency is an immunodeficiency or immunosuppressive state induced in the client by medical therapies or procedures

    1. Drug induced
    a. Cytotoxic drugs
    b. Corticosteroids
    c. Cyclosporine
    2. Radiation induced

For more information on these immunodeficiencies, see *Medical-Surgical Nursing: A Nursing Process Approach,* **pp. 647–650.**

Impotence

OVERVIEW

- Impotence is the inability to achieve or maintain an erection firm enough for sexual intercourse 25% of the time.
- Causes of psychogenic impotence include anxiety, fatigue, boredom, depression, guilt, and pressure to perform sexually.
- Causes of physiologic impotence include injury, disease, hormonal imbalance, or surgery.
- Impotence occurs in 50% to 60% of diabetic men.

COLLABORATIVE MANAGEMENT

- Assessment of sexual and medical history includes
  1. Psychologic impotence
     a. Acute onset
     b. Selectivity
     c. Periodicity
     d. Nocturnal erections and emissions
     e. Ability to masturbate
     f. Ability to have an erection and function sexually under certain circumstances
     g. Retention of testicular sensitivity
  2. Physiologic impotence
     a. Gradual loss of erectile dysfunction in all sexual circumstances
     b. Lack of nocturnal erections and emissions
     c. Some degree of erectile dysfunction in all sexual circumstances
  3. Medical history
     a. Family history of impotence
     b. Diabetes
     c. Hypertension
     d. Thyroid or adrenal disorders
     e. Stroke
     f. Arteriosclerosis
     g. Multiple sclerosis
     h. Amyotrophic lateral sclerosis
     i. Brain or spinal cord injury
     j. Surgical intervention of the prostate, bladder, or rectum
     k. Medications, including narcotics, barbiturates, tranquilizers, monoamine oxidase inhibitors,

and other antidepressants, estrogens, and antihistamines
    l. Alcohol, tobacco, and illicit drugs
- Nonsurgical management includes
    1. Psychosocial intervention
    2. Change or adjustment in medication
    3. Control of underlying disease
- Surgical interventions include
    1. Arterial bypass procedure to improve blood flow to the penis
    2. Penile prosthesis insertion if there is irreversible physiologic impotence demonstrated by history and diagnostic testing, a strong desire for sexual satisfaction, the presence of some penile sensation, and the absence of prostatic or genitourinary problems
- See Sexuality.

For more information on impotence, see *Medical-Surgical Nursing: A Nursing Process Approach*, **pp. 1754–1756.**

Incontinence, Urinary

OVERVIEW

- Urinary incontinence results when the bladder fails to contract at the appropriate time or when it contracts inappropriately.
- Types of urinary incontinence include
    1. *Stress incontinence*, caused by weakness of the urethra and/or surrounding muscles and tissues or alteration in the urethrovesical angle
    2. *Urge incontinence*, caused by a hypertonic bladder with stimulation of the detrusor muscle
    3. *Overflow incontinence*, which occurs when the bladder pressure exceeds urethral resistance
    4. *Functional incontinence*, caused by physical and environmental factors and psychologic causes such as depression and regression

5. *Total incontinence*, caused by neurologic disorders
- *Reversible* causes are correctable and include
  1. Symptomatic infections
  2. Fecal impaction
  3. Medications such as sedatives, anticholinergics, diuretics, and adrenergic agents
  4. Acute confusion
  5. Vaginal and urethral atrophy
  6. Prostatic enlargement
  7. Maladaptive emotional responses
- *Nonreversible organic* causes are permanent but may be improved with treatment and include
  1. Congenital defects
  2. Traumatic or surgical effects
  3. Neurogenic bladder
  4. Psychologic causes
- Incontinence is often associated with the aging process; contributing factors include
  1. Decreased mobility from disease
  2. Neurologic dysfunction
  3. Musculoskeletal degeneration
  4. Multiple medications
  5. Depression

COLLABORATIVE MANAGEMENT

Assessment

- The nurse records the client's
  1. Onset and circumstances surrounding urinary incontinence
  2. Sex and age
  3. Changes in voiding patterns
  4. Incontinence occurrences (during sleep or intermittently throughout the day)
  5. Contributing factors
  6. Perceptions of warning signals
  7. History of pregnancies or surgical procedures
  8. Menstrual pattern versus menopause
  9. Medication history
  10. Psychologic stressors
  11. Previous and concurrent health problems
- The nurse assesses for
  1. Bladder distention
  2. Bladder discomfort
  3. Apparent urethral or uterine prolapse or cystocele by inspecting external genitalia
  4. Secretions from genitourinary orifices
  5. Tactile sensation and rectal sphincter contraction during digital rectal examination

6. Fecal impaction
7. Prostatic enlargement

Planning and Implementation

NDx: STRESS INCONTINENCE
Nonsurgical Management

- The nurse
  1. Administers medications, as ordered, to increase the resistance of the urethra, such as ephedrine sulfate (Efedron), an adrenergic agent, and amitriptyline hydrochloride (Elavil), a tricyclic antidepressant
  2. Administers beta-adrenergic blocking agents, as ordered, such as propranolol hydrochloride (Inderal), to increase outlet resistance
  3. Teaches weight-reduction strategies in consultation with a dietitian, if necessary
  4. Teaches the client to avoid bladder stimulants such as alcohol and caffeine
  5. Teaches Kegel exercises to strengthen the muscles of the pelvic floor
  6. Recommends behavior modification and psychotherapy, as needed

- Electrical devices may be required for inhibition of bladder contraction.

Surgical Management

- Surgical procedures are performed to restore the normal urethrovesical angle (Pereyra's procedure or the Marshall-Marchetti-Krantz operation) or increase the urethral length (anterior urethropexy).

- For both men and women, the surgical implantation of an artificial urinary sphincter is done to treat stress incontinence.

- After surgery, the nurse secures the indwelling Foley catheter with adhesive tape to prevent unnecessary traction or movement on the neck of the bladder.

NDx: URGE INCONTINENCE

- The nurse
  1. Administers medications, as ordered, to control involuntary contraction of the hypertonic bladder, including anticholinergic agents, smooth muscle relaxants, and calcium channel blockers
  2. Implements an individualized bladder training program

NDx: REFLEX INCONTINENCE

- The nurse
  1. Administers cholinergic drugs, as ordered, to increase bladder pressure

2. Administers alpha-adrenergic blocking agents, as ordered, to decrease urethral resistance
3. Implements bladder training, including the Credé method, the Valsalva maneuver, and the double-voiding technique

NDx: TOTAL INCONTINENCE

- The nurse
  1. Maintains and reviews the use of applied devices, such as intravaginal devices for women and penile clamps for men
  2. Applies or teaches the client how to use incontinence pads and briefs
  3. Teaches intermittent self-catheterization
  4. Inserts an indwelling catheter (Foley) as a last-resort measure for incontinence

Discharge Planning

- The nurse teaches the client/family to
  1. Remove barriers that impede access to toileting facilities
  2. Use toilet seat extenders to provide the appropriate level of seating to provide maximal abdominal pressure for voiding
  3. Use a portable commode, if necessary
- The nurse teaches
  1. Prescribed medications, including purpose, dosage, method, routes of administration, desired effects, and side effects
  2. Weight reduction, as needed
  3. Importance of an adequate fluid intake to maintain renal function and overall health status
  4. Advantages and disadvantages of external devices or incontinence pads
  5. Bladder training exercises, with practice
  6. Intermittent catheterization technique to the client and family; the client or family member demonstrates the technique in practice sessions
  7. Importance of follow-up visits with the physician(s)

For more information on urinary incontinence, see *Medical-Surgical Nursing: A Nursing Process Approach*, **pp. 1843–1850.**

Infection/Infectious Disease

OVERVIEW

- Infection is caused by the invasion by a biological agent.

- Infectious diseases include those that are thought to be communicable (e.g., measles, hepatitis, and influenza) and those that are not contagious (e.g., nephritis, pancreatitis, and trichinosis).

- A *pathogen* is the causative agent; a *host* is the recipient of infection.

- *Pathogenicity* is the ability to cause disease.

- *Virulence* refers to the frequency with which the disease occurs in persons exposed to the organism (degree of communicability) and the ability to invade and damage a host; it also refers to the severity of the disease.

- In *colonization* the microorganisms are present in the tissues of the host yet cause neither symptomatic nor subclinical disease.

- A *nosocomial* infection is an infection acquired while in the hospital.

- Factors that must be present for transmission of infection are the host, pathogen, portal of entry, mode of transmission, and portal of exit.

- Host factors that increase the risk of infection include

    1. Congenital or acquired immunodeficiencies (e.g., AIDS)
    2. Alteration of normal flora by antibiotic therapy
    3. Age (especially infants and elderly clients)
    4. Pregnancy, diabetes, corticosteroid therapy, and adrenal insufficiency
    5. Defective phagocytic function, circulatory disturbances, and neutropenia
    6. Break in skin or mucous membrane integrity
    7. Interference with the flow of urine, tears, or saliva
    8. Impaired cough reflex or ciliary action
    9. Malnutrition
    10. Smoking, alcohol consumption, and inhalation of toxic chemicals
    11. Invasive therapy, chemotherapy, radiation therapy, steroid therapy, and surgery

- Modes of transmission of infection are commonly
  1. Direct contact
  2. Indirect contact
  3. Droplet spread
  4. Common vehicle
  5. Vectors

- The portal of exit is usually through the portal of entry.
- Human defenses against infection include
  1. Intact skin
  2. Mucous membranes
  3. Respiratory tract
  4. Gastrointestinal tract
  5. Genitourinary tract
  6. Phagocytosis
  7. Inflammation
  8. Humoral and cellular immune systems

- Certain diseases must be reported to the Centers for Disease Control.
- Isolation procedures that are commonly used, depending on the mode of transmission, are
  1. *Strict* isolation, to prevent the transmission of organisms that may spread by direct contact and by the airborne route
  2. *Contact* isolation, to prevent the transmission of organisms that are spread primarily by close or direct contact
  3. *Respiratory* precautions, to prevent the transmission of diseases spread by large droplets that travel only a short distance through the air
  4. *Acid-fast bacteria* isolation, to prevent the spread of tuberculosis
  5. *Enteric* precautions, to prevent infections that are transmitted by contact with feces
  6. *Drainage and secretion* precautions, to prevent infections that are spread by direct and indirect contact with infectious material
  7. *Blood and body fluid* precautions, to prevent infections (e.g., malaria, AIDS, hepatitis B) that are spread by contact with infectious blood or body fluids
  8. *Universal* precautions, to assume that all clients' blood and body fluids are potentially infectious and are handled in that manner

- Typical complications of infection are relapse, cellulitis, pneumonia, abscess formation, systemic complications, and systemic sepsis.

COLLABORATIVE MANAGEMENT

Assessment

- The nurse records the client's
    1. Exposure to a person with similar clinical symptoms or to contaminated food or water and date of exposure
    2. Contact with animals
    3. Travel history
    4. Intravenous (IV) drug use
    5. Transfusion history
    6. Sexual history
    7. Order of onset of symptoms

- Common clinical manifestations are associated with specific sites of infection; the nurse assesses for
    1. Gastrointestinal tract manifestations
        a. Fever
        b. Nausea and vomiting
        c. Diarrhea
        d. Abdominal distention
    2. Genitourinary tract manifestations
        a. Dysuria
        b. Frequency
        c. Urgency
        d. Hematuria
        e. Fever
        f. Purulent discharge
        g. Pelvic or flank pain
    3. Respiratory tract manifestations
        a. Cough
        b. Congestion
        c. Rhinitis
        d. Sore throat
        e. Fever
        f. Chest pain
    4. Skin manifestations
        a. Redness
        b. Warmth
        c. Swelling
        d. Drainage
        e. Pain
    5. Generalized infection manifestations
        a. Fever
        b. Malaise
        c. Fatigue
        d. Muscle aches
        e. Joint pain

6. Psychosocial dysfunction
    a. Anxiety and frustration
    b. Social isolation
    c. Coping mechanisms

Planning and Implementation
NDx: Potential Altered Body Temperature

• Antimicrobial therapy depends on the type of causative pathogen.
• Commonly used antimicrobial agents include
    1. Penicillin (penicillin G, procaine penicillin)
    2. Semisynthetic penicillins (methicillin, oxacillin, nafcillin)
    3. Extended-spectrum penicillin (ampicillin, carbenicillin, ticarcillin)
    4. Cephalosporins (cephalothin, cefazolin, cephapirin, cefoxitin, cefamandole, cefotaxime, moxalactam)
    5. Other beta-lactam agents (monobactams, aztreonam, penems)
    6. Tetracyclines (tetracycline, doxycycline, minocycline)
    7. Chloramphenicol
    8. Macrolides and lincosamides (erythromycin, lincomycin, clindamycin)
    9. Vancomycin
    10. Antituberculous agents (isoniazid, rifampin, ethambutol)
    11. Antifungal agents (amphotericin B, miconazole, ketoconazole, flucytosine)
    12. Antiviral agents (acyclovir, vidarabine)

• Aspirin and acetaminophen are generally not used until the client's temperature is 101° F or more; they may be used earlier in the client with heart failure or a history of febrile seizures.

• Aspirin and, perhaps, acetaminophen are not given in viral illness such as chicken pox and influenza because of their association with Reye's syndrome.

• The nurse
    1. Applies a hypothermia blanket and monitors frequently for shivering, which may further increase temperature
    2. Sponges the client with tepid water
    3. Places ice packs/cold compresses over pulse points
    4. Monitors for signs of dehydration, such as increased thirst, decreased skin turgor, and dry mucous membranes

5. Encourages fluid intake
6. Records strict measurement of intake and output

NDx: ACTIVITY INTOLERANCE
- The nurse
    1. Collaborates with the dietitian and client to identify a diet that the client can tolerate and meets calorie and protein requirements
    2. Ensures bed rest during the acute phase of the illness
    3. Collaborates with the client to develop a progressive program for return to a normal level of activity
    4. Encourages frequent rest periods

NDx: SOCIAL ISOLATION
- The nurse
    1. Educates the client/family about the mode of transmission of the infection and mechanisms that prevent the spread of organisms from the client to others
    2. Encourages family and friends to visit the client; provides information and instructions on isolation techniques and other precautions needed to prevent transmission of the disease
    3. Ensures that the client has access to a telephone and radio
    4. Visits with the client frequently (every hour or more if time permits), to say hello and check if the client needs anything

Discharge Planning
- The nurse
    1. Ensures that client who is discharged on IV medication has proper storage facilities for the medication(s)
    2. Emphasizes the importance of a clean home environment
    3. Provides drug information
        a. Taking all medications in the correct dosage, at the right time, and by the right route
        b. What to do if a dose is missed or if complications or side effects occur
        c. The importance of completing the entire drug prescription, as ordered
        d. Teaches care of the client with IV/intravascular devices for the administration of IV medications
            (1) Care of the device

358

(2) Indications of malfunction of the device
(3) Indications of infection of the device or site of insertion
(4) Method of drug administration
(5) Indications that the medication is not stored properly (for example, if the temperature of the storage area is too high, discoloration of the medication may occur)
(6) How to handle emergencies

5. Reviews the precautions necessary to prevent spread of the infection

For more information on infection/infectious disease, see *Medical-Surgical Nursing: A Nursing Process Approach,* **pp. 604–628.**

Influenza

- Influenza (flu) is a highly contagious, acute viral respiratory infection caused by one of several viruses.
- Typical symptoms include severe headache, muscle aches, fever, chills, fatigue, weakness, anorexia, and respiratory symptoms, such as sore throat, cough, and rhinorrhea.
- Treatment is symptomatic and includes
  1. Bed rest
  2. Increased oral fluid intake
  3. Acetaminophen (Tylenol) or aspirin
  4. Saline gargles
  5. Antihistamines
- As a preventive measure, it is recommended that

persons over the age of 65 and those with chronic illness or immune compromise receive the influenza vaccination annually.

For more information on influenza, see *Medical-Surgical Nursing: A Nursing Process Approach*, **p. 2060.**

Intestinal Obstruction

OVERVIEW

- Partial or total intestinal obstruction can be either mechanical or nonmechanical (paralytic).
- *Mechanical* obstruction can be due to
  1. Disorders outside the intestine (adhesions and hernias)
  2. Disturbances inside the intestine (tumors, diverticulitis, or strictures)
  3. Blockage of the intestinal lumen (gallstones or intussusception)
- The most common causes of mechanical obstruction include adhesions and hernias.
- *Nonmechanical* obstruction (paralytic or adynamic ileus) involves decreased muscular activity of the intestine, resulting in a slowing of the movement of intestinal contents.
- Distention results from the intestine's inability to absorb and mobilize intestinal contents.
- Paralytic, or adynamic, ileus is the most common cause of intestinal obstruction; as it can be caused by physiologic, neurogenic, or chemical imbalances.
- *Strangulated* obstruction results when there is obstruction with compromised blood flow.
- *Incarcerated* obstruction results from obstructed blood flow with necrosis.

COLLABORATIVE MANAGEMENT
Assessment
- The nurse records the client's
  1. Past medical history, including abdominal surgical procedures, radiation therapy, or bowel diseases such as Crohn's disease, ulcerative colitis, diverticular disease, gallstones, hernias, or tumors
  2. Diet history
  3. Bowel elimination patterns, including the presence of blood in the stool
  4. Familial history of colorectal cancer
- The nurse assesses (for mechanical intestinal obstruction)
  1. Intermittent mid-abdominal cramping (characteristic of mechanical obstruction)
  2. Peristaltic waves
  3. High-pitched bowel sounds (borborygmi) in *early* obstructive process
  4. Absent bowel sounds in *later* stages
  5. Abdominal distention caused by fatigue of the intestine (hallmark sign)
  6. Nausea and vomiting
     a. Obstruction above the ileum causes early and profuse vomiting of partially digested food and chyme changing to watery contents containing bile and mucus.
     b. Obstruction in the large intestine produces vomitus with orange-brown color and a foul odor due to bacterial overgrowth, which may be fecal contamination.
  7. Obstipation (characteristic of total small and large mechanical obstruction)
- The nurse assesses (for nonmechanical intestinal obstruction)
  1. Constant, diffuse abdominal discomfort; severe pain in intestinal vascular insufficiency or infarction
  2. Decreased bowel sounds in *early* obstruction
  3. Absent bowel sounds in *later* obstruction
  4. Vomiting of gastric contents and bile
  5. Shigultus (hiccups) (common with all types of intestinal obstruction)

Planning and Implementation
NDx: Altered (Gastrointestinal) Tissue Perfusion
Nonsurgical Management
- The nurse
  1. Maintains the client on nothing-by-mouth (NPO) status

2. Monitors drainage from the nasogastric tube, such as the Salem sump or Anderson suction tube, which sits distally in the stomach and is connected to low continuous suction (commonly used)
3. Monitors drainage from the intestinal tube, such as the Miller-Abbott, Cantor, or Harris tube, which are used for small intestine obstructions. (These tubes weighted with mercury-filled balloons act as a food bolus stimulating peristalsis advancing through the intestinal tract, and are less commonly used.)
4. Assists with intestinal tube progression by helping the client change position every 2 hours and by advancing the tube 3 to 4 inches at specified times, as ordered
5. Avoids taping the intestinal tube to the nose until the desired position is reached in the intestine
6. Monitors intestinal tube drainage, which occurs by gravity and instills 10 cc of air, as ordered, if the drainage stops; *does not* irrigate the tube with fluid
7. Maintains low intermittent suction, as ordered, when the tube has reached the desired location
8. Provides frequent mouth care for the client with an intestinal tube

• Obstruction caused by fecal impaction resolves after disimpaction and enema.

• Intussusception (telescoping of bowel) may resolve during hydrostatic pressure changes during a barium enema.

Surgical Management

• Surgical management is required for complete mechanical obstruction and for many cases of incomplete mechanical obstruction.

• An exploratory laparotomy is done to locate the obstruction and distinguish the nature of the problem.

• The specific surgical procedure performed is dependent on the etiology and location of the obstruction. Examples of procedures include lysis of adhesions; colon resection with anastamosis for obstruction due to tumor or diverticulitis; and embolectomy or thrombectomy for intestinal infarction.

• Nursing care for abdominal surgery is similar to that described under Colorectal Cancer.

- The nurse
    1. Administers IV fluid because of vascular fluid losses from lack of normal reabsorption in the intestine, increased intestinal secretions, nasogastric suction, and NPO status (normal saline solutions with potassium replacement are used based on electrolyte results)
    2. Provides blood products in case of strangulated obstruction because of blood loss into the bowel or peritoneal cavity
    3. Provides ice chips only with a physician's order

NDx: PAIN

- The nurse
    1. Reports changes in pain to the physician, including pain that significantly increases or changes from a colicky, intermittent type to constant discomfort (changes could indicate perforation or peritonitis)
    2. Usually withholds narcotic analgesics (if given, the drug is usually meperidine hydrochloride [Demerol], as ordered)
    3. Provides a position of comfort, including semi-Fowler's, which helps relieve the pressure of abdominal distention and facilitates thoracic excursion and normal breathing patterns

Discharge Planning

- Client/family education is dependent on the specific etiology and treatment for the obstruction.

- The nurse instructs the client to report signs that may indicate recurrent obstruction, including abdominal pain or distention, nausea, vomiting, or constipation (for nonmechanical obstruction after surgery or trauma).

- The nurse instructs the client to develop a structured bowel regime, including a high-fiber diet, daily exercise, and psyllium hydrophilic mucilloid (Metamucil) with copious amounts of water (for prevention of fecal impaction recurrence).

- The nurse provides written postoperative instructions for mechanical obstructions requiring surgical intervention
    1. Inspection of the incision for redness, tenderness, swelling, and drainage
    2. Dressing change procedure, if necessary

3. Pain management
4. Activity limitations, if indicated

For more information on intestinal obstruction, see *Medical-Surgical Nursing: A Nursing Process Approach*, **pp. 1393–1400.**

Intraoperative Care

OVERVIEW

• Intraoperative care begins when the client enters the surgical suite.

• An *anesthesiologist* is a physician who specializes in the administration of anesthesia.

• A *nurse anesthetist* is a registered nurse who administers anesthetics under the direct supervision of an anesthesiologist or a surgeon.

• A *circulating nurse* sets up the room, maintains the necessary supplies, checks that all equipment is safe and functional before surgery, positions the client, cleans the surgical field before draping, reviews the chart and assesses the client's physical and emotional status, and orients the client to the environment.

• A *scrub nurse* or *technologist* is responsible for setting up and handing surgical instruments to the surgeon and assistants and maintains an accurate count of sponges, needles, and instruments.

• There are multiple types of anesthesia
   1. *General anesthesia,* which induces depression of the central nervous system, causing analgesia, amnesia, and unconsciousness
   2. *Balanced anesthesia*, a combination of agents used to provide hypnosis, amnesia, analgesia, muscle relaxation, and relaxation of reflexes with minimal disturbance to the client's physiological function
   3. *Local* or *regional* anesthesia, which temporarily interrupts the transmission of nerve impulses to and from a specific area or region; motor function

may or may not be involved, and the client does not lose consciousness.

  a. *Topical anesthesia* involves the use of a regional anesthetic applied directly to the surface of the area to be anesthetized, usually in the form of an ointment or spray.
  b. *Local infiltration* is the injection of an anesthetic agent intracutaneously and subcutaneously into the tissue surrounding an incision, wound, or lesion.
  c. A *nerve block* involves the injection of a local anesthetic into or around a nerve or nerve supply.
  d. *Spinal* anesthesia is administered by injecting an anesthetic into the subarachnoid space at L2–3 or L3–4.
  e. A *caudal block* is the injection of the anesthetic agent into the epidural space through the sacral hiatus and caudal canal.
  f. An *epidural block* is the injection of the anesthetic agent into the epidural space through the interspace of the vertebrae.

- The four stages of general anesthesia include
  1. Relaxation
  2. Excitement
  3. Operative or surgical anesthesia
  4. Danger

COLLABORATIVE MANAGEMENT
Assessment
- The nurse validates
  1. For the correct client by checking the client's identification bracelet and chart using the client's name and hospital assigned number
  2. All aspects of the preoperative checklist are complete and information is on the chart
     a. Allergies are noted.
     b. Previous anesthesia and any reactions are documented.
     c. History of blood transfusions and reaction, if any, are noted.
     d. Reports on laboratory, radiographic, and diagnostic tests are complete.
     e. The client's history and physical examination are reported.
     f. Medications routinely taken by the client are noted.
  3. Correct attire and removal of items such as jewelry and dentures

Planning and Implementation

NDx: POTENTIAL FOR INJURY

• The surgical team observes for and treats complications of general anesthesia.

• *Difficult intubation* can result in broken or injured teeth or caps and/or trauma to vocal cords.

• *Overdosage* can cause the client to progress to the life-threatening *danger* stage of general anesthesia.

• *Malignant hyperthermia* is manifested by

1. Increase in metabolic rate
2. Body temperature as high as 46° C
3. Tachycardia
4. Cyanosis
5. Hypotension
6. Muscle rigidity
7. Darker color of blood at the surgical site
8. Dysrhythmias

• Treatment of malignant hyperthermia includes

1. Immediate discontinuance of surgery
2. Cooling of the client using iced IV solutions, iced nasogastric lavage, and packing the client in ice
3. Dantrolene sodium (Dantrium)
4. Steroids
5. Diuretics
6. 100% oxygen

• The nurse ensures proper *positioning* by assessing for

1. Physiologic alignment
2. Minimal interference with circulation
3. Protection of skeletal and neuromuscular structures
4. Optimal exposure of the operative site and IV line
5. Access for the anesthesiologist
6. Preservation of the client's dignity

• The nurse pads joints and places grounding pads as appropriate.

• The nurse observes for complications of special positioning, such as wrist or foot drop, loss of sensation, and inflammation.

NDx: IMPAIRED SKIN INTEGRITY

• The surgeon applies a plastic drape after the skin has been prepped and is dry.

• Skin closures include

1. Sutures

   a. Absorbable
   b. Nonabsorbable

2. Clamps

3. Staples
4. Steri-Strips

- After the wound is sutured, the plastic drape is carefully removed, and a sterile dressing is applied by the surgeon.

For more information on intraoperative care, see *Medical-Surgical Nursing: A Nursing Process Approach,* **pp. 454–472.**

Irritable Bowel Syndrome

OVERVIEW

- Irritable bowel syndrome (IBS), also known as spastic bowel and mucous colitis, is the most common digestive disorder facing Americans today, entailing a change in bowel habits without an inflammatory process or changes in bowel mucosa.
- Factors such as stress, diet, or anxiety may precipitate exacerbations.
- Changes in gastrointestinal motility result in diarrhea, constipation, or diarrhea alternating with constipation.

COLLABORATIVE MANAGEMENT

Assessment

- The nurse records the client's
  1. Age
  2. Race
  3. Sex
  4. Occupational stressors
  5. Cigarette, alcohol, and caffeine use
  6. Usual dietary patterns
  7. Usual bowel patterns
  8. Past medical history
- The nurse assesses for
  1. Diarrhea or constipation
  2. Abdominal cramping

3. Abdominal pain
4. Nausea associated with mealtime and defecation
5. Tympanic bowel sounds

Planning and Implementation

NDx: DIARRHEA; CONSTIPATION

- The nurse
  1. Administers bulk-forming laxatives such as psyllium hydrophilic mucilloid (Metamucil) or calcium polycarbophil (Mitrolan), as ordered
  2. Administers antidiarrheal agents such as diphenoxylate hydrochloride with atropine sulfate (Lomotil), loperamide (Imodium), or camphorated tincture of opium (Paregoric), as ordered, to decrease cramping and frequent stools
  3. Administers cholinergic receptor blocking agents such as dicyclomine hydrochloride (Bentyl) and propantheline bromide (Pro-Banthine), as ordered, to help relieve cramping and intestinal spasm
  4. Consults with the dietitian to teach the client to add 30 to 40 g of fiber to the diet daily
  5. Encourages the client to eat regular meals and chew food slowly
  6. Teaches the client to drink 8 to 10 cups of liquid per day
  7. Encourages the client to implement a regular exercise program to promote bowel elimination and reduce stress

Discharge Planning

- The nurse instructs the client
  1. To establish regular bowel patterns and to defecate regularly
  2. To implement a regular exercise program
  3. To follow a high-fiber diet with adequate liquid intake and regular mealtimes
  4. To avoid alcohol, caffeine, and other gastric irritants
  5. To follow instructions regarding medications

For more information on irritable bowel syndrome, see *Medical-Surgical Nursing: A Nursing Process Approach*, **pp. 1365–1368.**

Keloid

• A keloid is an overgrowth of a scar, resulting from an excess accumulation of collagen and ground substances after skin trauma.

• Keloids appear as an elevated, protuberant nodule extending beyond the boundaries of the original scar and are common in the black population.

• Treatment is difficult and often unsuccessful.

• Surgery may be performed in combination with intralesional steroid injections or low-dose radiation therapy.

K

For more information on keloids, see *Medical-Surgical Nursing: A Nursing Process Approach*, **p. 1207.**

Knee Injury

• *Menisci* injuries are characterized by pain, swelling, and tenderness in the knee and sometimes by a clicking or snapping sound when moving the knee.

• A common diagnostic technique is the McMurray test in which the examiner flexes and rotates the knee and then presses on the medial aspect while slowly extending the leg; the test is positive if a clicking sound is palpated or heard, but a negative finding does not rule out a tear.

• Treatment of *locked* knee is manipulation followed by casting for 3 to 6 weeks.

- A *meniscectomy*, or removal of all or part of the meniscus, may be required.
- Postoperative care includes
  1. Monitoring the dressing for drainage and bleeding
  2. Circulation checks: skin temperature and color, movement, sensation, pulses, capillary refill, pain
  3. Leg exercises: quadriceps setting, straight-leg raising
  4. Knee immobilizer
  5. Elevating the leg on pillows; applying ice
- Ligament injuries result in sprains.
- A *mild sprain* involves the tearing of a few fibers of a ligament and is treated by rest, ice, and a compression bandage for a few days.
- In a *moderate sprain*, more fibers are torn, but the stability of the joint remains intact; the treatment is casting for 4 to 6 weeks.
- *Severe sprains* cause marked instability of the joint; treatment includes surgical repair of the torn ligaments.
- For a *rupture* of the *patellar tendon,* the treatment is surgical repair and casting for 6 to 8 weeks or tendon transplant. (For care of the client in a cast, see also Fracture.)

For more information on knee injuries, see *Medical-Surgical Nursing: A Nursing Process Approach,* **pp. 819–821.**

Labyrinthitis

- Labyrinthitis is an infection of the labyrinth, part of the inner ear.
- Clinical manifestations include hearing loss, tinnitus, spontaneous nystagmus to the affected side, nausea, and vomiting.

- The most common complication is meningitis.
- Treatment includes
  1. Systemic antibiotics such as ampicillin (Omnipen)
  2. Bed rest in a darkened room
  3. Antiemetics such as chlorpromazine (Thorazine)
  4. Antivertiginous medications
  5. Psychological support to cope with hearing loss

For more information on labyrinthitis, see *Medical-Surgical Nursing: A Nursing Process Approach,* **pp. 1122–1123.**

Laryngeal Cancer

L

OVERVIEW

- Ninety percent of laryngeal tumors are squamous cell in origin, usually related to an injury.
- Laryngeal cancer presents as malignant ulcerations with underlying filtration.
- Metastasis to the lungs is common.

COLLABORATIVE MANAGEMENT

Assessment

- The nurse records the client's
  1. Tobacco and alcohol use
  2. Past history of acute or chronic laryngitis
  3. Exposure to environmental pollutants
  4. Family history of cancer
  5. Overuse of the voice
- The nurse assesses for
  1. Persistent hoarseness
  2. Persistent sore throat
  3. Painless neck mass

4. Feeling of a lump in the throat
5. Dysphagia
6. Change in voice quality
7. Burning in the throat
8. Dyspnea
9. Weight loss
10. Loss of appetite
11. Pain (a late symptom)

Planning and Implementation

NDx: POTENTIAL FOR INJURY

Nonsurgical Management

- The nurse
  1. Positions the client in the Fowler's position to promote optimal air exchange
  2. Monitors respiratory effort
  3. Observes for signs of aspiration of food and liquids

- Radiation therapy is the treatment of choice if the cancer is limited to a small area in one vocal cord, either done alone or in combination with surgery or chemotherapy.

Surgical Management

- Surgical interventions for cancer of the larynx include a *small tumor excision* or a *total laryngectomy* (removal of the larynx) for infiltrative tumors that involve vocal cord paralysis and for tumors that do not respond to radiation therapy.

- For lymph node involvement, a *radical neck dissection* with larygectomy and *tracheostomy* is performed, involving
  1. Removal of all tissues from the lower edge of the mandible to the clavicle and from the anterior edge of the trapezius muscle to the midline, except for the carotid arteries; the vagus, hypoglosseal, and phrenic nerves; and trunks of the brachial plexus
  2. Routinely involves the sternocleidomastoid muscle, the jugular vein, the eleventh cranial nerve, the submaxillary salivary gland, and surrounding soft tissue

- The nurse provides preoperative care
  1. Provides routine preoperative instruction and preparation
  2. Explains the procedure and cosmetic repair, if needed
  3. Explains the rehabilitation program
  4. Provides information about the tracheostomy,

suctioning, and compensatory methods of communication

5. Teaches the client about the critical care environment, including the mechanical ventilator

- The client usually spends the immediate postoperative period in the critical care unit.
- The nurse provides postoperative care

1. Provides routine postoperative care
2. Monitors for airway patency and provides frequent suctioning of the airway to remove bloody secretions
3. Maintains mechanical ventilator support, as needed, or a tracheostomy collar with humidification
4. Positions the client in a high-Fowler's position
5. Maintains the surgical drains in the neck area and the nasogastric tube
6. Monitors for postoperative hemorrhage
7. Maintains intravenous fluids or total parenteral nutrition, until nutrition is given via the nasogastric or gastrostomy/jejunostomy tube
8. Teaches the client the procedure for supraglottic swallowing, in consultation with the speech and language pathologist

- Rehabilitation/speech therapy is instituted with the use of an artificial larynx, followed by learning esophageal speech.

L

NDx: ANXIETY

- The nurse

1. Explores the specific reasons for the client's anxiety
2. Refers the client to support groups
3. Cautiously administers antianxiety agents such as diazepam (Valium), as ordered

NDx: BODY IMAGE DISTURBANCE

- The client with a total laryngectomy and/or radical neck dissection experiences a permanent change in body image because of deformity and the presence of the neck stoma. (See Body Image for a complete discussion.)
- The nurse

1. Assists the client in setting realistic goals
2. Teaches the client alternative communication methods
3. Recommends the client wear loose-fitting, high-collar shirts or sweaters to help hide the stoma

Discharge Planning

- Depending on the surgical intervention, the client/family are taught how to care for the stoma or tracheostomy or laryngectomy tube.
- The nurse
  1. Teaches clean suctioning technique
  2. Reviews the plan of care for radiation or chemotherapy
  3. Teaches the client how to clean the incision and provide stoma care, including cleaning and inspection for signs of infection
  4. Instructs the client to avoid swimming and to take showers with caution
  5. Teaches the client to wear a stoma guard to shield the stoma
  6. Advises the client to increase humidity in the home
  7. Tells the client to continue to use the alternative communication method
  8. Recommends that the client wear a Medic Alert bracelet or necklace

For more information on laryngeal cancer, see *Medical-Surgical Nursing: A Nursing Process Approach*, **pp. 1964–1972.**

Laryngeal Edema

- Acute laryngeal edema is a potential medical emergency.
- Etiologies include anaphylaxis, acute laryngitis, inflammation, trauma, difficult intubation, and radiation to the head and neck.
- Symptoms include hoarseness, dyspnea, and laryngeal stridor.

- Management includes
  1. Inhaled epinephrine
  2. Corticosteroids
  3. Emergency tracheostomy or endotracheal intubation

For more information on laryngeal edema, see *Medical-Surgical Nursing: A Nursing Process Approach*, **p. 1963.**

Laryngeal Nodule/ Laryngeal Polyp

- Nodules occurring on the vocal cords usually appear at the point at which the cords come together forcibly.
- *Nodules* are hypertrophied fibrous tissue that result from overuse of the voice and may appear after an infectious process.
- Vocal cord *polyps* are chronic edematous masses.
- Nodules and polyps are painless but produce hoarseness.
- The nurse
  1. Instructs the client about the hazards of tobacco use
  2. Stresses the importance of voice rest
- Treatment interventions include
  1. Providing humidification
  2. Voice rest
  3. Speech therapy
  4. Treatment of underlying allergen
- Surgical excision of the nodules and polyps with direct laryngoscopy may be required for persistent hoarseness.

- After surgery, the nurse ensures alternative communication methods to promote voice rest.

For more information on laryngeal nodules and polyps, see *Medical-Surgical Nursing: A Nursing Process Approach*, **p. 1963.**

Laryngeal Paralysis

- Laryngeal paralysis results from injury, trauma, metallic poisons, or disease processes that affect the laryngeal or vagus nerve.
- Vocal paralysis is unilateral or bilateral.
- The airway remains patent with unilateral involvement, but the voice is affected.
- Bilateral vocal cord paralysis results from traumatic injury or cerebral vascular accident; symptoms include dyspnea, hoarseness, stridor, and a weak voice.
- Treatment is aimed at maintaining a patent airway and preventing aspiration.

For more information on laryngeal paralysis, see *Medical-Surgical Nursing: A Nursing Process Approach*, **pp. 1962–1963.**

Laryngeal Trauma

- Laryngeal trauma consists of crushing injuries, fractures, or intrinsic injuries such as prolonged endotracheal intubation.
- Symptoms include hoarseness and aphonia; edema and bleeding also occur.
- Respiratory assessment includes monitoring for a patent airway and distress symptoms, which include tachypnea, anxiety, sternal retractions, nasal flaring, and stridor.
- Management is cause specific.
- Laceration of the cricoid cartilage requires surgical repair and tracheostomy.
- Extensive trauma requires total laryngectomy.

For more information on laryngeal trauma, see *Medical-Surgical Nursing: A Nursing Process Approach*, **pp. 1963–1964.**

L

Laryngitis

- Laryngitis is an inflammation of mucous membranes lining the larynx with or without edema of the vocal cords.
- Laryngitis is commonly associated with upper respiratory tract infections.
- Etiologic factors include exposure to irritating inhalants and pollutants, overuse of the voice, and inhalation of volatile gases.
- Clinical manifestations include acute hoarseness, dry cough, and dysphagia; aphonia may occur.
- Management includes
  1. Steam inhalation

2. Voice rest
3. Cool liquids
4. Topical throat lozenges
5. Antibiotics
6. Bronchodilators

• Recurrent bouts of laryngitis require further evaluation.

For more information on laryngitis, see *Medical-Surgical Nursing: A Nursing Process Approach*, **pp. 1960–1962.**

Leprosy

• Leprosy, or Hansen's disease, is a chronic, highly contagious, systemic mycobacterial infection of the peripheral nervous system complicated by secondary skin involvement.

• Clinical manifestations are directly related to the degree of individual resistance to mycobacteria.

• *Localized* leprosy (high immunity) is characterized by one or two isolated, erythematous, anesthetic plaques that are hairless and scaly in texture.

• *Generalized* leprosy (low immunity) involves widespread, faintly erythematous macules, papules, nodules, and plaques with concomitant peripheral nerve damage.

• Treatment is aimed at controlling bacterial proliferation and minimizing associated deformities and done as an outpatient to prevent spread.

• The drug of choice is dapsone, a sulfone.

For more information, see *Medical-Surgical Nursing: A Nursing Process Approach*, **p. 1211.**

Leukemia

OVERVIEW

- Leukemia is a group of malignant disorders involving abnormal overproduction of specific cell types, usually at the immature stage, in bone marrow.
- The two major types of leukemia include
  1. Lymphocytic or lymphoblastic, involving cells within the committed lymphoid maturational pathways (acute and chronic)
  2. Myelocytic or myelogenous, including cells within the myeloid maturational pathways (acute and chronic)
- The basic pathologic defect in leukemia is malignant transformation of stem cells or early committed precursor leukocytes, producing an abnormal proliferation of a specific type of leukocyte in the bone marrow that shuts down normal bone marrow production of erythrocytes, platelets, and functionally mature leukocytes.

COLLABORATIVE MANAGEMENT

Assessment

- The nurse records the client's
  1. Age
  2. Environmental exposure
  3. Previous illnesses and exposure to ionizing radiation or medications
  4. History of infections, including influenza, cold, pneumonia, bronchitis, and unexplained fever
  5. Overt bleeding episodes
  6. History of weakness or fatigue
  7. Associated symptoms
- The nurse assesses for
  1. Pale skin, mucous membranes, conjunctiva
  2. Petechiae
  3. Skin and/or oral infections
  4. Bleeding gums
  5. Tachycardia
  6. Increased respiratory rate
  7. Weight loss, nausea, and/or anorexia
  8. Hepatosplenomegaly
  9. Headaches
  10. Papilledema
  11. Hematuria
  12. Bone and joint pain

Planning and Implementation

NDx: Potential for Infection

- The nurse employs infection control measures
  1. Frequent, thorough hand washing between client contacts
  2. Wearing a mask (for persons with upper respiratory infections)
  3. Limiting the number of personnel entering the client's room
  4. Limiting visitors to healthy adults only
  5. Placing the client in a private room, if able
  6. Using aseptic technique for dressing changes
- The nurse
  1. Monitors for signs of infection
  2. Provides meticulous skin care to maintain skin integrity
  3. Provides pulmonary toilet to prevent respiratory infections
  4. Administers chemotherapeutic drugs, as ordered, aimed at interrupting or halting infectious processes and controlling infection
     a. Induction chemotherapy includes administration with agents such as cytosine arabinoside with daunorubicin.
     b. Consolidation therapy consists of another course of the same drugs or a different combination of chemotherapeutic agents.
     c. Maintenance therapy includes transfusion of red blood cells, platelets, and granulocytes.
- The nurse administers
  1. Antibacterial agents (antibiotics including aminoglycosides and a systemic penicillin), as ordered
  2. Antifungal agents when fungal infections are present (amphotericin B and ketoconazole), as ordered
  3. Antiviral agents used prophylactically (e.g., acyclovir), as ordered
- A bone marrow transplant may be required if other measures are ineffective. A suitable donor is identified after human leukocyte antigen (HLA) typing. The marrow is harvested from the donor and administered by intravenous infusion via a Hickman catheter to the client.
- The nurse monitors for post–bone marrow complications
  1. Infection due to loss of natural immunity
  2. Severe thrombocytopenia

3. Failure to engraft
4. Graft versus host disease (GVHD)

• The immunosuppressive agents required to prevent GVHD increase the client's susceptibilty to infection.

• Isolation procedures are required for bone marrow recipients.

NDx: POTENTIAL FOR INJURY

• The nurse
1. Avoids intramuscular or subcutaneous injections
2. Avoids using razors
3. Avoids inserting rectal suppositories and/or a thermometer
4. Protects the client from harmful situations; provides careful turning and/or movement
5. Uses only silk and/or paper tape
6. Avoids aspirin
7. Avoids diets high in roughage and/or spicy foods
8. Monitors for evidence of bleeding

• A client with decreased platelets (less than 20,000/mm^3) may require platelet transfusions.

NDx: FATIGUE

• The nurse
1. Increases dietary intake with small, frequent meals high in protein and carbohydrates
2. Administers oxygen, as ordered
3. Provides blood transfusions, as ordered, to increase the oxygen-carrying capacity of the blood
4. Conserves the client's energy by providing rest periods for him or her

Discharge Planning

• The nurse teaches the client/family
1. Measures to protect the client from infection
2. The importance of meticulous mouth care
3. The need to report signs of infection immediately to the physician
4. The necessity of maintaining a healthy diet
5. The importance of maintaining medical follow-up despite unpleasant side effects
6. Resources for psychosocial support for role and self-esteem adjustment

For more information on leukemia, see *Medical-Surgical Nursing: A Nursing Process Approach*, **pp. 2260–2271.**

Liver Cancer

- Liver cancer usually develops as a metastatic process from primary cancer sites such as the esophagus, stomach, colon, rectum, breasts, and/or lungs or from malignant melanoma.

- Elevated serum alkaline phosphatase levels are common, and a needle biopsy confirms metastasis.

- Surgery is indicated for a single metastatic lesion; a hepatic lobe resection is performed.

- High-dose hepatic chemotherapy may be given, and hepatic artery ligation deprives the metastatic lesion of oxygen.

- Primary hepatic carcinoma is rare in the United States.

- The most common form is hepatoma, and signs include jaundice, ascites, bleeding, and encephalopathy.

For more information on liver cancer, see *Medical-Surgical Nursing: A Nursing Process Approach*, **p. 1506.**

Liver Transplantation

- Liver transplantation is done to treat diseases including
  1. End-stage cirrhosis from chronic active hepatitis or primary biliary cirrhosis

2. Hepatic metabolic diseases, such as protoporphyria and Wilson's disease
3. Budd-Chiari syndrome
4. Sclerosing cholangitis

● Extensive physiologic and psychologic assessment of the client is required.

● After a donor organ is retrieved, the liver transplant surgical procedure requires 8 to 16 hours to complete.

● Liver transplantation involves five anastamoses between recipient and donor organs, including the suprahepatic inferior vena cava, infrahepatic vena cava, portal vein, hepatic artery, and biliary anastamoses.

● Immunosuppression therapy with cyclosporin A is given to prevent organ rejection.

● Clinical manifestations of rejection include
1. Tachycardia
2. Fever
3. Right upper quadrant or flank pain
4. Diminished bile flow through the T tube
5. Change in bile color
6. Increased jaundice

● Immunosuppression increases the client's susceptibility and risk for infection.

● Other complications include hemorrhage, fluid and electrolyte imbalances, atelectasis, acute renal failure, hypothermia, and psychologic maladjustment.

● The nurse monitors for signs of complications
1. Fever
2. Increased abdominal pain, distention, and rigidity
3. Change in neurologic status
4. Coagulopathy

For more information on liver transplantation, see *Medical-Surgical Nursing: A Nursing Process Approach,* **pp. 1506–1507.**

Liver Trauma

- Liver trauma is the most common organ injury in penetrating abdominal trauma and the second most common organ injury after blunt abdominal trauma.

- Common injuries to the liver include simple lacerations, multiple lacerations, avulsions, and crush injuries.

- The liver is a vascular organ; therefore, blood loss is massive.

- Signs of hemorrhagic shock include hypotension, tachycardia, tachypnea, pallor, diaphoresis, cool, clammy skin, and confusion.

- Clinical manifestations include right upper quadrant pain with abdominal tenderness, distention, guarding, and rigidity and abdominal pain aggravated by deep breathing and referred to the left shoulder.

- Peritoneal lavage confirms injury.

- Exploratory laparotomy with either simple suture closure and/or packing or extensive hepatic resection may be performed depending on the extent of trauma.

- The client requires infusion of multiple blood products and massive volume to maintain hydration.

For more information on liver trauma, see *Medical-Surgical Nursing: A Nursing Process Approach*, **pp. 1505–1506.**

Loss, Response to

OVERVIEW

- *Loss* is the state of being deprived of or being without something valued that one once had; synonyms are *detriment, impairment, injury,* and *incapacitation.*

- The types of loss include
  1. Loss of a loved one
  2. Loss of self (the overall mental representation each person has of his or her body and personality
  3. Loss of objects
- *Grieving* is the psychologic, social, and somatic reaction to the perception of significant loss.
- Effective grieving is achieved by facing the pain of the loss and by living through its full range of feelings and their expression.
- Common responses to loss are shock and disbelief; yearning and protest, or anger and guilt; anguish, disorganization, and despair; identification with the deceased; and/or reorganization and restitution.
- In *atypical* grief, the client is unable to resolve a particular loss.
- In *delayed* grief, the survivor goes on with life for more than a few weeks after a major loss as if nothing serious had happened.
- Delayed grief may be indicated by exaggerated expressions of guilt and self-reproach, prolonged anger and hostility, alcohol abuse, heavy reliance on medications for inducing sleep, and/or use of tranquilizers.
- Death from suicide is a real danger.

COLLABORATIVE MANAGEMENT
- The nurse records the client's description of
  1. The last illness of the deceased
  2. Timeliness of the death
  3. Age of the deceased
  4. Relationship of the deceased to the survivor
  5. Characteristics of the survivor
     a. Age, ages of his or her children
     b. Education and employment
     c. Economic status
     d. Past depressions and/or personality problems
     e. Diagnosed mental health problems
     f. Substance abuse history
     g. Past major losses and how they were handled
  6. Coping strategies used in the past with previous losses and setbacks
  7. Characteristics of the relationship with the deceased
  8. Relevant cultural and family factors
  9. Spiritual aspects of the client's life
  10. Source of strength and hope in time of crisis

11. Ties to the wider community
12. Source of sense of meaning and purpose in life
- The nurse assesses for
    1. Physical responses associated with loss
        a. Headache
        b. Appetite (increase or decrease)
        c. Changes in bowel and/or bladder habits
        d. Changes in sleep and dream pattern
        e. Tightness in the throat and/or chest
        f. Breathlessness
        g. Sighing
        h. Dry mouth
        i. Muscle weakness
        j. General malaise
    2. Anger and hostility
    3. Guilt and self-reproach
- The nurse
    1. Encourages the client to talk about feelings and loss; permits the client to express feelings (crying, anger)
    2. Actively listens to the client
    3. Provides guidance and information, as needed
    4. Reassures the client that grieving is a normal process
    5. Respects the religious, cultural, and social mores of the client

For more information on loss, see *Medical-Surgical Nursing: A Nursing Process Approach,* **pp. 196–208.**

Lung Cancer

OVERVIEW

- Lung cancer is the leading cause of cancer-related mortality.
- Bronchiogenic carcinoma spreads through direct extension and lymphatic dissemination.

- The four major types of lung cancer include
  1. Small cell (oat cell)
  2. Epidermal (squamous cell)
  3. Adenocarcinoma
  4. Large cell anaplastic carcinoma

COLLABORATIVE MANAGEMENT
Assessment
- The nurse records the client's
  1. Smoking history
  2. Environmental exposure to carcinogens
  3. Hoarseness
  4. Complaints of pain or vague discomfort
  5. Ill-defined sensations in the chest
  6. Dyspnea and related respiratory symptoms
- The nurse assesses for
  1. Sputum quantity and quality
  2. Breathing patterns
  3. Abnormal retractions, stridor, and/or use of accessory muscles
  4. Asymmetry of diaphragmatic movement
  5. Chest wall tenderness and/or masses
  6. Decreased tactile fremitus over areas of consolidation
  7. Tracheal deviation
  8. Dullness or obvious masses on percussion of the chest wall
  9. Decreased or absent breath sounds over the tumor
  10. Increased vocal fremitus, which indicates consolidation
  11. Pleural friction rub
  12. Distant heart sounds
  13. Cardiac dysrhythmias
  14. Skin ecchymosis
  15. Lethargy and somnolence
  16. Pain radiating to the shoulder

Planning and Implementation
NDx: PAIN

- The nurse administers analgesics (parenteral or oral meperidine hydrochloride or morphine sulfate), as ordered.

NDx: INEFFECTIVE AIRWAY CLEARANCE; IMPAIRED GAS EXCHANGE
Nonsurgical Management

- The nurse
  1. Provides humidification to moisten and loosen secretions

2. Provides symptomatic relief with medications, as ordered, especially bronchodilators and/or steroids to decrease bronchospasm, inflammation, and edema
3. Positions the client in an upright position for ease of breathing
4. Provides supplemental oxygen, as ordered
5. Administers chemotherapy to promote tumor regression, as ordered
6. Administers immunotherapy, with tumor extracts, irradiated whole tumor cells, or cells killed by other methods; and/or nonspecific immune therapy with Bacille Calmette-Guérin vaccine and levamisole, as ordered

• Radiation therapy may be used for localized intrathoracic lung cancers.

Surgical Management

• Surgical management includes
    1. *Laser therapy*, to relieve endobronchial obstructions
    2. *Thoracotomy* with *pneumonectomy* (removal of the lung), for bronchiogenic carcinoma
    3. *Thoracotomy* with *lobectomy* (removal of a lobe), for tumors confined to a single lobe
    4. *Thoracotomy* with *segmental resection* (removal of a lobe segment), for clients unable to tolerate lobectomy or pneumonectomy

• The nurse provides routine preoperative care and instructions on what to expect postoperatively.
• The nurse provides postoperative care
    1. Provides routine postoperative care
    2. Maintains chest tubes and the closed chest drainage system(s), which drain air and/or blood that accumulates in the pleural space
    3. Monitors for excess bleeding in the drainage system
    4. Monitors for an air leak in the underwater seal chamber
    5. Checks for the rise and fall of fluid in the column as the client breathes in and out
    6. Assesses for the absence or presence of lung sounds
    7. Provides oxygen therapy, as ordered

Discharge Planning

• The nurse provides the client/family education
    1. Physical activity limitations
    2. Coping with dyspnea
    3. Pain relief measures, including prescriptions

4. Written postsurgical instructions
   a. Incision care
   b. Inspection of the thorocotomy incision for redness, tenderness, swelling, and drainage
5. Follow-up appointments for chemotherapy or radiation therapy
6. Psychosocial preparations, depending on prognosis
7. Importance of follow-up visits with the physician(s)

For more information on lung cancer, see *Medical-Surgical Nursing: A Nursing Process Approach,* **pp. 2046–2054.**

L

Lupus Erythematous

OVERVIEW

- *Systemic* lupus erythematosus (SLE) is a chronic progressive, systemic, inflammatory disease that can cause major body organs and systems to fail; it has no cure.
- *Discoid* lupus erythematosus (DLE) affects only the skin, and its occurrence is infrequent.
- Lupus is thought to be an autoimmune process.

COLLABORATIVE MANAGEMENT

Assessment

- The nurse assesses for
  1. Family history of the disease
  2. Triggering mechanisms, such as sunlight, physical and emotional stress, adverse reaction to medications (procainamide, hydralazine)
  3. Dry, scaly, raised rash on the face and/or upper body (may be the only indicator of DLE)

4. Articular involvement; *initial* joint changes are similar to rheumatoid arthritis, but deformities are not uncommon
5. Avascular necrosis
6. Muscle atrophy
7. Myalgia
8. Fever
9. Various degrees of weakness, fatigue, anorexia, and weight loss
10. Renal involvement, such as changes in urinary output, proteinuria, hematuria, and fluid retention
11. Pulmonary effusions
12. Pericarditis
13. Neurologic changes, such as psychoses, seizures, paresis, migraine headaches, and cranial nerve palsies
14. Raynaud's phenomenon
15. Abdominal pain
16. Liver enlargement
17. Sjögren's syndrome
18. Body image changes
19. Social isolation

Planning and Implementation

NDx: IMPAIRED SKIN INTEGRITY

- The nurse administers drug therapy, as ordered
  1. Topical steroid preparations
  2. Hydroxychloroquine (Plaquenil) to decrease inflammatory response
  3. Chronic steroid therapy to treat the systemic disease process
- The nurse teaches measures for skin protection
  1. Avoiding exposure to sunlight and other forms of ultraviolet light
     a. Long sleeves, wide-brim hats
     b. Sun-blocking agents with a sun protection factor of 25 or higher
  2. Cleaning skin with a mild soap, avoiding harsh, perfumed substances
  3. Using cosmetics with moisturizers
  4. Using a mild shampoo, with women avoiding permanents and frosting

NDx: SELF-ESTEEM DISTURBANCE

- The nurse
  1. Determines the client's reaction to changes
  2. Communicates his or her acceptance of the client by establishing a trusting relationship

3. Encourages the client to verbalize his or her feelings
4. Encourages the client to wear street clothes, his or her own night clothes, and/or a bathrobe
5. Assists with grooming, such as shaving and makeup
6. Emphasizes the client's strengths
7. Treats the client with patience and understanding (the client often appears to be manipulative and demanding)

NDx: ACTIVITY INTOLERANCE
- The nurse identifies factors contributing to fatigue
  1. Anemia
     a. Treats with iron, folic acid, and/or vitamin supplements
     b. Assesses the client for drug-related blood loss, such as that caused by salicylate therapy, by testing the stool for occult blood
  2. Muscle atrophy, treated with a daily exercise program
  3. Inadequate rest, treated with a quiet environment and a warm beverage before bed
- The nurse teaches the principles of energy conservation
  1. Pacing activities
  2. Setting priorities
  3. Allowing rest periods
  4. Obtaining assistance when possible and delegating to family and friends

NDx: PAIN
- The nurse administers drug therapy, as ordered
  1. Salicylates
     a. The daily dosage is 3 to 6 g.
     b. Toxicity is manifested by tinnitus; other side effects include nausea, vomiting, and ulcers.
     c. Give with meals or a snack.
     d. The drug may interfere with clotting ability; the client needs observation for abnormal bleeding and bruising.
  2. Nonsteroidal anti-inflammatory drugs (NSAID), which may cause retention of fluids and sodium and require observation of the client for hypertension, changes in renal function, and fluid retention
  3. Steroids (systemic)
     a. Prednisone (Deltasone) is commonly given methylprednisolone (Solu-Medrol) may be

L

given intravenously for acute
exacerbations.
  b. Complications include diabetes mellitus,
     infection, hypertension, osteoporosis, and
     glaucoma.
  c. Observe for cushingoid changes (moon-face,
     acne, etc.).
4. Antineoplastic agents
  a. Agents include cyclophosphamide (Cytoxan),
     azathioprine (Imuran), and methotrexate.
  b. Monitor the client for pancytopenia,
     gastrointestinal distress, and hepatic toxicity.
5. Antimalarial infective agents
  a. Agents include hydroxychloroquine
     (Plaquenil) and chloroquine.
  b. They are given in conjunction with NSAIDs.
  c. The client needs monitoring for
     gastrointestinal distress.

Discharge Planning
- The nurse provides the client/family education
  1. Protection of the skin (see "Impaired Skin
     Integrity")
  2. Importance of monitoring for fever (the first sign
     of exacerbation)
  3. Importance of joint protection and energy
     conservation
  4. Importance of follow-up visits with the
     physician(s)
  5. Use of the Lupus Foundation as a resource
  6. Drug information, as needed

For more information on lupus erythematosus, see
*Medical-Surgical Nursing: A Nursing Process
Approach,* **pp. 700–704.**

Lyme Disease

- Lyme disease is transmitted by infected deer ticks.

- The disease can be prevented by avoiding heavily wooded areas or those with thick underbrush, wearing long-sleeved tops and long pants, and using an insect repellent on skin and clothes when in an area where infected ticks are likely to be found.

- The disease is manifested by a spreading circular rash, malaise, fever, chills, swollen glands, headache, and muscle and/or joint aches.

- Cardiac symptoms may include low-grade heart block, bradycardia, tachycardia, chest pains, and/or syncope.

- Neurologic manifestations include meningitis, cranial neuropathy, and/or encephalitis.

- Lyme disease is treated with oral antibiotics such as doxycycline (Vibramycin), tetracycline (Achromycin), and amoxicillin (Amoxil); intravenous cefotaxime (Claforan); or pencillin G (Bicillin C-R), which may alleviate arthritic, cardiac and neurologic manifestations.

- Testing for Lyme disease should not be done until 4 to 6 weeks after being bitten by a tick because testing is not reliable before that time.

For more information on Lyme disease, see *Medical-Surgical Nursing: A Nursing Process Approach,* **p. 710.**

Lymphadenopathy

- Lymphadenopathy is a swelling or enlargement of one or more lymph nodes.
- Lymphadenopathy can result from infection, inflammation, or neoplasms.
- Common causes of bacterial infections are streptococcal or staphylococcal organisms.
- Viral infections occur with influenza, measles, and/or mononucleosis.
- Lymphadenopathy also occurs with neoplasms such as Hodgkin's disease and leukemia.

For more information on lymphadenopathy, see *Medical-Surgical Nursing: A Nursing Process Approach,* **p. 2229.**

Lymphangitis

- Lymphangitis is an inflammation of the peripheral lymphatic channels or vessels.
- Lymphangitis is usually caused by infection with beta-hemolytic streptococci; infection enters body from a break in the skin.
- Other causes include influenza, tuberculosis, and septicemia.
- Lymphangitis is characterized by
  1. Red streaks that extend up the arm and/or leg,

outlining the course of the lymphatics as they
drain
2. Enlarged, red, and tender lymph nodes
- Interventions include
1. Rest
2. Immobilization of the affected part
3. Local heat application
4. Elevation of the extremity
5. Antibiotics

For more information on lymphangitis, see *Medical-Surgical Nursing: A Nursing Process Approach*, **p. 2228.**

For more information on lymphangitis, see *Medical-Surgical Nursing: A Nursing Process Approach*, **p. 2228.**

L

Lymphedema

- Lymphedema is a swelling of soft tissues due to an increase in lymph.
- Two types of lymphedema are
1. *Primary*, which results from abnormal development of the lymph vessels
2. *Secondary*, which occurs as a result of obstruction or destruction of normal lymphatic channels
- Causes include radiation, trauma or excision of lymph pathways, inflammation, parasitic invasion, and/or malignant disease.
- Clinical manifestations include
1. Elephantine distribution of limb swelling
2. Failure of the skin over the dorsum of the toes or fingers to tent when pinched
- Conservative treatment management includes
1. Elevating the affected limb

2. Compression therapy with elastic wraps or pneumatic compression devices
- Surgical treatment is seldom employed.

For more information on lymphedema, see *Medical-Surgical Nursing: A Nursing Process Approach*, **pp. 2228–2229.**

Malabsorption Syndrome

- Malabsorption syndrome is associated with a variety of disorders and intestinal surgical procedures in which one or multiple nutrients are not digested or absorbed.
- Physiologic mechanisms limit absorption because of one or more abnormalities.
  1. Bile salt deficiencies
  2. Enzyme deficiencies
  3. Bacteria
  4. Disruption of the mucosal lining of the small intestine
  5. Alteration in lymphatic or vascular circulation
  6. Decreased gastric or intestinal surface area
- Interventions focus on avoiding dietary substances that aggravate malabsorption and supplementing nutrients and surgical or nonsurgical management of the primary causative disease.

For more information on malabsorption syndrome, see *Medical-Surgical Nursing: A Nursing Process Approach*, **pp. 1409–1410.**

Mastoiditis

- Mastoiditis is a secondary disorder resulting from an untreated or inadequately treated chronic or acute otitis media.
- *Chronic* mastoiditis occurs when an acute infection is superimposed over a chronic infection that has invaded the mastoid cells, often secondary to cholesteatoma production.
- Clinical manifestations include swelling behind the ear and pain with minimal movement of the tragus, pinna, and/or head.
- Otoscopic examination reveals a reddened, dull, thick, immobile tympanic membrane with or without perforation, low-grade fever, malaise, and anorexia.
- Treatment includes antibiotics and/or surgical removal of the infected tissue, such as a *tympanoplasty*, or a simple or modified radical *mastoidectomy*.
- Complications of surgery include damage to the abducens and facial nerves (cranial nerves VI and VII, respectively), meningitis, brain abscess, chronic purulent otitis media, and wound infection.

M

For more information on mastoiditis, see *Medical-Surgical Nursing: A Nursing Process Approach,* pp. 1115–1116.

Melanoma, Ocular

- Melanoma of the eye is a unilateral tumor that occurs most frequently in the choroid.
- Symptoms are not readily obvious, and the lesion may be found during a routine eye exam.

- The problem is manifested by blurred vision, changes in visual acuity, increased intraocular pressure, change in color of the iris, and sudden change in peripheral vision.
- Treatment includes
  1. *Enucleation* (removal of the entire eyeball) and insertion of a ball implant to maintain conformity of the eye until a prosthesis is fitted (approximately 1 month)
  2. Radiation therapy
     a. Complications include radiation tumor vasculopathy, radiation retinopathy, and cataract formation.
     b. Cycloplegic eyedrops (Cyclogyl) and an antibiotic-steroid combination (neomycin sulfate, polymyxin B sulfate, dexamethasone) are ordered.
- Nursing management includes
  1. Closely monitoring the client for hemorrhage, reporting any change in vital signs and/or the presence of bright red drainage on the dressing to the physician
  2. Teaching the client strategies to compensate for loss of vision
     a. A scanning (turning head side to side) type of vision must is used.
     b. Judging distances and depth perception are altered.
  3. Cleaning the eye, generally by rinsing the eye socket with an irrigating solution daily and the artificial eye only with warm water or saline

For more information on ocular melanoma, see *Medical-Surgical Nursing: A Nursing Process Approach,* **pp. 1069–1072.**

Meniere's Syndrome

OVERVIEW

- Meniere's syndrome, also called *endolymphatic hydrops*, refers to dilation of the endolymphatic system, either by overproduction or decreased reabsorption of endolymphatic fluid.

COLLABORATIVE MANAGEMENT

Assessment

- The nurse records the client's
  1. History of viral and bacterial infections
  2. Allergies, especially to environmental antigens
  3. Exposure to drugs and/or chemicals
- The nurse assesses for
  1. Duration, intensity, and time between episodes of the classic triad of symptoms
     a. Tinnitus, a continuous, low-pitched roar or a humming sound, is present much of the time but worsens just before and during a severe attack.
     b. Unilateral sensorineural hearing loss, initially for low-frequency tones, worsens to include all levels after repeated episodes. Permanent hearing loss develops as the number of attacks increases.
     c. Vertigo, described as periods of whirling that might cause the client to fall to the ground, may be so intense that even while lying down, the client holds the bed or ground in an attempt to prevent the whirling. The severe vertigo usually lasts only 3 to 4 hours and is followed by a sense of dizziness.
  2. Presence of a feeling of fullness in the ear before an attack
  3. Nausea and vomiting
  4. Nystagmus (rapid eye movements)
  5. Severe headache
  6. Stress
  7. Powerlessness

Planning and Implementation

NDx: POTENTIAL FOR INJURY

- The nurse
  1. Collaborates with the client to develop strategies to cope with vertigo

399

a. The client determines factors that warn of an impending attack.
b. The client lies down in a quiet, calm, stress-free environment.
c. The client uses slow head movements.

2. Teaches dietary changes such as salt and fluid restriction
3. Teaches the importance of smoking cessation
4. Administers nicotinic acid, as ordered, which is useful for its vasodilator effect
5. Administers antihistamines, as ordered, such as diphenhydramamine (Benedryl) and dimenhydrinate (Dramamine)
6. Administers antiemetics, as ordered, such as chlorpromazine (Thorazine), droperidol (Inapsine), and trimethobenzamide (Tigan)
7. Administers diazepam (Valium), as ordered, to calm the anxious client and help control vertigo, nausea, and vomiting

Surgical Management

- Surgical treatment is controversial because the remaining hearing in the affected ear is sacrificed.

- *Labyrinthectomy* involves the resection of the vestibular nerve or total removal of the labyrinth.

- An endolymphatic drainage and shunt may be performed early in the course of the disease to relieve vertigo.

- The nurse provides routine preoperative care.

- The nurse provides postoperative care, which varies depending on the type of surgical procedure

1. Keeps the dressing clean and dry
2. Speaks to the side of the unaffected ear
3. Performs frequent neurologic assessments if a cranial surgical approach was used
4. Keeps the side rails up at all times; assists the client to ambulate until vertigo is relieved
5. Administers antivertiginous and antiemetic drugs, as ordered

NDx: SENSORY/PERCEPTUAL ALTERATION (AUDITORY)

- See Hearing Loss.

Discharge Planning

- The nurse

1. Identifies and suggests corrections for hazards in the home prior to discharge
2. Ensures that the client can use assistive devices such as a cane or walker if vertigo is present

3. Refers the client to a local support group
4. Provides drug information as needed

For more information on Meniere's syndrome, see *Medical-Surgical Nursing: A Nursing Process Approach,* **pp. 1123–1126.**

Meningitis

OVERVIEW

• Meningitis is an inflammation of the arachnoid and pia mater (leptomeninges) of the brain and spinal cord).

• Bacterial meningitis occurs most frequently; viral meningitis is usually self-limiting.

COLLABORATIVE MANAGEMENT

Assessment

• The nurse records the client's
  1. Signs and symptoms
  2. Progression of symptoms
  3. Factors that aggravate and relieve symptoms
  4. Past medical history, including information about viral or respiratory diseases; head trauma; ear, nose, and/or sinus infection; heart disease; diabetes mellitus; cancer; immunosuppressive therapy; neurologic surgery and/or procedures
  5. Exposure to communicable disease

• The nurse assesses for
  1. Level of consciousness, orientation, cognition, memory
  2. Pupil size and reaction to light, photophobia, nystagmus, abnormal eye movement
  3. Motor strength
  4. Severity of headache
  5. Nuchal rigidity: positive Kernig's sign and Brudzinski reflex
  6. Dysfunction of cranial nerves I, III, IV, VI, and VIII

7. Nausea, vomiting
8. Fever, chills
9. Generalized aches and pains
10. Seizure activity
11. Syndrome of inappropriate antidiuretic hormone (SIADH) production
12. Fluid and electrolyte imbalance, particularly hyponatremia
13. Changes in color and temperature of extremities
14. Presence of all peripheral pulses
15. Abnormal bleeding

Planning and Implementation

NDx: ALTERED CEREBRAL AND PERIPHERAL TISSUE PERFUSION

• The nurse performs a neurologic assessment a minimum of every 4 hours or more often if clinically indicated
1. Verbal response, orientation
2. Eye opening, pupil size and reaction to light
3. Motor response
4. Cranial nerves, with particular attention to cranial nerves I, III, IV, VI, and VIII
• The nurse
1. Avoids flexion of the client's neck as this may cause severe pain
2. Elevates the head of the bed 30 to 45 degrees
3. Performs a vascular assessment (circulation, especially to hands, may be compromised from septic emboli)
   a. Checks the color of nail beds
   b. Checks peripheral pulses; notifies the physician immediately if absent
• The nurse administers drug therapy, as ordered
1. Bacterial meningitis
   a. Broad-spectrum antibiotics (ampicillin) are administered until Gram stain results are available.
   b. Penicillin G is used to treat *pneumococci, meningococci,* and *streptococci* organisms.
   c. Gentamicin is used to treat *Klebsiella, Pseudomonas,* and *Proteus* organisms.
   d. Chloramphenicol is used to treat *Hemophilus influenzae.*
   e. Antibiotics are begun within 2 to 4 hours, and the nurse monitors for allergic reactions.
   f. Isolation precautions are in effect only for the first 24 to 48 hours after the start of antibiotics.
2. Viral meningitis
   a. The disease is generally self-limiting.

b. Isolation precautions are usually taken for urine and stool only and depend on the associated viral disease.

NDx: PAIN

- The nurse
  1. Administers analgesics such as acetaminophen or narcotics such as codeine, as ordered
  2. Provides frequent position changes, moist heat, and back rubs
  3. Maintains a dark, quiet environment
  4. Plans client care activities to allow for periods of uninterrupted rest
  5. Restricts visitors

NDx: POTENTIAL FOR INJURY

- The nurse
  1. Implements seizure precautions
  2. Keeps the side rails up at all times and the bed in a low position
  3. Keeps oxygen and suction apparatus at the bedside
  4. Records seizure activity
     a. Description of event
     b. Length of event
     c. Head and eye deviations
     d. Intervention to treat seizure
     e. Postictal status

M

Discharge Planning

- Most clients are discharged with few neurologic problems.

- The nurse provides drug information, including the importance of taking all medications until the supply is completely depleted.

- Family and other close contacts of the client with meningococcal or *H. influenzae* meningitis may be required to take rifampin (rifamycin) as a preventive measure. Side effects include orange-colored urine, permanent orange discoloration of contact lenses, and interference with the effectiveness of birth control pills.

For more information on meningitis, see *Medical-Surgical Nursing: A Nursing Process Approach,* **pp. 897–902.**

Metabolic Acidosis

OVERVIEW

- Metabolic acidosis is characterized by a low pH, low bicarbonate level, normal carbon dioxide partial pressure, normal oxygen tension, elevated serum potassium level, elevated serum chloride level, and elevated anion gap.
- Common causes include
  1. Overproduction of hydrogen ions
     a. Diabetic ketoacidosis
     b. Starvation
     c. Heavy skeletal muscle exercise
     d. Fever
     e. Hypoxia, ischemia
     f. Ethanol, methanol, and/or ethylene glycol intoxication
     g. Salicylate intoxication
  2. Underelimination of hydrogen ions (renal failure)
  3. Underproduction of bicarbonate ions (decreased pancreatic and hepatic functions)
  4. Overelimination of bicarbonate ions
     a. Diarrhea
     b. Dehydration
     c. Buffering of organic acids

COLLABORATIVE MANAGEMENT

Assessment

- The nurse records the client's
  1. Age
  2. Use of prescribed and over-the-counter medications, especially those containing aspirin or alcohol
  3. Current and past medical history
     a. Respiratory problems
     b. Renal failure
     c. Diabetes mellitus
     d. Pancreatitis
     e. Persistent diarrhea
     f. Fever
  4. Diet history
  5. Behavior and/or personality changes
- The nurse assesses for

1. Central nervous system changes
   a. Lethargy, confusion, stupor
   b. Reduced attention span
2. Neuromuscular changes
   a. Hyporeflexia
   b. Skeletal muscle weakness
   c. Flaccid paralysis
3. Cardiac changes
   a. Delayed electrical conduction
      (1) Bradycardia
      (2) Tall T waves
      (3) Widened QRS complex
      (4) Prolonged PR interval
   b. Hypotension
   c. Thready peripheral pulses
4. Respiratory changes
   a. Kussmaul's respiration (respirations deep, rapid, and not under voluntary control)
   b. Difficulty talking or eating because of the energy expended on these respiratory efforts
5. Integumentary changes (warm, flushed, dry)

Planning and Implementation

- Metabolic acidosis is managed by treating the underlying cause of the acid imbalance.

M

For more information on metabolic acidosis, see *Medical-Surgical Nursing: A Nursing Process Approach,* **pp. 337–340.**

Metabolic Alkalosis

OVERVIEW

- Metabolic alkalosis is characterized by a high pH, elevated bicarbonate (above 28 mEq/L), normal oxygen tension, rising carbon dioxide partial pressure, reduced serum potassium level, reduced serum calcium level, and reduced serum chloride level.

- Common causes include
  1. Increase of base components
     a. Oral ingestion of antacids
     b. Milk-alkali syndrome
     c. Blood transfusion
     d. Sodium bicarbonate given to correct metabolic acidosis
     e. Total parenteral nutrition (TPN)
     f. Excess Ringer's lactate
  2. Decrease of acid components
     a. Prolonged vomiting
     b. Nasogastric suctioning
     c. Cushing's syndrome
     d. Bartter's syndrome
     e. Hyperaldosteronism
     f. Use of thiazide diuretics

COLLABORATIVE MANAGEMENT

Assessment

- The nurse records the client's
  1. Age
  2. Use of prescribed and over-the-counter medications
     a. Antacids
     b. Diuretics
     c. Antihypertensive agents
     d. Products containing aspirin or other salicylates
  3. Current and past medical history
     a. Nausea and vomiting
     b. Fever
     c. Severe pain
     d. Excessive licorice ingestion
     e. Problems with respirations
  4. Urinary output, including the frequency and quantity
  5. Actual fluid intake over the previous 24 hours
  6. Recent weight loss
  7. Disturbance in sleep pattern or insomnia
- The nurse assesses for
  1. Central nervous system changes
     a. Memory changes
     b. Changes in the ability to concentrate
     c. Anxiety, irritability
     d. Tetany, seizures
     e. Positive Chvostek's sign
     f. Positive Trousseau's sign
     g. Paresthesia

2. Neuromuscular changes
   a. Hyperreflexia
   b. Muscle cramping and twitching
   c. Skeletal muscle weakness
3. Cardiac changes
   a. Increased heart rate
   b. Normal or low blood pressure
   c. Increased digitalis toxicity
4. Respiratory changes (decreased respiratory effort associated with skeletal muscle weakness)

Planning and Implementation

NDx: ALTERED THOUGHT PROCESSES

- The nurse
  1. Performs neurologic checks every 4 hours
     a. Level of consciousness
     b. Orientation
     c. Past and recent memory
     d. Ability to concentrate and other cognitive functions
  2. Administers medications, as ordered, to treat underlying cause, such as discontinuing diuretics, administering antiemetics, and administering specific agents to restore fluid, electrolyte, and acid-base balance
  3. Maintains a hazard-free environment
  4. Implements seizure precautions
  5. Orients the client to time and place with every interaction
  6. Places large clocks and calendars where the client can see them
  7. Ensures that the client who needs adaptive-assistive devices such as glasses or a hearing aid wears them
  8. Reduces environmental stimuli
  9. Ambulates the client with assistance
  10. Maintains the bed in a low position with the side rails up
  11. Assesses the need for a chest or jacket restraint; strictly adheres to facility policy regarding the use of restraints

NDx: POTENTIAL FROM INJURY

- See interventions 3–11 from "Altered Thought Processes."

Discharge Planning

- The nurse
  1. Instructs the client/family about the pathologic

condition and the treatment for the chronic underlying problem that leads to the development of alkalosis

2. Reviews signs and symptoms of alkalosis

For more information on metabolic alkalosis, see *Medical-Surgical Nursing: A Nursing Process Approach,* **pp. 351–352.**

Mitral Insufficiency/ Regurgitation

- Mitral insufficiency is a pathologic process that occurs from thickening of the mitral valve in the left heart.
- The fibrotic and calcific changes cause the valve to fail to close completely, allowing backflow of blood from the left ventricle into the left atrium during ventricular systole.
- During diastole, regurgitant output is returned from the left atrium to the left ventricle, in addition to the normal blood amount, increasing the volume of blood to be ejected during systole.
- Rheumatic heart disease is the predominant etiologic factor, usually coexisting with mitral stenosis.
- Signs and symptoms include
  1. Fatigue
  2. Dyspnea on exertion
  3. Orthopnea
  4. Palpitations
  5. Atrial tachycardia
  6. Neck vein distention
  7. Pitting edema
  8. High-pitched, holosystolic murmur

• The reparative surgical procedure is mitral annuloplasty, which is performed during cardiopulmonary bypass surgery; mitral valve leaflets and annulus are reconstructed to narrow the valve orifice.

• The postoperative client requires lifetime anticoagulation therapy to prevent thrombus formation on the valve.

• For preoperative and postoperative care, see care of the client undergoing a coronary artery bypass grafting procedure under Coronary Artery Disease.

For more information on mitral insufficiency/ regurgitation, see *Medical-Surgical Nursing: A Nursing Process Approach,* **pp. 2171–2178.**

M

Mitral Stenosis

• Mitral stenosis is the thickening of the mitral valve by fibrosis and calcification.

• Valve leaflets fuse together, becoming stiff; the chordae tendinae contract and shorten; the valvular orifice narrows, preventing normal blood flow from the left atrium to the left ventricle; and as a result, the left atrial pressure rises, the left ventricle dilates, pulmonary artery pressures increase, and the right ventricle hypertrophies.

• Pulmonary congestion and right-sided heart failure occur.

• Rheumatic fever is most often the cause of mitral stenosis.

• Nonrheumatic causes include atrial myxoma, calcium accumulation, and thrombus formation.

- Signs and symptoms include
    1. Fatigue
    2. Dyspnea on exertion
    3. Orthopnea
    4. Paroxysmal nocturnal dyspnea
    5. Hemoptysis
    6. Hepatomegaly
    7. Neck vein distention
    8. Pitting edema
    9. Atrial fibrillation
    10. Rumbling, apical diastolic murmur

- *Mitral commissurotomy*, the procedure of choice for pure mitral stenosis, is performed during cardiopulmonary bypass surgery by incising the fused commissures, widening the orifice.

- *Mitral valve replacement* is indicated if the leaflets are calcified and immobile; the valve is excised during cardiopulmonary bypass surgery, and a new valve is sutured into place.

- The postoperative client requires lifetime anticoagulant therapy to prevent thrombus formation on the valve.

- For preoperative and postoperative care, see care of the client undergoing a coronary artery bypass grafting procedure under Coronary Artery Disease.

For more information on mitral stenosis, see *Medical-Surgical Nursing: A Nursing Process Approach*, **pp. 2171–2178.**

Mitral Valve Prolapse

- Mitral valve prolapse occurs due to mitral valve leaflet enlargement, prolapsing into the left atrium during systole.
- Mitral valve prolapse is usually benign but may progress to a stage of pronounced mitral regurgitation.

- The etiology is associated with endocarditis, myocarditis, and acute or chronic rheumatic heart disease.
- A familial occurrence is well established.
- Signs and symptoms include
  1. Atypical chest pain
  2. Dizziness and syncope
  3. Palpitations
  4. Atrial tachycardia
  5. Ventricular tachycardia
  6. Nonejection systolic click
- Valve replacement surgery is indicated only when pronounced mitral regurgitation follows.

For more information on mitral valve prolapse, see *Medical-Surgical Nursing: A Nursing Process Approach*, **pp. 2172–2178.**

M

Mononucleosis

- Mononucleosis is an acute, infectious, systemic process caused by the *Epstein-Barr* virus.
- The disease is common in the adolescent to young adult population between the ages of 15 and 25 years.
- Mononucleosis is mildly contagious and is spread by close intimate contact; the incubation period is 2 to 6 weeks after exposure.
- Clinical manifestations include sore throat, fever, chills, diaphoresis, malaise or fatigue, headache, generalized aches and pains, tender lymphadenopathy, and anorexia.
- Symptoms last about 2 weeks, and fatigue can persist for several months.
- Physical examination reveals generalized

lymphadenopathy; a grayish-white exudate on the tonsils; pharyngeal inflammation and swelling; a red, raised rash on the trunk and extremities; abdominal discomfort; splenomegaly; hepatomegaly; and jaundice.

- Symptomatic relief includes
  1. Saline throat gargles
  2. Aspirin for fever, headaches, pain, and myalgias
  3. Bed rest for the first 3 to 5 days and while febrile
- Client/family teaching includes
  1. Prevention of infection spread
  2. Avoidance of heavy lifting, intense exercise, or contact sports for 4 to 6 weeks
  3. Avoidance of alcoholic beverages
  4. Seeking medical intervention for abdominal pain to rule out spleen rupture

For more information on mononucleosis, see *Medical-Surgical Nursing: A Nursing Process Approach*, **pp. 1972–1973.**

Multiple Myeloma

- Multiple myeloma is a malignant condition in which a clone of transformed plasma cells proliferates in bone marrow.

- Essentially, an excess number of abnormal plasma cells infiltrates the bone marrow and develops into tumors, ultimately destroying bone; they then invade lymph nodes, liver, spleen, and kidneys.

- The onset of multiple myeloma is generally slow and insidious, and most clients remain asymptomatic until the disease is somewhat advanced.

- Clinical manifestations include
  1. Skeletal pain, especially in the pelvis, spine, and ribs

2. Weakness and fatigue
3. Recurrent infections
4. Osteoporosis and hypercalcemia related to destruction of bone
5. Spinal cord compression and paraplegia
6. Pathologic fractures
7. Anemia, thrombocytopenia, and granulocytopenia
8. Renal failure (occurs in approximately 20% of the clients)

- Treatment of multiple myeloma includes

1. Systemic chemotherapy with melphalan (Alkeran), which is often given with corticosteroids and cyclophosphamide
2. Supportive care
   a. Hydration (approximately 3 to 4 L/day) helps to offset the potential problems of hypercalcemia and proteinuria.
   b. Intravenous sodium chloride and furosemide (Lasix) or other potent diuretics help to increase renal excretion of calcium.
3. Encouraging the client to ambulate to slow down bone resorption
4. Promptly recognizing and treating low back pain and the development of symptoms in the lower extremities, which may indicate impending spinal cord compression and are treated with surgery or radiation to prevent paraplegia
5. Teaching the client to recognize symptoms of infection so that infections can be treated early and efficiently
6. Blood transfusions required for anemia
7. Pain control with analgesics
8. Orthopedic supports, local radiation, and relaxation techniques

M

For more information on multiple myeloma, see *Medical-Surgical Nursing: A Nursing Process Approach,* **pp. 669–670.**

Multiple Sclerosis

OVERVIEW

- Multiple sclerosis (MS) is a progressive degenerative disease that affects the myelin sheath and conduction pathway of the central nervous system.
- MS is one of the leading causes of disability in persons 20 to 40 years of age.
- The three types are
  1. Classic, with exacerbations followed by remission
  2. Progressive, with absence of periods of remission
  3. Combined, which begins with classic presentation and at some point converts to a progressive course

COLLABORATIVE MANAGEMENT

Assessment

- The nurse assesses for
  1. Progression of symptoms (often the client reports noticing symptoms several years previously but they disappeared and medical attention was not sought)
  2. Factors that aggravate symptoms
     a. Stress
     b. Fatigue
     c. Overexertion
     d. Temperature extremes
     e. Hot shower or bath
  3. Personality or behavior changes (the nurse verifies this information with family or friends of the client)
  4. Changes in neurologic status
     a. Vision: acuity, visual fields, blurred vision, diplopia, scotoma, nystagmus
     b. Motor: weakness, fatigue, stiffness of legs, flexor spasms, increased deep-tendon reflexes, clonus, positive Babinski's reflex, absent abdominal reflexes
     c. Cerebellar: ataxic gait, tinnitus, vertigo
     d. Cranial nerve: hearing loss, facial weakness, swallowing difficulties
     e. Speech pattern: dysarthria; slow, scanning speech
     f. Sensation: hypalgesia, paresthesia, facial pain
     g. Changes in mental status (late in the disease

process): memory loss, decreased ability to perform calculations, inattention

5. Changes in bowel and bladder function
6. Changes in sexuality: impotence, frigidity
7. Apathy, emotional lability, and depression
8. Body image disturbance

Planning and Implementation

NDx: SENSORY/PERCEPTUAL ALTERATION

- The nurse
  1. Applies an eye patch to relieve diplopia and switches the eye patch every few hours
  2. Teaches scanning techniques to compensate for peripheral vision deficits
  3. Provides a hazard-free and standardized environment
  4. Tests the temperature of the water before bathing (teaches the client to do this at home before placing hands in hot water)
  5. Administers carbamazepine (Tegretal) or acetaminophen (Tylenol) for pain and paresthesia

NDx: IMPAIRED PHYSICAL MOBILITY; TOTAL SELF-CARE DEFICIT

- Due to weakness and fatigue the client requires more time to complete activities of daily living (ADL).

- The nurse teaches, in collaboration with physical and occupational therapy,
  1. Exercise program to strengthen and stretch muscles
  2. Ambulation as tolerated, with assistive devices as appropriate such as a cane, walker, or electric (Amigo) cart
  3. How to use assistive-adaptive devices to help the client remain independent in ADL

NDx: BODY IMAGE DISTURBANCE; ALTERED ROLE PERFORMANCE

- The nurse
  1. Encourages the client to remain independent in ADLs for as long as possible
  2. Encourages the client to maintain work and social activities
  3. Refers the client for vocational counseling, if necessary
  4. Encourages the client to ventilate feelings of frustration and/or anger

NDx: KNOWLEDGE DEFICIT

- The nurse teaches information about drug therapy
  1. Adrenocorticotropic hormone (ACTH) and

corticosteroids (prednisone, dexamethasone) used
to reduce edema and inflammatory response

   a. Observe for adverse effects, including
      hyponatremia or hypernatremia, fluid
      retention, and pedal edema; congestive heart
      failure and hypertension; gastric ulceration;
      hyperglycemia; increased risk of infection;
      and/or personality changes.
   b. Monitor fluid and electrolytes.
   c. The client takes dietary or supplemental
      potassium.
   d. Observe for gastrointestinal bleeding (blood in
      stool, abdominal pain).

2. Immunosuppressive therapy with a combination
   of cyclophosphamide (Cytoxan) and ACTH

   a. The client recognizes that alopecia occurs 4 to
      5 weeks after initiation of therapy; hair growth
      returns in 2 to 3 months.
   b. The nurse observes for side effects, which
      include nausea, vomiting, anorexia, and
      hemorrhagic cystitis; gives antiemetics; checks
      urine for blood; monitors strict intake and
      output; forces fluids; and weighs the client
      daily.

Discharge Planning

- The nurse
   1. Ensures that the client can correctly use all
      adaptive-assistive devices ordered for home use
   2. Provides drug information, as needed
   3. Provides the name of a resource person to call to
      answer questions
   4. Teaches an exercise program in collaboration
      with physical and occupational therapy

      a. ADL and the use of adaptive equipment
      b. Strengthening and stretching exercises
      c. Positioning techniques

   5. Reviews the established bowel and bladder
      program
   6. Refers the client to a support group

For more information on multiple sclerosis, see
*Medical-Surgical Nursing: A Nursing Process
Approach,* **pp. 906–910.**

Muscular Dystrophy, Progressive

- There are five types of muscular dystrophy (MD) frequently seen in adults

1. *Duchenne*
   a. Sex-linked recessive variety seen in males
   b. Manifested by symmetric pelvic and shoulder girdle weakness, waddling gait, cardiac involvement, and possible mental retardation
   c. Death from respiratory or cardiac failure usually occurring in the second or third decade

2. *Becker*
   a. Sex-linked recessive variety also seen exclusively in males
   b. Manifested by wasting of pelvic and shoulder muscles and normal cardiac and mental function; slowly progressive; inability to walk seen 25 years after onset
   c. Normal life span

3. *Limb-girdle*
   a. Usually autosomal dominant and can occur in either sex
   b. Manifested by upper-extremity and neck muscles and lower-extremity and hip muscle weakness; severe disability within 10 to 20 years
   c. Shortened life span by 10 to 20 years

4. *Facioscapulohumeral* or Landouzy-Dejerine
   a. Autosomal dominant and seen in either sex
   b. Manifested by facial and shoulder girdle muscle involvement
   c. Normal life span

5. *Myotonic*
   a. Autosomal dominant and seen in either sex
   b. Manifested by muscle atrophy with multiple organ involvement (heart, lungs, smooth muscles, and endocrine system)
   c. Gradual progression if onset in adulthood

- Management and nursing care is supportive. (Also see Rehabilitation.)

For more information on muscular dystrophy, see *Medical-Surgical Nursing: A Nursing Process Approach,* **pp. 775–776.**

Myasthenia Gravis

OVERVIEW
- Myasthenia gravis (MG) is a chronic, neuromuscular, autoimmune disease that involves a decrease in the number and effectiveness of acetylcholine (ACh) receptors at the neuromuscular junction.

COLLABORATIVE MANAGEMENT
Assessment
- The nurse records the client's
  1. Rapid onset of fatigue
  2. Muscular weakness that increases on exertion or as the day wears on and improves with rest (with a temporary increase in weakness sometimes noted after vaccination, menstruation, and exposure to extremes in environmental temperature)
  3. Inability to perform activities of daily living (ADLs)
  4. Ptosis, diplopia
  5. Respiratory distress
  6. Choking, dysphagia
  7. Weakness of voice
  8. Difficulty holding head up
  9. Paresthesia or aching in weakened muscles

- The nurse assesses for
  1. Progressive paresis of affected muscle groups that is resolved by rest, at least in part
  2. Symptoms related to involvement of the levator palpebrae or extraocular muscles
     a. Ocular palsies
     b. Ptosis
     c. Diplopia
     d. Weak or incomplete eye closure
  3. Involvement of muscles for facial expression, chewing, and speech
     a. The client's smile may turn into a snarl.
     b. The jaw hangs.
     c. Difficulty chewing and swallowing may lead to severe nutritional deficits.
  4. Proximal limb weakness; client has difficulty climbing stairs, lifting heavy objects, and/or raising arms overhead
  5. Mild or severe neck weakness
  6. Difficulty sustaining a sitting and/or walking posture
  7. Respiratory distress
  8. Bowel and bladder incontinence
  9. Weakness of the pelvic and shoulder girdles (seen in Eaton-Lambert syndrome, a special form of MG often observed in combination with small cell carcinoma of the lung)
  10. Body image disturbance
  11. Feelings of loss, fear, helplessness, and grief
  12. Usual coping methods

M

Planning and Implementation

NDx: INEFFECTIVE AIRWAY CLEARANCE; INEFFECTIVE BREATHING PATTERN; IMPAIRED GAS EXCHANGE

- The nurse
  1. Performs a respiratory assessment at least every 8 hours
  2. Monitors for respiratory distress: dyspnea, shortness of breath, air hunger, confusion
  3. Assesses tidal volume and vital capacity every 2 to 4 hours
  4. Encourages the client to turn, cough, and deep breathe every 2 hours
  5. Monitors arterial blood gases as the client's condition indicates
  6. Performs chest physiotherapy, including postural drainage, percussion, and vibration
  7. Has intubation equipment readily available

Nonsurgical Management

- The nurse
  1. Assesses motor strength before and after periods of activity
  2. Provides assistance with mobilization as necessary
  3. Teaches the client to plan activities early in the day or during the energy peaks that follow the administration of medications
  4. Plans rest periods for the client to avoid excessive fatigue
  5. Performs active and passive range-of-motion (ROM) exercises
  6. Uses heel and elbow protectors as needed
  7. Assesses the need for an eggcrate or alternating pressure mattress
  8. Recognizes that medications MUST be given on time to maintain blood levels
  9. Administers anticholinesterase drugs such as neostigmine, pyridostigmine (Mestinon), or ambenonium (Mytelase), as ordered, to increase the response of muscles to nerve impulses, thus improving strength
     a. The drug is given with a small amount of food to minimize gastrointestinal (GI) side effects; meals are provided 45 minutes to 1 hour after taking medication.
     b. Drugs containing magnesium, morphine or its derivatives, curare, quinine, quinidine, procainamide, hypnotics, and sedatives are avoided because they may increase weakness.
  10. Avoids antibiotics such as neomycin, kanamycin, streptomycin, polymyxin B, and certain tetracyclines that have been shown to increase myasthenic symptoms
  11. Recognizes that edrophonium produces a temporary improvement in myasthenic crisis but no improvement or a worsening of symptoms in cholinergic crisis
  12. Administers corticosteroids, such as prednisone (Deltasone), used in conjunction with anticholinesterase drugs; worsening of symptoms may be seen for the first 7 to 10 days
  13. Observes for side effects of corticosteroids, such as electrolyte imbalance, weight gain, acne, GI upset, and hyperglycemia
  14. Administers immunosuppressives with drugs

420

such as azathioprine (Imuran), methotrexate (Mexate), and cyclophosphamide (Cytoxan), as ordered, which have resulted in some clinical improvement

• Plasmapheresis is a method by which autoantibodies are removed from the plasma. Immunosuppressive drugs are administered concurrently to decrease the formation of additional antibodies. Nursing management includes maintaining the intravenous line or shunt, monitoring vital signs, and assessing neurologic signs.

• The nurse observes for myasthenic crisis, an exacerbation of the myasthenic symptoms caused by undermedication with anticholinergic drugs

1. Increased pulse and respiration
2. Rise in blood pressure
3. Anoxia, cyanosis
4. Bowel and bladder incontinence
5. Decreased urinary output
6. Absence of cough and swallow reflex

• The nurse monitors for respiratory compromise; anticholinesterase drugs may be withheld.

• The nurse observes for cholinergic crisis, an acute exacerbation of muscle weakness caused by overmedication with cholinergic (anticholinesterase) drugs

1. Nausea, vomiting, diarrhea
2. Abdominal cramps
3. Blurred vision
4. Pallor
5. Facial muscle twitching
6. Pupillary miosis
7. Hypotension

Surgical Management

• Thymectomy is an alternative method of treatment.
• The nurse provides preoperative care

1. Provides routine preoperative care
2. Administers pyridostigmine (Mestinon), as ordered, to keep the client stable throughout surgery
3. Gives steroids before surgery but tapers them postoperatively

• The nurse provides postoperative care

1. Monitors the client in the intensive care unit
2. Provides routine postoperative care
3. Observes for signs of pneumothorax or hemothorax, such as chest pain, sudden shortness of breath, diminished or absent breath sounds, and restlessness or a change in vital signs

4. Provides routine chest tube care
5. Observes for signs and symptoms of wound infection

NDx: Total Self-Care Deficit

- The nurse
  1. Assesses the client's ability to perform ADLs to establish his or her abilities and limitations
  2. Encourages the client to perform activities as independently as possible; provides assistance as needed
  3. Plans activities to follow the administration of medication to maximize independence and successful attempts at self-care
  4. Documents and monitors the client's response to or tolerance of activity
  5. Collaborates with physical and occupational therapy to identify the need for adaptive-assistive devices

NDx: Potential for Injury; Sensory/Perceptual Alterations

- The nurse
  1. Assesses cranial nerves III, IV, VI, and VII to determine deficits and abilities
  2. Provides orientation to the surroundings and explains the need for assistance with ADLs and mobility if the client has visual impairments
  3. Applies artificial tears to the client's eyes to keep the corneas moist and free from abrasion
  4. Alternates patches on each eye to treat diplopia

NDx: Impaired Verbal Communication

- The nurse
  1. Assesses cranial nerves V, VII, IX, X, and XII to determine the client's ability to communicate
  2. Instructs the client to speak slowly; attempts to lip read; repeats information to verify that it is correct
  3. Collaborates with the speech therapist to develop a communication system that the client can use, such as eye blinking, use of flash cards, and/or a word board

NDx: Altered Nutrition: Less Than Body Requirements

- The nurse
  1. Weighs the client daily
  2. Maintains a calorie count
  3. Assesses the client's gag reflex and ability to chew and swallow without undue fatigue or aspiration
  4. Provides frequent oral hygiene

5. Obtains a dietary consultation to identify food preferences and dislikes
6. Provides small, frequent meals and high-calorie snacks
7. Administers anticholinesterase medications 45 minutes to 1 hour before meals, as ordered
8. Observes the client for choking, nasal regurgitation, and aspiration
9. Gives tube feedings, if necessary

NDx: Body Image Disturbance; Self-Esteem Disturbance; Anticipatory Grieving

- The nurse
  1. Establishes a trusting and therapeutic relationship with the client/family by listening, providing emotional support, and just "being there" for them
  2. Reinforces the client's abilities
  3. Keeps the client/family informed of progress
  4. Encourages the client/family to talk about the future

Discharge Planning

- The nurse
  1. Identifies and suggests correction of hazards in the home prior to discharge
  2. Ensures that the client can correctly use all assistive-adaptive devices ordered for home use
  3. Provides drug information, including informing the client to avoid such medications as morphine, quinine, quinidine, procainamide, mycin-type antibiotics, and drugs containing magnesium

M

- The nurse emphasizes specific points concerning the disease process
  1. Its episodic nature
  2. Factors that predispose the client to exacerbation, such as infection, stress, surgery, and hard physical exercise
  3. Symptoms of myasthenic crisis and cholinergic crisis
  4. Life-style adaptations that may be indicated, such as avoiding heat (sauna, sunbathing), crowds, overeating, and erratic changes in sleep habits

For more information on myasthenia gravis, see *Medical-Surgical Nursing: A Nursing Process Approach,* **pp. 968–980.**

Nasal Fracture

- A nasal fracture commonly occurs from minor injuries received during falls and sports or from violence or motor vehicle trauma.
- Bone or cartilage displacement can cause airway obstruction and cosmetic deformity.
- Assessment includes deviation of the nose to one side, and/or malaligned bridge, and drainage of blood or clear fluid (CSF).
- Treatment includes
  1. Simple, closed reduction with local anesthesia (the treatment of choice)
  2. Rhinoplasty, or surgical reconstruction, for severe fractures
- Postoperative assessment includes
  1. Checking for edema, bleeding, increased swallowing of blood
  2. Maintaining the client in a semi-Fowler's position
  3. Applying ice to the nose and cool compresses to the eyes and face
- The client is instructed to
  1. Avoid the Valsalva maneuver
  2. Use laxatives or stool softeners
  3. Avoid aspirin
  4. Take the full antibiotic prescription

For more information on nasal fracture, see *Medical-Surgical Nursing: A Nursing Process Approach*, **p. 1955.**

Nasal Polyp

- Nasal polyps are benign grapelike clusters of mucous membrane and loose connective tissue.
- Nasal polyps occur bilaterally.
- If polyps are very large, airway obstruction can occur.
- Nasal polyps are caused by irritation to the mucosa of the nose or sinuses from allergies or infection (chronic sinusitis).
- Nasal polyps are removed surgically (*polypectomy*) with local or general anesthesia.

For more information on nasal polyps, see *Medical-Surgical Nursing: A Nursing Process Approach*, **p. 1956.**

Nasal Septal Deviation

N

- Slight deviations in the nasal septum are present in most adults and do not cause symptoms.
- Major nasal septal deviations may obstruct nasal passages and/or interfere with sinus drainage.
- *Nasoseptoplasty* or *submucous resection* (SMR) is done to straighten the septum.
- For nursing care, see Nasal Fracture.

For more information on nasal septal deviation, see *Medical-Surgical Nursing: A Nursing Process Approach*, **pp. 1954–1955.**

Nephrosclerosis

• Changes in the afferent and efferent arterioles and glomerular capillary loops of the kidney nephron cause nephrosclerosis.

• Changes include thickening of the vessel walls and narrowing of the vessel lumen, resulting in decreased renal blood flow and interstitial tissue changes.

• Ischemia and fibrosis develop over time.

• Nephrosclerosis is associated with benign essential hypertension or malignant hypertension, atherosclerosis, and diabetes mellitus.

• Control of blood pressure and preserving renal function are goals of treatment, which includes antihypertensive agents.

For more information on nephrosclerosis, see *Medical-Surgical Nursing: A Nursing Process Approach*, **pp. 1855–1856.**

Nephrotic Syndrome

• Nephrotic syndrome is a clinical entity occurring as a consequence of severe proteinuria.

• Causes include diseases that alter the glomerular membrane, allowing the loss of protein in the urine
   1. Primary glomerular disease
   2. Neoplastic disease
   3. Multisystem disease
   4. Exposure to viral, bacterial, or fungal pathogens

- The primary feature of the disorder is severe proteinuria (greater than 3.5 g/day).
- Other features include
  1. Hypoalbuminemia
  2. Hyperlipidemia
  3. Edema
  4. Renal vein thrombosis
  5. Thromboembolytic phenomena
- Nephrotic syndrome may progress to end-stage renal disease.
- Treatment varies depending on the specifics of glomerulopathy
  1. Immunologic processes may respond to steroids or cytotoxic agents.
  2. If the glomerular filtration rate is decreased, dietary protein will be decreased.
  3. Mild diuretics and dietary sodium restrictions are prescribed to control edema and hypertension.

For more information on nephrotic syndrome, see *Medical-Surgical Nursing: A Nursing Process Approach*, **p. 1855.**

N

The Nursing Process

OVERVIEW

- The nursing process provides the framework for nursing practice; it is the organized, comprehensive, and systematic approach used by nurses to meet the health care needs of the client.
- The nursing process is used to
  1. Collect information about the client
  2. Identify client problems
  3. Specify plans for solutions to the problems

4. Implement nursing actions
5. Evaluate the effectiveness of the actions taken to resolve the identified problems

• The client can be an individual, family, group, community or society.

• Steps of the nursing process are interrelated; once the process is begun, it is continuous or cyclic.

FIVE STEPS OF THE NURSING PROCESS

Assessment

• Assessment is the systematic method of collecting data about the client for the purpose of identifying actual and potential problems.

• *Subjective* data are not directly observable or measurable by persons other than the person to whom the data relate.

• *Objective* data are observable pieces of information about the client that are measurable and are gathered by the nurse or other members of the health team.

• The nurse
   1. Recalls that the approach to the client and family greatly affects the amount and quality of the information received during an interview to collect data
   2. Does not ask a series of routine questions and answers; an interview should flow in a natural progression, with cues that the client provides used to elicit further information
   3. Provides privacy during the interview
   4. Assesses factors such as lighting, temperature, background noise, and odors that can distract the client
   5. Plans the interview with consideration of the client's physical and emotional state

• Observation involves the use of the senses of sight, hearing, smell, and touch to elicit additional information.

• The nurse
   1. Observes the client's general appearance, facial expressions, posture, body gestures, movements, and gait to validate findings from the interview
   2. Observes the interactions of the client with family and significant others

• The nurse uses four techniques to collect data during a physical examination
   1. *Inspection*, which refers to the visual examination of the client

2. *Palpation*, which is the use of touch to examine the client's body and to determine characteristics of body structures under the skin
3. *Percussion*, which involves tapping of a body surface with a finger or fingers to produce sounds
4. *Auscultation*, which is the act of listening for sounds produced by organs in the body either directly with the ear or indirectly with a stethoscope

• Records such as the medical history, laboratory data, and previous medical records provide additional information for the assessment phase of the nursing process.

• Consultation with other members of the health care team (e.g., the physician, social worker, community health nurse) is an excellent way to obtain supplemental information about the client.

Analysis: Problem Identification (Nursing Diagnosis)

• The nurse summarizes the data that have been collected, organizes the data into a logical framework, and analyzes and draws conclusions from the data to determine what health problems the client may have.

• Client findings are compared with normal parameters.

• The nurse categorizes the client's problems as *potential*, requiring prevention, or *actual*, those being managed, requiring intervention, and/or requiring further investigation.

• Problems may be physiologic, psychologic, and/or sociologic.

• A *nursing diagnosis* is a conclusion about the client that indicates the need for nursing care.

• A nursing diagnosis is a clinical diagnosis made by a professional nurse that describes actual or potential health problems that the nurse, by virtue of her or his education and experience, is capable and licensed to treat.

• A nursing diagnosis is not a diagnostic test, equipment for implementation of medical therapy, or problem experienced by the nurse while caring for the client; it identifies the client's response to illness.

• A nursing diagnosis statement consists of two parts

1. Actual or potential problem of the client (indicates what needs to change)
2. Probable cause/etiology and/or risk factors (reflects the environmental, psychologic, sociologic, physiologic, and/or spiritual factors

thought to be related or contributing to the problem).

- Goals are established with the client/family after priorities are established.

Planning

- A *goal* is a desired client behavior to meet the individual's optimal level of wellness (also referred to as the long-term goal)

- *Expected outcomes* are interim or sequential steps needed to reach the goal (may be used interchangeably with *short-term goal*).

- Goals should be realistic in terms of the client's potential for achievement and the nurse's ability to help the client achieve them.

- Anyone caring for the client should be able to determine whether the goals have been achieved.

- After goals have been determined, strategies to accomplish these behaviors are developed.

- The nurse

1. Records these strategies in the client care plan
2. Includes information about prescribed nursing actions that correspond to the client's preferences, problems, priorities, complications to be prevented, and expected outcomes
3. Develops a plan that is comprehensive and incorporates interventions performed by other members of the health care team
4. Recognizes that the care plan serves as a communication vehicle to inform health care team members about the client's problems
5. Revises the care plan as new data indicate a need for modification
6. Identifies nursing orders that are interventions or actions designed to assist the client in achieving outcomes

   a. Consistent with the therapeutic plan of health care
   b. Based on scientific rationale
   c. Specific for the individual client
   d. Use the teaching-learning process

- The nurse determines what resources are necessary to implement the actions after planning the interventions.

- The nurse establishes mechanisms to determine goal achievement and the effectiveness of nursing interventions before actions are implemented.

Implementation

- The actual carrying out of the specific, individualized care plan is the implementation step of the nursing process.
- Selection of appropriate nursing interventions is based on

  1. Characteristics of the nursing diagnosis
  2. Research knowledge associated with the intervention
  3. Greatest possibility of success
  4. The client's acceptance of the intervention
  5. Least amount of risk and discomfort for the client
  6. Capability of the nurse

- Actions that are implemented may be

  1. Independent (activities performed by the nurse without a physician's order)
  2. Collaborative (refer to carrying out the physician's orders by using sound nursing judgment and working with other health team members to produce a specific outcome)

- The nurse documents the client's status to

  1. Provide evidence of goal achievement
  2. Summarize the client's reactions
  3. Provide guidance and direction for continued interventions
  4. Meet the legal perspective of "if it was not documented, it was not done"

Evaluation

- Evaluation is an intellectual activity that completes the nursing process by indicating the degree to which the nursing diagnosis, plans, and actions have been successful.
- Evaluation is used to detect omissions that occurred during the assessment, analysis, planning, and implementation phases of the nursing process.
- Outcome evaluation may be one or a combination of the following

  1. The client responded as expected and the problem is resolved; no further action is needed.
  2. The problem has not been resolved; expected outcomes have been accomplished but the overall goal has not been achieved; re-evaluation will continue.
  3. Little evidence is available to show that the problem has been resolved; reassessment and replanning are needed

4. There is a new problem; assessment, planning, and implementation of an additional plan of action are needed to resolve the problem

For more information on the nursing process, see *Medical-Surgical Nursing: A Nursing Process Approach,* **pp. 22–33.**

Obesity

- Obesity is defined as more than a 20% increase in body weight for height and body build standards of ideal weight.
- Obesity results when caloric intake is greater than metabolic demands.
- There are multiple causes of obesity, including heredity, individual body build and metabolism, the presence of fat cells, and psychosocial factors.
- Traditional management combines dieting, exercise, psychologic support, and behavior modification; short-term appetite-suppressant drugs may be required.
- Clients who do not respond to traditional measures may be considered for surgical procedures aimed at allowing for permanent weight reduction.
- Treatments include jaw wiring to reduce food intake drastically; lipectomy to excise subcutaneous fat; and other surgical interventions aimed at permanent weight reduction, including gastric bypass, gastroplasty (gastric stapling), and jejunoileal bypass.
- Criteria for surgery typically include massive or morbid obesity (e.g., more than two times ideal weight) that has not responded to traditional weight-reduction methods; absence of cardiac, kidney, or inflammatory bowel disease; emotional stability and a commitment to comply with postoperative care; and age less than 50 years.
- The nurse provides postoperative instructions to the client following *jejunoileal bypass*
    1. The occurrence of diarrhea with resultant potassium loss

2. Potential complications, such as polyarthritis, malnutrition, renal failure, renal calculi, cholelithiasis, hepatic dysfunction, and cirrhosis
3. For excessive weight loss, inadequate weight loss, or severe complications, a possible revision of the bypass

● The nurse provides postoperative instructions to the client following *gastric bypass* and *gastroplasty*
   1. The need for a nasogastric tube for at least 3 days after surgery (this tube should not be repositioned, which could cause disruption of the suture line)
   2. When liquids are started, only 1-oz amounts for consumption, with the liquids advanced from water to clear liquids, as tolerated
   3. Signs and symptoms of intolerance such as nausea, vomiting, or discomfort
   4. The need to take liquid or chewable vitamins daily
   5. The need to drink high-protein liquids to promote healing

For more information on obesity, see *Medical-Surgical Nursing: A Nursing Process Approach*, **pp. 1401–1402.**

Occupational Pulmonary Disease

● There are several occupational pulmonary diseases.
● *Pneumoconiosis* refers to chronic respiratory diseases related to occupation or environmental exposure.
● *Acute occupational diseases* include
   1. *Byssinosis*, a pulmonary disease of textile workers

caused by excess inhalation of certain vegetable fibers and characterized by chest tightness, coughing, weakness, and dyspnea, especially prominent on the first day back to work following an absence
2. *Toxic pneumonitis*, caused by excess exposure to irritant gases such as ammonia, sulfur dioxide, ozone, and nitrogen dioxide, which cause inflammation or edema of respiratory system
- *Chronic occupational diseases* include
    1. *Silicosis*, a chronic fibrosing disease of the lungs caused by excess inhalation of free crystalline silica dust over a long period. Hazardous exposure includes mines and quarries, foundries, tunneling, sandblasting, pottery making, stone masonry, and the manufacture of glass, tile, and bricks. The disease is characterized by the formation of selective nodules in the pulmonary parenchyma accompanied by massive fibrosis. Clients experience dyspnea on exertion and marked reduction in lung volumes.
    2. *Asbestosis*, diffuse interstitial fibrosis with diffuse pleural thickening and diaphragmatic calcification caused by exposure to asbestos. At risk are asbestos miners and millers and building trade and shipyard workers, including loggers, insulation workers, pipe fitters, steam fitters, sheet metal workers, and welders. Restrictive ventilatory defects result, and frequent respiratory infections are common
    3. *Talcosis*, a fibrosis occurring after years of exposure to high concentrations of talc dust in the production of paints, ceramics, asphalt, roofing materials, cosmetics, and rubber goods
    4. *Pneumoconiosis and chronic bronchitis,* caused by coal workers' chronic excess exposure to coal dust
    5. *Berylliosis*, caused by exposure to beryllium in an operation in which metals are heated to fumes or machined to dust; higher likelihood of progression of advanced irreversible diseases

- Preventive measures include wearing special masks and adequate ventilation.

- Interventions are based on the fact that restrictive pulmonary disease is present (deficits in chest wall compliance, vital capacity, and total lung volume).

- Oxygen therapy is indicated for the hypoxemic client.

- Respiratory therapy treatments to promote sputum clearance are essential.

For more information on occupational pulmonary diseases, see *Medical-Surgical Nursing: Nursing Process Approach*, **pp. 2054–2055.**

Orchitis

- Orchitis is an acute testicular inflammation, caused by trauma or the direct spread of bacteria through the urethra or from an infection elsewhere in the body.
- Orchitis usually occurs along with an epididymis infection.
- Orchitis can be a unilateral or bilateral, with the latter increasing the risk for infertility.
- Clinical manifestations include
    1. Scrotal pain
    2. Scrotal edema
    3. Nausea and vomiting
    4. Pain radiating to the inguinal canal
- Treatment measures include
    1. Bed rest with scrotal elevation
    2. Ice application
    3. Analgesia
    4. Antibiotics

For more information on orchitis, see *Medical-Surgical Nursing: A Nursing Process Approach*, **p. 1770.**

Osteomalacia

OVERVIEW

- Osteomalacia is a metabolic disease in which there is a defect in the mineralization of bone as a result of vitamin D deficiency.

COLLABORATIVE MANAGEMENT

Assessment

- The nurse records the client's
  1. Age
  2. Exposure to sunlight
  3. Skin pigmentation
  4. Dietary habits
  5. Current medical problems and prescribed and over-the-counter medications
  6. History of fracture(s) and when the fracture occurred
- The nurse assesses for
  1. Muscle weakness in the lower extremities, which may progress to a waddling and unsteady gait
  2. Bone pain and muscle cramps
  3. Bone tenderness
  4. Skeletal malalignment, such as long-bone bowing or spinal deformity
  5. Indications of hypocalcemia or hypophosphatemia
  6. Anxiety regarding the suspected diagnosis or possible occurrence of fracture or deformity

Planning and Implementation

NDx: POTENTIAL FOR INJURY

- The nurse
  1. Administers vitamin D; provides the client with information about the correct dosage and side effects of the medication
  2. Encourages increased dietary intake of vitamin D through dietary intake, sun exposure, and drug supplementation
  3. Teaches the client to avoid alcohol and caffeine

NDx: IMPAIRED PHYSICAL MOBILITY

- The nurse
  1. Teaches exercises to strengthen the abdominal and back muscles to improve posture and provide

support for the spine (in collaboration with physical therapy)

2. Teaches abdominal isometrics, deep breathing, and pectoral stretching to increase pulmonary capacity
3. Encourages extremity exercises
   a. Isometric
   b. Resistive
   c. Active range of motion (ROM) to improve joint mobility and increase muscle tone
4. Encourages daily walking, both slow and fast, and bicycling
5. Teaches the client to avoid recreational activities that could cause vertebral compression, such as bowling and horseback riding

NDx: PAIN
- The nurse
  1. Administers analgesics, narcotics, and nonnarcotics for the acute phase of the disease, as ordered
  2. Administers muscle relaxants to ease the discomfort of muscle spasms, as ordered
  3. Administers anti-inflammatory agents, as ordered, for pain and spinal nerve root inflammation
  4. Applies a back brace to immobilize the spine during the acute phase and to provide spinal column support (because many clients tolerate these devices poorly, the nurse carefully ensures proper fit and assesses client tolerance, in collaboration with physical therapy)

- If known, the underlying cause of the disease, such as malabsorption or chronic renal failure, is treated.

Discharge Planning

- Recovery is usually complete if the diagnosis is made before severe fractures and deformity occur.

- The client is most often discharged to the home setting and assessed periodically to ensure compliance with therapy.

For more information on osteomalacia, see *Medical-Surgical Nursing: A Nursing Process Approach,* **pp. 745–748.**

Osteomyelitis

OVERVIEW

- Osteomyelitis is the term used to describe any infection of the bone.

COLLABORATIVE MANAGEMENT

Assessment

- The nurse records the client's
  1. Risk factors
  2. History of drug abuse, previous infections anywhere in the body
  3. Past medical history, such as sickle cell anemia, diabetes mellitus, nonpenetrating trauma, penetrating wounds, surgical procedures, and radiation therapy
  4. Overall health status
- The nurse assesses for
  1. Fever
  2. Swelling, tenderness, and erythema around the site of infection
  3. Draining ulcers on the feet or hands
  4. Bone pain that is described as a constant, localized, pulsating sensation that intensifies with movement
  5. Anxiety and fear
  6. Impact of prolonged hospitalization or home care treatment on the client's family, work, and financial situation
  7. Impaired social interactions, secondary to isolation, depending on the type of organism involved

Planning and Implementation

NDx: POTENTIAL FOR INJURY

Nonsurgical Management

- The nurse
  1. Administers intravenous (IV) antibiotic(s) specific for the involved organism(s) for 4 to 6 weeks (may require up to 3 months of oral antibiotics)
  2. Administers ciprofloxacin (Cipro), a potent oral antibiotic used as an alternative to IV drug therapy (the client is cautioned not to take antacids as they decrease absorption of the antibiotic)

3. Implements drainage precautions for all open wounds
4. Covers the wound and uses strict aseptic technique when changing dressings

- Wounds may be managed through the window of a cast, which must remain dry during dressing or irrigation procedures.

Surgical Management

- *Sequestrectomy* is performed to débride the infected bone and allow revascularization of tissue.

- *Bone grafts* are used to obliterate bone defects.

- *Bone segment transfers* are used when the infected bone is extensively resected and consist of reconstruction with microvascular bone transfers.

- *Muscle flaps* are used to treat relatively small bony defects.

- *Amputation* of the affected limb may be required if the surgical procedure is ineffective or inappropriate.

NDx: PAIN

- The nurse administers potent analgesics and nonsteroidal anti-inflammatory drugs (NSAID) such as ibuprofen (Motrin), as ordered.
- See Pain for further information.

NDx: IMPAIRED PHYSICAL MOBILITY

- The nurse
  1. Collaborates with the physical therapist to assess the need for assistive-adaptive devices
  2. Provides instruction on transfer techniques and the use of ambulatory aids
  3. Encourages strengthening and range-of-motion exercises

NDx: ALTERED (PERIPHERAL) TISSUE PERFUSION

- The nurse
  1. Assesses the extremity for neurovascular status at least every 4 hours
  2. Elevates the affected extremity on two pillows
- A hyperbaric chamber may be used to increase the flow of oxygen to the tissues to promote healing.

NDx: IMPAIRED SKIN INTEGRITY

- The nurse
  1. Observes the skin carefully for changes in color, temperature, size of lesion, and drainage
  2. Increases the client's caloric, protein, calcium, and vitamin C and D intake

439

Discharge Planning

- The nurse
  1. Arranges for a home health nurse to assist with care in the home if the client is discharged on IV antibiotics
  2. Provides a detailed plan of care at the time of discharge for clients to be transferred to a long-term-care facility or who will receive home care nursing
  3. Provides drug information
     a. Taking all medications in the correct dosage, at the right time, and by the right route
     b. What to do if a dose is missed or if complications or side effects occur
  4. Reviews dressing change information
     a. Sterile technique
     b. Proper disposal of contaminated dressings
     c. Proper handling of contaminated linen and clothing
     d. Wound or contact isolation
  5. Teaches signs and symptoms of surgical wound infection
  6. Obtains a dietary consultation to help the client select personal food preferences that are high in calories, protein, and vitamins C and D
  7. Encourages a fluid intake of 3000 mL per day

For more information on osteomyelitis, see *Medical-Surgical Nursing: A Nursing Process Approach,* **pp. 753–759.**

Osteoporosis

OVERVIEW

- Osteoporosis is an age-related metabolic disease in which bone demineralization results in decreased density and subsequent fractures, most commonly in the wrist, hip, and vertebral column.

- There are two types of osteoporosis
  1. Postmenopausal, or type I, caused by a decrease in the serum estrogen level and a consequent rapid decrease in bone mass in postmenopausal women
  2. Senile, or type II, which occurs mainly in women over 65 but also in men
- Vertebral fractures occur in both types.
- Wrist fractures are associated with postmenopausal osteoporosis; hip fractures are seen more frequently with senile osteoporosis.

COLLABORATIVE MANAGEMENT

Assessment
- The nurse records the client's
  1. Height, including any history of changes (clients often report being 2 to 3 inches shorter than they were years ago)
  2. Usual exposure to sunlight
  3. Cigarette, alcohol, and caffeine use
  4. Daily calcium and vitamin D intake
  5. Usual exercise pattern
  6. Current medical problems and prescribed and over-the-counter medications
  7. History of falls, fractures, and/or other injuries
  8. Family history of osteoporosis
- The nurse assesses for
  1. Classic dowager's hump (kyphosis of the dorsal spine) by inspection and palpation of the vertebral column
  2. Back pain after lifting, bending, or stooping
  3. Back pain that increases with palpation, particularly of the lower thoracic and lumbar vertebrae
  4. Back pain with tenderness and voluntary restriction of spinal movement, which indicates compression fracture(s), usually of T8-L3
  5. Fractures in the distal end of the radius or at the upper third of the femur
  6. Constipation, abdominal distention, and respiratory compromise from movement restriction and spinal deformity
  7. Body image disturbance, especially if the client is severely kyphotic
  8. Impaired social interactions, which may have been self-curtailed because of changes in appearance or an inability to sit in restaurants, theaters, and so forth

O

Planning and Implementation

NDx: POTENTIAL FOR INJURY

- The nurse administers drug therapy, as ordered
    1. Estrogens, calcium supplements, and vitamin D, if necessary, for prevention and treatment
    2. Sodium fluoride, used clinically or investigationally with extreme caution, with estrogen and calcium, to stimulate new bone formation and to inhibit bone loss
    3. Androgens to decrease bone resorption (may cause masculinization and/or liver disease in postmenopausal women)
    4. Calcitonin to inhibit bone loss (expensive and must be administered by injection)
- The nurse
    1. Teaches the client to increase his or her dietary intake of calcium and vitamin D
    2. Teaches the client to avoid alcohol and caffeine
    3. Teaches the client to increase dietary protein, vitamin C, and iron to promote bone healing in clients with fractures
    4. Creates a hazard-free environment, including glare-free lighting to prevent falls and fractures in clients who experience dizziness, drowsiness, and weakness caused by such drugs as diuretics, phenothiazines, and tranquilizers

NDx: IMPAIRED PHYSICAL MOBILITY

- The nurse
    1. Teaches exercises to strengthen the abdominal and back muscles to improve posture and provide support for the spine (in collaboration with physical therapy)
    2. Encourages abdominal isometrics, deep breathing, and pectoral stretching to increase pulmonary capacity
    3. Encourages extremity exercises
        a. Isometric
        b. Resistive
        c. Active range of motion to improve joint mobility and increase muscle tone
    4. Encourages daily walking, both slow and fast, and bicycling
    5. Teaches the client to avoid recreational activities that could cause vertebral compression, such as bowling and horseback riding

NDx: PAIN

- The nurse administers drug therapy, as ordered

1. Analgesics, narcotics, and nonnarcotics for the acute phase
2. Muscle relaxants to ease the discomfort of muscle spasms
3. Anti-inflammatory agents for pain and spinal nerve root inflammation

• Back braces may be used to immobilize the spine during the acute phase and to provide spinal column support. (Because elderly clients tolerate these devices poorly, the nurse carefully ensures proper fit and assesses client tolerance.)

• Surgery may be needed to reduce or alleviate pain when medications and orthotics are ineffective.

Discharge Planning

• The nurse
1. Helps the client/family to identify and correct hazards in the home prior to discharge
2. Ensures that the client can correctly use all assistive-adaptive devices ordered for home use
3. Provides a detailed plan of care at the time of discharge for clients to be transferred to a long-term-care facility
4. Teaches measures to prevent falls
   a. Situations where extra care may be required (icy or slippery walkways, unfamiliar surroundings)
   b. Use of orthotic and ambulatory aids
5. Reviews the prescribed exercise regimen (client mastery is ensured by observing correct performance on return demonstration)
6. Obtains a dietary consultation to help the client select personal food preferences high in essential nutrients
7. Provides drug information,
   a. Using sunlight exposure as a source of vitamin D
   b. Taking all medication in the correct dosage, at the right time, and by the right route
   c. What to do if a dose is missed or if complications or side-effects occur
8. Emphasizes the importance of follow-up visits with the physician(s)

For more information on osteoporosis, see *Medical-Surgical Nursing: A Nursing Process Approach,* **pp. 733–745.**

Otitis Media

OVERVIEW

- Otitis media is an infection in the middle ear that causes an inflammatory process within the mucosa.
- This inflammatory process leads to swelling and irritation of the bones, or ossicles, within the middle ear, resulting in the formation of purulent inflammatory exudate.
- Otitis media may be *acute* or *chronic*.
- *Serous* otitis media is characterized by an accumulation of sterile fluid behind the tympanic membrane, can precede or be a long-term complication of acute otitis media, and, if the fluid remains in the ear longer than 3 months, it begins to thicken, and a complication called *adhesive* otitis media results.

COLLABORATIVE MANAGEMENT

Assessment

- The nurse records the client's
  1. Recent upper respiratory tract infection
  2. Allergies affecting the upper respiratory system
  3. Episodes of otitis, the treatment prescribed, and the effectiveness of the treatment
- The nurse assesses for (for acute or chronic otitis media)
  1. Ear pain (is relieved if the tympanic membrane ruptures)
  2. Feeling of fullness in the ear
  3. Slightly retracted tympanic membrane initially; later is red, thickened, and bulging, with a loss of landmarks; exudate may be seen behind the membrane; if the disease progresses, the membrane spontaneously perforates, and pus or blood drains from the ear
  4. Conductive hearing loss
  5. Headache
  6. Malaise
  7. Fever
  8. Nausea and vomiting
  9. Slight dizziness or vertigo
- The nurse assesses for (for serous otitis media)
  1. Fullness and change in sounds within the ear
  2. Absence of pain, fever, and systemic symptoms such as malaise and nausea

3. Characteristic ground glass, amber discoloration of the tympanic membrane; impaired mobility of the membrane; clear fluid behind the membrane
4. Conductive hearing loss

Planning and Implementation

NDx: Pain

Nonsurgical Management

• Treatment is directed toward decreasing the amount of fluid in the middle ear and local inflammation.

• The nurse
1. Ensures bed rest to limit head movement and thereby decrease pain
2. Applies localized heat and occasionally the application of cold
3. Administers systemic antibiotic therapy, as ordered, such as penicillin V potassium (Pen Vee K), erythromycin (E-Mycin), cephalexin monhydrate (Keflex), and amoxicillin (Larotid)
4. Administers analgesics, as ordered, such as acetylsalicylic acid (aspirin) or acetaminophen (Tylenol) or treats severe pain with narcotics such as meperidine (Demerol)
5. Administers oral and nasal decongestants, as ordered

Surgical Management

• *Myringotomy* is the surgical procedure performed to reduce pain and when fever persists, hearing loss worsens, or the client complains of vertigo; it is usually performed with anesthesia, often in the physician's office.

• Postoperative care consists of antibiotic eardrops, such as neomycin sulfate or bacitracin.

• Care must be taken to keep the external ear and canal free from other substances while the incision is healing; the client should avoid showering and washing his or her hair.

NDx: Potential for Injury

• The nurse
1. Encourages the client to eat a balanced diet and drink plenty of fluids to supply the proper nutrients for tissue repair and production of antibodies to fight infection
2. Stresses the importance of adequate rest; nonstrenuous activities such as walking are allowed
3. Places a cotton ball coated with petroleum jelly in the client's ear to provide an effective barrier

against water if the tympanic membrane is perforated
4. Monitors for complications, including meningitis, brain abscess, or destruction of certain cranial nerves, especially the facial nerve (cranial nerve VII)

NDx: Sensory/Perceptual Alterations (Auditory)
Nonsurgical Management
• The nurse ensures that the environment is quiet and without additional distractions when giving instructions to the client and gives information in a soft voice.

• The nurse uses written information/instructions if the client is able to read.

Surgical Management
• *Tympanoplasty*, or reconstruction of the middle ear, may be done to improve the conduction hearing loss.
• The nurse provides preoperative care
  1. Administers or teaches the client how to administer antibiotic eardrops to eliminate any remaining infecting organisms
  2. Irrigates the ear to restore its normal pH with a solution of equal parts of vinegar and sterile water
• The nurse provides postoperative care
  1. Keeps the dressing clean and dry
  2. Keeps the client flat with the operative ear up for at least 12 hours
  3. Administers prophylactic antibiotics, as ordered

Discharge Planning
• The nurse instructs the client to avoid
  1. Straining when having a bowel movement
  2. People with colds
  3. Washing his or her hair, showering, and getting the head wet for 1 week
  4. Rapid head movements, bouncing, and bending over for 3 weeks
  5. Blowing the nose through both nostrils at the same time
• The nurse teaches the client/family
  1. To change the ear dressing every 24 hours as directed using aseptic technique
  2. To report excessive drainage to the physician

3. How to instill eardrops
4. Drug information, as needed

For more information on otitis media, see *Medical-Surgical Nursing: A Nursing Process Approach,* **pp. 1108–1115.**

Otosclerosis

OVERVIEW

● Otosclerosis is a disease of the labyrinthine capsule of the middle ear that results in a bony overgrowth of the tissue surrounding the ossicles.

COLLABORATIVE MANAGEMENT

Assessment

● The nurse records the client's
  1. Time of onset of hearing loss (usually begins early in adulthood but is not noticeable until middle age)
  2. Family history of otosclerosis
  3. Race, sex, and age
  4. History of ear infections
● The nurse assesses for
  1. Slowly progressive conductive hearing loss

     a. The loss is bilateral, although the progression of the disease is different in each ear, which gives the effect of one "good" ear and one "bad" ear.

     b. Hearing loss on an audiogram may be quite severe, although the client is able to discriminate the spoken word well enough for daily conversation.

c. Initial hearing loss is of the lower frequencies but progresses to all frequencies.

2. Roaring or ringing type of constant tinnitus loud enough to disturb the rest and communication abilities of the client
3. Normal tympanic membrane; occasionally the eardrum has a pinkish discoloration
4. Negative Rinne's test result (bone conduction is greater than or equal to air conduction)
5. Weber's test that reveals lateralization of the sound to the ear with the most conductive hearing loss
6. Anxiety and fear

Planning and Implementation

NDx: SENSORY/PERCEPTUAL ALTERATION (AUDITORY)

Nonsurgical Management

• The nurse initiates strategies to promote better hearing

1. Provides an environment with few distractions (background noises) when communicating
2. Validates the client's understanding of information presented by having the client repeat the instructions or give a return demonstration
3. Uses written words or computerized communication devices if the client is able to read
4. Uses flash cards with pictures if the client is unable to read

• The nurse assists the client to adjust to a hearing aid.

Surgical Management

• Surgical procedures used to correct hearing loss include a partial or complete *stapedectomy* (removal of stapes) with a prosthesis.
• The nurse provides preoperative care

1. Instructs the client to follow measures to prevent infection

a. Avoid excessive nose blowing.
b. Do not place objects in the ear canal for cleaning.
c. Do not wear a hearing aid for 2 weeks prior to surgery.

2. Reminds the client that hearing is usually worse for a period of time after the surgical procedure

• The nurse provides postoperative care

1. Administers antibiotics such as neomycin (Miciguent) prophylactically, as ordered

2. Administers analgesics for pain secondary to swelling, as ordered
3. Administers antivertiginous drugs such as meclizine hydrochloride (Antivert) and antiemetics such as droperidol (Inapsine), as ordered
4. Monitors for complications, which include complete hearing loss, prolonged vertigo, infection, and damage to cranial nerves (VII, VIII, X)

Discharge Planning

- The nurse instructs the client to avoid
  1. Persons with upper respiratory infections
  2. Showering or getting the head and wound wet
  3. Using small objects such as cotton tip applicators for cleaning the external canal
  4. Quick head movements
  5. Sneezing, coughing, and blowing the nose
  6. Straining during a bowel movement
  7. Changes in altitude

- The nurse instructs the client in the use of a hearing aid (if ordered).

For more information on otosclerosis, see *Medical-Surgical Nursing: A Nursing Process Approach,* **pp. 1116–1120.**

o

Ovarian Cancer

OVERVIEW

- Ovarian cancer is the leading cause of death from female reproductive organ malignancies.

- The most common tumor is the serous adenocarcinoma.

- Tumors grow rapidly, spread fast, and are often

bilateral with the worst prognosis of all other epithelial tumors.

• Cancer spreads by several mechanisms: direct spread to other organs in the pelvis, distal spread through lymphatic drainage, and peritoneal seeding.

COLLABORATIVE MANAGEMENT

• The nurse records the client's
   1. Family history of ovarian cancer
   2. History of breast, bowel, or endometrial cancer
   3. Nulliparity
   4. Infertility
   5. History of dysmenorrhea or heavy bleeding
   6. Diet high in animal fat
• The nurse assesses for
   1. Abdominal pain or swelling
   2. Dyspepsia
   3. Indigestion
   4. Gas and distention
   5. Heavy menstrual flow
   6. Dysfunctional bleeding
   7. Premenstrual tension
   8. Abdominal mass

• Exploratory laparotomy is performed to diagnose and stage ovarian tumors.

• For nursing care, see Cervical Cancer and Endometrial Cancer.

• The options for treatment depend on the stage of the cancer and include
   1. Chemotherapy agents (used postoperatively for all stages, although their purpose is usually palliative for stage IV tumors)
   2. Intraperitoneal chemotherapy (involves the instillation of chemotherapy agents into the abdominal cavity)
   3. Immunotherapy (alters the immunologic response of the ovary and promotes tumor resistance)
   4. External radiation therapy (used if the tumor has invaded other organs)
   5. Total abdominal hysterectomy and bilateral salpingo-oophorectomy (the surgical procedure for all stages of ovarian cancer)
• The nurse
   1. Encourages the client to ventilate feelings about death and dying
   2. Provides information about ovarian cancer and treatment options

3. Provides encouragement and support to the client/family

For more information on ovarian cancer, see *Medical-Surgical Nursing: A Nursing Process Approach*, **pp. 1726–1728.**

Ovarian Cyst

- There are several types of ovarian cysts.
- *Follicular cysts*
    1. Follicular cysts develop in young menstruating females, are nonneoplastic, and do not grow without hormonal influences.
    2. They develop when a mature follicle fails to rupture or an immature follicle fails to reabsorb follicular fluid.
    3. The cyst is usually small (6 to 8 cm) and may be asymptomatic unless it ruptures, causing acute, severe pelvic pain, which usually resolves following bed rest and administration of mild analgesics.
    4. If the cyst does not rupture, it usually disappears in two to three menstrual cycles without medical intervention.
    5. Oral contraceptives may be prescribed for one or two menstrual cycles to depress ovulation, resulting in cyst shrinkage.
    6. Surgery is recommended only before puberty, after menopause, or when cysts are larger than 8 cm.
    7. Cystectomy (removal of cyst) is recommended instead of oophorectomy (removal of an ovary).
- *Corpus luteum cysts*
    1. Corpus luteum cysts occur after ovulation and are often associated with increased secretion of progesterone.

O

2. The cysts are small, averaging 4 cm, and are purplish-red due to hemorrhage within the corpus luteum.
3. The cysts are associated with delay in the onset of menses, and irregular or prolonged flow and may be accompanied by unilateral, low abdominal, or pelvic pain.
4. Cyst rupture may cause intraperitoneal hemorrhage.
5. Corpus luteum cysts may disappear in one or two menstrual cycles or with suppression of ovulation.
6. The treatment is the same as for follicular cysts.

- *Theca-lutein cysts*
  1. Theca-lutein cysts, the least common of the functional ovarian cysts, are associated with hydatidiform mole and develop as a result of prolonged stimulation of the ovaries by excessive amounts of human chorionic gonadotropin (hCG).
  2. The cysts regress spontaneously within 3 months with the removal of the molar pregnancy or source of the excess hCG.

- *Polycystic ovary* (Stein-Leventhal) *syndrome*
  1. The syndrome results when elevated levels of luteinizing hormone cause hyperstimulation of the ovaries; endometrial hyperplasia or carcinoma may result.
  2. The typical client is obese, is hirsute, has irregular menses, and may be infertile due to anovulation.
  3. The best treatment is administration of oral contraceptives because of lutein production inhibition.

- Bilateral *salpingo-oophorectomy* (removal of both tubes and ovaries) and *hysterectomy* (removal of uterus) are advised for women over 35 who no longer desire childbearing.

- Women desiring fertility can be treated with drugs to stimulate ovulation.

For more information on ovarian cysts, see *Medical-Surgical Nursing: A Nursing Process Approach*, **pp. 1707–1708.**

Ovarian Fibroma

- Ovarian fibromas are the most common benign, solid ovarian neoplasms.
- The fibromas appear as pearly white tumors of connective tissue origin with low malignancy potential.
- Fibroma size ranges from a small nodule to masses weighing more than 50 lb; the average size is 6 cm.
- The fibromas tend to have a unilateral occurrence and on examination present with slightly irregular contour and are mobile.
- Fibromas greater than 6 cm may be associated with ascites and may cause feelings of pelvic pressure or abdominal enlargement.
- Fibromas often occur postmenopausally.
- Management is surgical removal of the tumor; oophorectomy (removal of ovary) may be performed.

For more information on ovarian fibroma, see *Medical-Surgical Nursing: A Nursing Process Approach*, **p. 1708.**

Ovarian Tumor, Epithelial

- Epithelial ovarian tumors are serous or mucinous cystadenomas that occur in women between the ages of 30 and 50.
- Serous cystadenomas usually occur bilaterally and have greater potential for malignancy than mucinous cystadenomas.

- Both tumors can be irregular and smooth, but mucinous adenomas grow to large sizes (up to 45 kg, or 100 lb).
- Management includes surgical unilateral salpingo-oophorectomy; small cystadenomas may be removed by cystectomy.

For more information on epithelial ovarian tumor, see *Medical-Surgical Nursing: A Nursing Process Approach*, **pp. 1708–1709.**

Overhydration

OVERVIEW

- Overhydration is not an actual disease but a clinical state or manifestation of a physiologic problem in which fluid intake exceeds fluid loss.
- There are two types of overhydration
  1. *Isotonic*, or hypervolemia, which occurs as a result of excess fluid in the extracellular fluid compartment (ECF) and rarely has serious consequences if mild to moderate; may result in circulatory overload and interstitial edema if severe
  2. *Hypotonic*, or water intoxication, in which all body fluid compartments experience expansion, with effects related to circulatory overload, interstitial edema, cellular edema, and specific electrolyte dilution

COLLABORATIVE MANAGEMENT
Assessment
- The nurse records the client's
  1. Age
     a. Both the very young and the elderly are more prone to fluid disturbances.

    b. The elderly are more likely to have chronic conditions that can lead to fluid imbalance and also more likely to be taking medications that influence fluid and electrolyte balance.

2. Height and weight
    a. Fluid increases are reflected in weight increases.
    b. Smaller-statured individuals are at increased risk.
    c. Changes in weight, especially sudden weight gain, have occurred.
3. Description of noticeable swelling or tightening of rings, shoes, clothes
4. Urinary output, including frequency and amount of voiding
5. Actual fluid intake and output in general and specifically during the previous 24 hours
6. Use of over-the-counter and prescribed medications, especially diuretics, antacids, laxatives, and morphine
7. Previous medical history
8. Detailed dietary history to determine approximate levels of sodium, protein, and sugar intake
9. History of any psychiatric disorder involving compulsive behavior and excessive fluid intake

- The nurse assesses for

1. Cardiovascular changes
    a. Increased pulse rate, bounding pulse
    b. Full peripheral pulses
    c. Elevated blood pressure, decreased pulse pressure
    d. Elevated central venous pressure
    e. Distended neck and hand veins
    f. Engorged venous varicosities

2. Respiratory changes
    a. Increased respiratory rate with shallow respirations
    b. Dyspnea that increases with exertion or in the supine position
    c. Moist rales or crackles on auscultation

3. Integumentary changes
    a. Pitting edema
    b. Skin pale and cool to touch

4. Neuromuscular changes
    a. Altered level of consciousness
    b. Headache
    c. Visual disturbances

d. Skeletal muscle weakness
e. Paresthesia

5. Gastrointestinal changes (increased motility)
6. Manifestations of isotonic overhydration

    a. Liver enlargement
    b. Ascites formation

7. Manifestations of hypotonic overhydration

    a. Polyuria
    b. Diarrhea
    c. Nonpitting edema
    d. Cardiac dysrhythmias associated with electrolyte dilution
    e. Projectile vomiting

Planning and Implementation

NDx: FLUID VOLUME EXCESS

- The nurse administers drug therapy, as ordered
    1. Diuretics (provided that renal failure is not the cause of the overhydration)
        a. Osmotic diuretics are used first to avoid initiating or exacerbating electrolyte disturbances.
        b. High-ceiling (loop) diuretics are given if osmotic diuretics are not effective.

- The nurse administers drug therapy, as ordered, for overhydration as a result of inappropriate or excessive secretion of antidiuretic hormone (ADH)
    1. ADH antagonizers (demeclocycline, lithium)
    2. Agents that block ADH receptors

- The nurse follows the physician's orders to treat the underlying causes of overhydration
    1. Digoxin, amrinone, or deslanoside is used to treat poor cardiac output.
    2. Dexamethasone or urea is used to treat cerebral edema.

- The nurse
    1. Recognizes that diet therapy may be of value in controlling fluid volume through restrictions of both fluids and sodium
    2. Measures intake and output
    3. Explains dietary restrictions to the client/family

- The nurse observes the client for pulmonary edema and depression of vital organ function.

NDx: INEFFECTIVE BREATHING PATTERN

- The nurse
    1. Administers bronchodilators, as ordered, to dilate

the upper and lower airways so that ventilation is not impaired
2. Avoids drugs that induce drowsiness, including diazepam (Valium) and diphenhydramine (Benadryl)
3. Administers oxygen, as ordered
4. Places the client in a semi-Fowler's position to increase ventilation to the available alveolar surfaces
5. Assesses respiratory status frequently
   a. Observes and records the rate and depth of respirations
   b. Auscultates breath sounds
   c. Examines the color of nail beds and mucous membranes
6. Encourages the client to turn, cough, and deep breathe at least every 2 hours

Discharge Planning

- The nurse
  1. Teaches the client about specific food or fluid restrictions
  2. Reviews the signs and symptoms of the specific imbalance for which the client is at risk, as well as what specific information should be reported immediately to the primary health care provider

O

P

For more information on overhydration, see *Medical-Surgical Nursing: A Nursing Process Approach,* **pp. 260–268.**

Paget's Disease

OVERVIEW

- Paget's disease is a metabolic disorder of bone remodeling, or turnover, in which increased reabsorption or loss results in bone deposits that are weak, enlarged, and disorganized.

- Three phases of the disease are
  1. *Active*, in which a prolific increase in osteoclasts causes massive bone destruction and deformity
  2. *Mixed*, in which the osteoblasts react in a compensatory manner to form new bone, and bone is disorganized and chaotic in structure
  3. *Inactive*, in which the newly formed bone becomes sclerotic and ivory hard

- Common sites include the vertebrae, the femur, the skull, the sternum, and the pelvis.

COLLABORATIVE MANAGEMENT
Assessment
- The nurse assesses for
  1. Bone pain, described as aching, deep, and aggravated by weight bearing and pressure; severe bone pain may indicate complications such as osteogenic sarcoma
  2. Back pain and headache
  3. Arthritis at the joints of affected bones
  4. Nerve impingement, particularly in the lumbosacral area of the vertebral column
  5. Posture, stance, and gait to identify gross bony deformities
  6. Flexion contracture of the hips
  7. Size and shape of the skull, which is soft, thick, and enlarged
  8. Deafness and vertigo
  9. Cranial nerve compression
  10. Warm and flushed skin
  11. Apathy, lethargy, and fatigue
  12. Pathological fractures
  13. Hyperparathyroidism and gout
  14. Congestive heart failure
  15. Ability to cope with pain and the effects of having a chronic disorder
  16. Fear associated with the potential development of bone cancer

Planning and Implementation
NDx: PAIN
- The nurse administers drug therapy, as ordered
  1. Nonsteroidal anti-inflammatory drugs (NSAID) such as ibuprofen (Motrin) and indomethacin (Indocin) given for pain
  2. Calcitonin (calcitonin-salmon [Calcimar]) effective in initiating a remission of the disease, with the usual duration of therapy as 6 months

followed by a 6-month course of etidronate disodium (EHDP) (Didronel)
3. Mithramycin (Mithracin), a potent anticarcinogen and antibiotic reserved for clients with marked hypercalcemia or severe disease with neurologic compromise
- The nurse
  1. Applies heat and massage
  2. Reviews the exercise program developed in collaboration with physical therapy
  3. Applies and teaches the application of orthotic devices for support and immobilization

NDx: Impaired Physical Mobility

- The nurse collaborates with the physical therapist to develop a structured exercise program.

- One or more *osteotomies* (bone resection) may be indicated.

NDx: Activity Intolerance

- The nurse
  1. Plans care in an organized fashion to promote rest
  2. Distributes activities throughout the day
  3. Allows the client time to nap in the afternoon and sleep uninterrupted for 8 to 10 hours at night

NDx: Body Image Disturbance

- The nurse
  1. Implements measures to promote pain reduction and improve mobility and activity tolerance to help improve the client's body image
  2. Encourages the client to verbalize her or his feelings of concern and anger and other emotions

NDx: Potential for Injury

- The nurse
  1. Notifies the physician of any client complaints of severe pain, hearing or feeling that a bone has cracked, or increased difficulty weight bearing
  2. Ensures a hazard-free environment

Discharge Planning

- The nurse
  1. Helps the client/family to identify and correct hazards in the home prior to discharge
  2. Ensures that the client can correctly use all adaptive-assistive devices ordered for home use
  3. Provides a detailed plan of care at the time of

discharge for clients to be transferred to a long-term-care facility

- Client/family education is determined by the extent of the disease.
- The nurse
  1. Provides drug information as needed
  2. Recommends nondrug pain relief measures, such as heat and massage
  3. Reviews the prescribed exercise program (ensures client mastery by observing correct performance on return demonstration)
  4. Emphasizes the importance of follow-up visits with the physician(s) and other therapists

For more information on Paget's disease, see *Medical-Surgical Nursing: A Nursing Process Approach,* **pp. 748–753.**

Pain

OVERVIEW

- Pain has both sensory and behavioral components and is strongly influenced by various physiologic, psychologic, and sociologic factors.

- One's pain threshold or sensation of pain is the amount or degree of noxious stimulus that leads an individual to interpret a sensation as painful.

- *Pain tolerance* refers to the ability of the client to endure the intensity of pain; it is more a function of psychologic and social variables than biologic characteristics.

- The factors that tend to *decrease* the threshold for and tolerance of pain include discomfort, insomnia, fatigue, anxiety, fear, anger, sadness, depression, and past experience with pain.

- Factors that tend to *increase* the threshold for and tolerance for pain are typically relief of symptoms, sleep/rest, understanding, diversion, and elevation of mood.

- *Psychogenic* or *psychosomatic* pain is pain that is believed to arise from mental and/or emotional factors.
- Pain is generally classified into three types
  1. *Acute* pain, usually temporary, of sudden onset, easily localized, and confined to the affected area (e.g., wound abscess)
  2. *Postoperative* pain, which is poorly understood and not always well managed
     a. It has a sensory component related to tissue destruction and also a major psychosocial component.
     b. Intrathoracic and upper intra-abdominal surgical approaches are generally associated with severe pain.
     c. Superficial surgery of the head and neck, chest wall, or limb are often associated with minimal pain.
  3. *Chronic* pain
     a. It affects an estimated 25% of the population and is defined as pain that persists or reoccurs for indefinite periods, usually for more than 6 months.
     b. It frequently involves deep somatic and visceral structures and is usually diffuse, poorly localized, and often difficult to describe.
     c. It is associated with cancer, connective tissue diseases, peripheral vascular diseases, musculoskeletal disorders, and posttraumatic insults.
     d. It has physiologic and psychosocial ramifications, which are influenced by the client's ability to cope, the availability of family support and social resources, and the severity of the physiologic and emotional consequences.
     e. It may interfere with activities of daily living (ADL) and personal relationships and may cause emotional and financial burdens

COLLABORATIVE MANAGEMENT

Assessment
- The nurse records
  1. Chronology of events
     a. Length of time the client has experienced pain
     b. Precipitating factors

    c. Aggravating factors
    d. Localization of pain
    e. Character and quality of pain
    f. Duration of pain
2. Adjustments in the client's life or that of the family
3. The client's beliefs about the cause of the pain and what should be done about it

- The nurse assesses for
  1. Changes in vital signs
     a. Tachycardia
     b. Increased heart rate
     c. Increased respiratory rate, tachypnea
     d. Peripheral vasoconstriction resulting in an elevation of blood pressure and cold, clammy skin
  2. Diaphoresis
  3. Restlessness, apprehension
  4. Splinting or holding painful body parts while moving
  5. Location of pain
     a. Localized (confined to site of origin)
     b. Projected (along a specific nerve or nerves)
     c. Radiating (diffuse around the site of origin, not well localized)
     d. Referred (perceived in an area distant from the site of painful stimuli)
     e. Superficial or deep
  6. Character and quality of pain
  7. Intensity of pain
  8. Pattern of pain
  9. Psychosocial factors

Planning and Implementation

NDx: PAIN

- The nurse
  1. Assesses the location, intensity, character, and quality of pain
  2. Assists the client to determine the duration and precipitating and alleviating factors
  3. Assists the client to discuss emotions associated with pain
  4. Administers an appropriate drug therapy, as ordered
     a. Codeine
     b. Hydromorphone (Dilaudid)
     c. Oxycodone (Percodan, Tylox, Percocet)
     d. Acetylsalicylic acid (aspirin)

    e. Acetaminophen (Tylenol)

    f. Nonsteroidal anti-inflammatory agents

  5. Assesses and evaluates the effectiveness of drug therapy

• Intraspinal analgesics are generally used during surgery and in the immediate postoperative period

  1. *Epidural analgesia*, the instillation of a pain-blocking agent, usually a local anesthetic or narcotic, into the epidural space, with the nurse observing for signs of complications, including infection, dislodging of the catheter, and respiratory depression

  2. *Intrathecal analgesia*, the instillation of a pain-blocking agent into the space between the arachnoid mater and pia mater of the spinal cord

• Patient-controlled analgesia (PCA) allows the client to control the dosage of analgesia received.

• PCA is achieved through the use of a PCA infusion pump, which delivers the desired amount of medication through a conventional intravenous route or via an implantable intravenous catheter inserted in subcutaneous tissue.

• Drug security with PCA is ensured through a locked syringe pump system or drug reservoir system programmed to deliver a certain amount of drug within a specified interval.

• The nurse implements methods of cutaneous stimulation, i.e., transcutaneous electrical nerve stimulation (TENS), hot and cold compresses when appropriate, as ordered. These methods may be used for acute or chronic pain.

• The nurse teaches the client that

  1. Benefits of cutaneous stimulation techniques are highly unpredictable

  2. Pain relief is generally sustained only as long as the stimulation continues

  3. Trials may be necessary to establish the desired effects

  4. Stimulation itself may aggravate preexisting pain or may produce new pain

  5. TENS involves the use of a battery-operated device capable of delivering small electrical current to the skin and underlying tissues

    a. Electrodes connected to a small box are placed over the painful sites.

    b. Voltage or current is regulated by adjusting a dial to the point at which the client perceives a prickly, pins-and-needles sensation.

    c. The client can continue to participate in ADL.
    d. The client's skin at the electrode sites may become irritated, and sites should be rotated.

- Alternative methods to relieve pain such as cognitive and behavioral strategies may be helpful (visual, auditory, or environmental distractions).

NDx: Chronic Pain
Nonsurgical Management

- The nurse
  1. Assesses the location, intensity, character, and quality of pain
  2. Assists the client to determine the duration and precipitating and alleviating factors
  3. Assists the client to discuss emotions associated with pain
  4. Encourages the client to record factors related to the onset, duration, and relief of pain
  5. Administers drug therapy, as ordered
     a. Nonnarcotic analgesics
        (1) Acetylsalicylic acid (aspirin)
        (2) Acetaminophen (Tylenol)
        (3) Nonsteroidal antiinflammatory drugs such as ibuprofen (Motrin)
        (4) Carbamazepine (Tegretol) and phenytoin (Dilantin) to treat certain neuralgias
     b. Narcotic analgesics
        (1) Meperidine (Demerol)
        (2) Codeine
        (3) Pentazocine (Talwin)
        (4) Morphine sulfate
        (5) Oxycodone (Percodan, Tylox)
        (6) Diacetylmorphine (Heroin)
        (7) Hydromorphone (Dilaudid)

- *Physical dependency* is associated with the administration of long-term narcotics; it is a physiologic adaptation of the body tissue so that continued administration of the drug is necessary for normal tissue function.

- *Drug tolerance* is characterized by a gradual resistance of the body to the effects of a narcotic, including its pain-relieving properties.

- *Addiction* is a term used to describe persistent drug craving and abuse of a drug for recreational purposes.

- *Adjuvant therapy* involves the use of medication and additional therapies such as TENS and cognitive-behavioral strategies.

- Long-acting narcotics are recommended for the management of cancer-related pain and other progressive pain syndromes.
- The nurse
    1. Monitors for side effects of narcotic analgesics (sedation, nausea, constipation, respiratory depression, urinary retention, and hypotension)
    2. Identifies the client at risk for adverse reactions to narcotic analgesics
    3. Reassures the client that frequent administration of narcotics rarely leads to addiction
    4. Educates the family and client that if physical dependence does occur with continued use of narcotics, tapering schedules will be devised to wean the client, if appropriate

- The nurse teaches the client about cognitive and behavioral strategies to help reduce the pain

    1. Imagery
    2. Relaxation
    3. Hypnosis
    4. Biofeedback
    5. Acupuncture

Surgical Management
- The purpose of surgery is to interrupt the pain pathways in situations in which pain is intractable or severely debilitating.
- *Nerve blocks* are usually indicated for pain that is confined to a specific area or nerve distribution. The procedure involves the destruction of a nerve root or roots by the use of a chemical agent such as phenol or alcohol.
- *Rhizotomy* involves the destruction of sensory nerve roots where they enter the spinal cord

P

    1. A *closed* rhizotomy is performed by inserting a percutaneous catheter to destroy the sensory nerve roots with neurolytic chemical, coagulation, or cryodestruction.
    2. *Open* rhizotomy requires a laminectomy; the nerve roots are isolated and destroyed.

- *Cordotomy* involves transection of the pain pathways at the midline portion of the spinal cord before nerve impulses ascend to the spinothalamic tract.
- The nurse provides postoperative care, including assessing the neurologic deficit and teaching the client how to protect the surgical area from harm.

Discharge Planning

- The nurse
    1. Involves the client/family in continuing health care behaviors that will relieve pain and improve psychological well-being and overall functional status.
    2. Teaches administration of drug therapy and other pain-reduction modalities

For more information on pain, see *Medical-Surgical Nursing: A Nursing Process Approach,* **pp. 107–145.**

Pancreatic Abscess

- A pancreatic abscess consists of infected, necrotic pancreatic tissue.
- Pancreatic abscess usually occurs after severe acute pancreatitis, exacerbations of chronic pancreatitis, and biliary tract surgery.
- The problem may occur as a single abscess or multiloculated abscesses resulting from extensive inflammatory necrosis of the pancreas readily invaded by infectious organisms, such as *Eschericia coli, Klebsiella, Bacteroides, Staphylococcus,* and *Proteus.*
- Temperature spikes may be as high as 104° F (40° C).
- There is 100% mortality if the abscess is not surgically drained; multiple drainage procedures are often required.
- Antibiotic therapy alone does not resolve the abscess.

For more information on pancreatic abscess, see *Medical-Surgical Nursing: A Nursing Process Approach,* **p. 1479.**

Pancreatic Carcinoma

OVERVIEW

• Pancreatic tumors are most often adenomas occurring in the exocrine portion of the pancreas.

• Pancreatic tumors are highly malignant; they originate in the epithelial cells of the pancreatic ductal system.

• Primary tumors are generally adenocarcinomas and grow in well-differentiated glandular patterns.

• Pancreatic tumors are highly metastatic, with rapid growth and spread to surrounding organs by direct extension and invasion of the lymphatic and vascular systems.

COLLABORATIVE MANAGEMENT

Assessment

• The nurse records the client's

1. Past medical history, including diabetes and pancreatitis
2. Smoking history
3. Coffee intake
4. Employment history to determine exposure to known environmental carcinogens
5. Skin color if jaundice is present
6. Ethnic group
7. Weight loss

• The nurse assesses for

1. Jaundice (yellow discoloration associated with obstruction) and pruritis (itching)
2. Clay-colored stool and dark, frothy urine
3. Enlarged gallbladder and liver
4. Firm, fixed mass in the left upper abdominal quadrant or epigastric area
5. Abdominal pain, constant dullness in the right upper quadrant or related to eating or activity
6. Referred back pain
7. Leg and/or calf pain with swelling or redness
8. Weight loss
9. Anorexia accompanied by early satiety, nausea, flatulence, and vomiting
10. Dull sound on abdominal percussion indicating ascites

Planning and Implementation

NDx: Pain

Nonsurgical Management

• The nurse provides narcotic analgesia with meperidine hydrochloride (Demerol), morphine, or hydromorphone hydrochloride (Dilaudid), as ordered; dependency is not a consideration due to the poor prognosis.

• Chemotherapy has limited success; combining agents such as fluorouarcil (5-FU) and carmustine (BCNU) has better results than single-agent chemotherapy.

• External radiation therapy to shrink pancreatic tumor cells may provide pain relief but has not increased survival rates.

• Implantation of radon seeds, in combination with systemic or intra-arterial administration of floxuridine (FUDR), has also been used.

Surgical Management

• Surgical management is the most effective management.

• The classic surgery, or *Whipple procedure*, entails extensive surgical manipulation, including resection of the proximal head of the pancreas, the duodenum, portion of the jejunum, the stomach (partial or total gastrectomy), and the gallbladder with anastamosis of the pancreatic duct (pancreatojejunostomy), the common bile duct (choledochojejunostomy), and the stomach (gastrojejunostomy) to the jejunum; the spleen may also be removed (splenectomy).

• Palliative measures to relieve obstruction such as cholecystojejunostomy may be done as a bypass procedure.

• The nurse provides routine preoperative care.

• The nurse provides intensive postoperative care and monitoring

1. Maintenance of the patency of nasogastric (NG) tube drainage to reduce gastric suture line stress and stimulation of the remaining pancreas
2. Assessment of drainage tubes for patency and drainage, undue stress or kinking, and dependent drainage position; monitoring of the suction device to maintain desired suction level
3. Assessment of drainage for color, consistency, and amount
4. Observation for fistula formation (drainage of pancreatic fluids are corrosive and irritating to the skin, and internal leakage causes peritonitis)
5. Positioning in a semi-Fowler's position to reduce suture line and anastamosis stress

6. Maintenance of fluid and electrolyte balance
7. Assessment of changes in vital signs, including decreased blood pressure and increased heart rate, decreased vascular pressures, decreased hemoglobin and hematocrit levels, and electrolyte imbalances
8. Assessment of blood glucose levels for transient hyperglycemia or hypoglycemia due to surgical manipulation of the pancreas

NDx: ALTERED NUTRITION: LESS THAN BODY REQUIREMENTS

- Enteral feeding with commercially prepared tube feeding is used while intestinal function is intact.

- A jejunostomy tube is inserted for late stages of pancreatic carcinoma; this method preferred to lessen reflux and facilitate absorption.

- Hyperalimentation by total parenteral nutrition to optimize nutrition may be used as a single measure or in combination with tube feedings; a Hickman or other type of catheter may be required for long-term use.

NDx: IMPAIRED SKIN INTEGRITY

- The nurse
  1. Clips the client's fingernails to avoid scratching of the skin as excess bile salts cause pruritis
  2. Uses soothing bath oil and avoids soap
  3. Provides emollient lotion to keep the skin soft and relieve itching
  4. Monitors drainage sites for excoriation and utilizes preventive skin barriers

Discharge Planning

- Many clients are end stage and die in the hospital or long-term-care facility.

- Client/family education is aimed at relief of symptoms and pain. See Pancreatitis, Chronic.

- The nurse emphasizes the importance of follow-up visits with the physician(s) and teaches the client to report any increase in pain and complications immediately to the physician.

For more information on pancreatic carcinoma, see *Medical-Surgical Nursing: A Nursing Process Approach*, **pp. 1474–1479.**

Pancreatic Pseudocyst

- Pancreatic pseudocysts develop as a complication of acute or chronic pancreatitis.
- Two percent of clients with pancreatitis develop pseudocysts, with a 15% mortality.
- These "false cysts" do not have an epithelial lining and are encapsulated saclike structures that form on or surround the pancreas.
- The pancreatic wall is inflamed, vascular, and fibrotic, containing large amounts of straw-colored or dark brown viscous fluid (enzyme exudate from the pancreas).
- The pseudocyst may be palpated as an epigastric mass in 50% of cases.
- The primary symptom is epigastric pain radiating to the back.
- A pseudocyst may spontaneously resolve or may rupture and cause hemorrhage.
- Surgical intervention with internal drainage is accomplished by creating an ostomy between the pseudocyst and the stomach, jejunum, or duodenum; external drainage is provided by insertion of a sump drainage tube to remove pancreatic exudate and secretions.
- Pancreatic fistulas are common postoperative complications, with skin breakdown.

For more information on pancreatic pseudocyst, see *Medical-Surgical Nursing: A Nursing Process Approach*, **p. 1479.**

Pancreatitis, Acute

OVERVIEW

- Acute pancreatitis is an inflammatory process of the pancreas resulting in autodigestion of the organ by its own enzymes, including trypsin, elastase, phospholipase A, lipase, and kallikrein.
- The extent of the inflammation and tissue destruction ranges from mild involvement, resulting in edema and inflammation, to severe, necrotizing hemorrhagic pancreatitis, characterized by diffusely bleeding pancreatic tissue with fibrosis and tissue death.
- Activation of the inflammatory process occurs after insult or injury, causing obstruction of the pancreatic duct and resulting in the production and release of pancreatic enzymes.
- Following pancreatic duct obstruction, increased pressure within the pancreas and the pancreatic ducts may cause the duct to rupture, allowing spillage of trypsin and other enzymes into the pancreas parenchymal tissue.
- Many factors can cause injury to the pancreas, including alcohol; biliary tract disease with gallstones; postoperative trauma from surgical manipulation; drug toxicities, including opiates, sulfonamides, thiazides, steroids, and oral contraceptives; and other medical diseases.

COLLABORATIVE MANAGEMENT

Assessment

- The nurse records the client's
  1. History of abdominal pain related to alcohol ingestion or high-fat meal intake
  2. Individual and family history of alcoholism, pancreatitis, and/or biliary tract disease
  3. Previous abdominal surgeries and/or diagnostic procedures
  4. Medical history, including peptic ulcer disease, renal failure, vascular disorders, hyperparathyroidism, and/or hyperlipedemia
  5. Recent viral infections
  6. Use of prescription and over-the-counter drugs
- The nurse assesses for
  1. Abdominal pain (the most frequent symptom), including a sudden onset, mid-epigastric, or left upper quadrant location with radiation to the

P

back; aggravated by a fatty meal, ingestion of a
large amount of alcohol, and/or lying in the
recumbent position
2. Weight loss, with nausea and vomiting
3. Jaundice
4. Discoloration of the abdomen and periumbilical
area (Cullen's sign)
5. Bluish discoloration of the flanks (Turner's sign)
6. Absent or decreased bowel sounds
7. Abdominal tenderness, rigidity, and guarding
8. Dull sound on abdominal percussion indicating
ascites
9. Elevated temperature with tachycardia and
decreased blood pressure

Planning and Implementation

NDx: Pain
Nonsurgical Management
- The nurse
  1. Withholds food and fluids in the acute period;
     hydration is maintained with intravenous fluids
  2. Maintains nasogastric intubation to decrease
     gastric distention and suppress pancreatic
     secretion
  3. Administers meperidine hydrochloride
     (Demerol), as ordered, the drug of choice for pain
     because it causes less incidence of spasm of the
     smooth musculature of the pancreatic ducts and
     the sphincter of Oddi
  4. Administers antacids, as ordered, to neutralize
     gastric secretions
  5. Administers histamine receptor-blocking drugs,
     as ordered, such as ranitidine (Zantac) and
     cimetidine (Tagamet), to decrease hydrochloric
     acid production
  6. Administers anticholinergics, as ordered, such as
     atropine and propantheline bromide (Pro-
     Banthine), to decrease vagal stimulation and
     decrease gastrointestinal motility

Surgical Management
- Surgical management is usually not indicated for
acute pancreatitis.
- Complications such as pancreatic pseudocyst and
abscess may require surgical drainage.

NDx: Altered Nutrition: Less Than Body Requirements
- The nurse
  1. Withholds food and fluids in the early stages of
     the disease

2. Administers total parenteral nutrition (TPN), as ordered, for severe nutritional depletion
3. Provides small, frequent, high-carbohydrate, and high-protein feedings with limited fats, when tolerated
4. Provides supplemental liquid diet preparations and vitamins and minerals to boost caloric intake, if needed

Discharge Planning

- Client/family education is aimed at preventing further episodes and preventing disease progression to chronic pancreatitis.
- The nurse
  1. Encourages alcohol abstinence to prevent further pain and extension of the inflammation and insufficiency
  2. Teaches the client to notify the physician for acute abdominal pain or symptoms of biliary tract disease, such as jaundice, clay-colored stools, and/or dark urine
  3. Emphasizes the importance of follow-up visits with the physician(s)

For more information on acute pancreatitis, see *Medical-Surgical Nursing: A Nursing Process Approach*, **pp. 1461–1469.**

P

Pancreatitis, Chronic

OVERVIEW

- Chronic pancreatitis is a progressive, destructive disease of the pancreas.
- Inflammation and fibrosis of the tissue contribute to pancreatic insufficiency and diminished organ function.

- The disease usually develops after repeated episodes of alcohol-induced acute pancreatitis, also known as *chronic calcifying* pancreatitis.
- Chronic pancreatitis is characterized by protein precipitates that plug the ducts and lead to ductal obstruction, atrophy, and dilation, causing metaplasia and ulceration, resulting in fibrosis of the pancreatic tissue.
- The pancreas becomes hard and firm due to cell atrophy and pancreatic insufficiency.
- *Chronic obstructive* pancreatitis develops from inflammation, spasm, and obstruction of the sphincter of Oddi.
- Inflammatory and sclerotic lesions develop in the head of the pancreas and around the ducts, causing an obstruction and backflow of pancreatic secretions/enzymes.
- *Pancreatic insufficiency* is characterized by the loss of exocrine function, which causes a decreased output of enzymes and bicarbonate; loss of endocrine function results in diabetes mellitus.

COLLABORATIVE MANAGEMENT

Assessment

- The nurse records the client's
  1. History of abdominal pain related to alcohol ingestion or high-fat meal intake, with specific information about alcohol intake, including time, amount, and relationship of alcohol to pain development
  2. Individual and family history of alcoholism, pancreatitis, and/or biliary tract disease
  3. Previous abdominal surgeries and/or diagnostic procedures
  4. Medical history, including peptic ulcer disease, renal failure, vascular disorders, hyperparathyroidism, and/or hyperlipedemia
  5. Recent viral infections
  6. Use of prescription or over-the-counter drugs
- The nurse assesses for
  1. Abdominal pain (major clinical manifestation)—continuous, burning, or gnawing dullness with intense and relentless exacerbations
  2. Abdominal tenderness
  3. Left upper quadrant mass, indicating a pseudocyst or abscess
  4. Dullness on percussion, indicating pancreatic ascites
  5. Steatorrhea, foul-smelling stools that may

increase in volume as pancreatic insufficiency
progresses
6. Weight loss and muscle wasting
7. Jaundice and dark urine
8. Signs and symptoms of diabetes

Planning and Implementation

NDx: CHRONIC PAIN

Nonsurgical Management

- The nurse
    1. Administers narcotic analgesia with meperidine
    hydrochloride (Demerol), as ordered, (the drug
    most often used); the client may develop a
    narcotic dependency with long-term use
    2. Administers nonnarcotic drugs, as ordered;
    pentazocine (Talwin) is also prescribed

Surgical Management

- Surgical management is not the primary intervention
for chronic pancreatitis; surgery may be indicated for
intractable pain, incapacitating pain relapses, or
complications such as pseudocyst and abscess.
- Surgical procedures include
    1. *Incision and drainage* for abscesses or
    pseudocysts
    2. *Cholecystectomy* or *choledochotomy* for
    underlying biliary tract disease
    3. *Sphincterotomy* (incision of the sphincter) for
    fibrosis
    4. *Pancreatojejunostomy* (the pancreatic duct
    opened and anastamosed to the jejunum relieving
    obstruction) to relieve pain and preserve
    pancreatic tissue and function
- For preoperative and postoperative care, see
Pancreatic Carcinoma for care of the client undergoing
Whipple procedure.

NDx: ALTERED NUTRITION: LESS THAN BODY
REQUIREMENTS

- The nurse
    1. Withholds food and fluids to avoid recurrent pain
    exacerbated by eating
    2. Administers total parenteral nutrition (TPN), as
    ordered, for severe nutritional depletion
    3. Provides small, frequent, high-carbohydrate, and
    high-protein feedings with limited fats, when
    tolerated
    4. Provides supplemental liquid diet preparations
    and vitamins and minerals to boost caloric
    intake, as needed
    5. Administers pancreatic enzyme replacement, as

ordered, such as pancreatin (Viokase) and
pancrelipase (Cotazym or Pancrease) given to aid
in digestion and absorption of fat and protein
6. Administers insulin or oral hypoglycemic agents
to control diabetes

NDx: Diarrhea

- The nurse
  1. Provides a low-fat diet to limit fat intake,
     decreasing the incidence of fatty stools
  2. Provides nutritional support with TPN, as
     ordered
  3. Administers intravenous fluids to maintain
     hydration with fat-soluble vitamin replacement,
     as ordered
  4. Cleanses the skin after each stool
  5. Applies soothing emollient or barrier protection,
     such as Sween products, to the skin to prevent
     breakdown and maintain skin integrity

Discharge Planning

- Client/family education is aimed at preventing
  further exacerbations.
- The nurse teaches the client to
  1. Avoid known precipitating factors such as
     alcohol, caffeinated beverages, and irritating foods
  2. Comply with diet instructions: bland, low-fat,
     frequent meals with avoidance of rich, fatty foods
  3. Follow written instructions and prescriptions for
     pancreatic enzyme therapy
     a. How and when to take enzymes
     b. Importance of maintaining therapy
     c. Importance of notifying the physician for
        increased steatorrhea, abdominal distention,
        cramping, and skin breakdown
  4. Follow prescribed pain management program
  5. Comply with elevated glucose management,
     including either oral hypoglycemic drugs or
     insulin injections and monitoring of blood
     glucose levels
  6. Keep follow-up visits with the physician(s)

For more information on chronic pancreatitis, see
*Medical-Surgical Nursing: A Nursing Process
Approach*, **pp. 1469–1474.**

Parkinson's Disease

OVERVIEW

- Parkinson's disease, also referred to as paralysis agitans, is a movement disorder involving the basal ganglia and substantia nigra.
- The disease is characterized by resting tremors, decreased postural reflexes, rigidity, bradykinesia, masklike facies, and slow, shuffling gait.

COLLABORATIVE MANAGEMENT

Assessment

- The nurse records the client's
    1. Time and progression of symptoms
    2. Bradykinesia, problems performing two activities at once
    3. Bowel and bladder incontinence
    4. Changes in handwriting, which typically becomes small and can be accomplished only slowly
- The nurse assesses for
    1. Rigidity, which is present early in the disease process and progresses over time
        a. Cogwheel rigidity, manifested by a rhythmic interruption of the muscles of movement
        b. Plastic rigidity, mildly restrictive movements
        c. Lead-pipe rigidity, total resistance to movement
    2. Masklike facies (wide-open, fixed, staring eyes caused by rigidity of the facial muscles)
    3. Difficulty chewing and swallowing
    4. Respiratory compromise
        a. Restricted chest wall expansion
        b. Decreased breath sounds
        c. Labored breath sounds
    5. Changes in the client's speech pattern
        a. Soft, low-pitched voice
        b. Dysarthria
        c. Echolalia (automatic repetition of what another person says)
        d. Repetition of sentences
    6. Changes in posture and gait
        a. Stooped posture with a flexed trunk
        b. Truncal rigidity
        c. Movement of the body as a unit

P

d. When standing, fingers abducted and flexed at the metacarpophalangeal joint and the wrist slightly dorsiflexed
e. When walking, arms that tend not to move and absent characteristic mannerisms such as "talking with the hands"
f. Slow and shuffling gait, with short, hesitant steps; propulsive gait (slow to initiate but accelerating almost to a trot)
g. Bradykinesia to the point at which the client is unable to move
h. Tremors at rest, absent during sleep
7. Orthostatic hypotension
8. Excessive perspiration
9. Oily skin
10. Seborrhea
11. Flushing, changes in skin texture
12. Gastrointestinal dysfunction, such as severe constipation
13. Emotional lability, depression, and paranoia

Planning and Implementation

NDx: TOTAL SELF-CARE DEFICIT
- The nurse
  1. Assesses the client's ability to perform activities of daily living (ADLs) to establish his or her abilities and limitations
  2. Encourages the client to perform activities as independently as possible; provides assistance as needed
  3. Allows sufficient time for the client to complete activities
  4. Documents and monitors the client's response to or tolerance of activity
  5. Collaborates with physical and occupational therapy to identify the need for assistive-adaptive devices

NDx: IMPAIRED PHYSICAL MOBILITY
- The nurse
  1. Collaborates with physical and occupational therapy to plan and implement an active and passive range-of-motion and muscle-stretching program
  2. Encourages the client to ambulate as tolerated, to avoid sitting for long periods of time, and to reposition the body frequently
  3. Teaches the client to perform breathing exercises
  4. Instructs the client with orthostatic hypotension

to change position slowly, especially when moving from a sitting to a standing position

- The nurse administers drug therapy, as ordered
  1. Levodopa (L-dopa), carbidopa-levodopa combination (Sinemet), or amantadine hydrochloride (Symmetrel)
  2. Biperiden (Akineton), trihexyphenidyl (Artane), and benztropine mesylate (Cogentin)

- Experimental surgical treatment consists of transplanting small pieces of the client's own adrenal gland into the caudate nucleus of the brain. The treatment is currently considered palliative.

NDx: IMPAIRED VERBAL COMMUNICATION

- The nurse
  1. Encourages the client to speak slowly and clearly and to pause and take deep breaths at appropriate intervals during each sentence
  2. Eliminates unnecessary environmental noise to maximize the listener's ability to hear and understand the client
  3. Asks the client to repeat words not understood; watches the client's lips and nonverbal expressions for cues to meaning of conversations
  4. Instructs the client to organize his or her thoughts before speaking
  5. Encourages the client to use facial expressions and gestures (if possible) to augment communication
  6. Collaborates with speech-language pathology to obtain a communication board for a client unable to communicate verbally

NDx: SELF-ESTEEM DISTURBANCE; BODY IMAGE DISTURBANCE

- The nurse
  1. Emphasizes the client's abilities or strengths and provides positive reinforcement
  2. Assists the client to set realistic goals that can be achieved
  3. Assists the client with grooming and hygiene

Discharge Planning

- The nurse identifies and suggests corrections for hazards in the home.
- The nurse teaches the client/family in collaboration with other health team members
  1. Training in ADL
  2. Structured exercise program

3. Correct use of adaptive-assistive equipment
4. Drug information as needed

For more information on Parkinson's disease, see *Medical-Surgical Nursing: A Nursing Process Approach,* **pp. 910–915.**

Pediculosis

- Pediculosis is infestation by human lice and includes *pediculosis capitis* (head lice), *pediculosis corporis* (body lice), and *pediculosis pubis* (pubic or crab lice).
- The oval-shaped lice measure approximately 2 to 4 mm in length.
- The female louse lays hundreds of eggs called *nits*, which are deposited at the base of the hair shaft.
- The most common symptom is pruritis, which may or may not be accompanied by excoriation.
- The treatment is chemical killing with agents such as lindane (Kwell) or topical malathion.
- Clothing and bed linens must be thoroughly washed in hot water.

For more information on pediculosis, see *Medical-Surgical Nursing: A Nursing Process Approach,* **pp. 1208–1209, 1792.**

Pelvic Inflammatory Disease

OVERVIEW

- Pelvic inflammatory disease (PID) is an infectious process that involves one or more pelvic structures, although the most common site is the fallopian tubes.
- PID is the leading cause of infertility.
- Acute PID is a complex disease in which organisms from the lower genital tract migrate from the endocervix through the endometrial cavity to the fallopian tubes.
- Resultant infections include endometritis, salpingitis, oophoritis, parametritis, and peritonitis, causing adhesions and strictures.
- Three sexually transmitted disease (STD) organisms most often cause PID and include *Neisseria gonorrhoeae*, *Chlamydia trachomatis*, and *Mycoplasma hominis*.
- Sexually active women with multiple partners may have increased risk.

COLLABORATIVE MANAGEMENT

Assessment

- The nurse records the client's
  1. Medical history
  2. Menstrual history
  3. Obstetrical history
  4. Sexual history
  5. Previous episodes of PID or other STDs
  6. Contraceptive use such as intrauterine devices
  7. History of reproductive surgeries
- The nurse assesses for
  1. Lower abdominal tenderness with rigidity or rebound pain
  2. Chills
  3. Fever
  4. Malaise
  5. Purulent vaginal discharge
  6. Tachycardia
  7. Dysuria
  8. Irregular vaginal bleeding
  9. Uterine or cervical tenderness on pelvic exam

P

Planning and Implementation

NDx: PAIN

Nonsurgical Management

- The nurse
  1. Provides analgesia, as ordered
  2. Provides sitz baths
  3. Applies heat to the lower back or abdomen
  4. Maintains bed rest in a semi-Fowler's position
  5. Administers antibiotic therapy, as ordered

Surgical Management

- Surgical intervention is an abdominal laparotomy to remove an abscess or pelvic mass.

Discharge Planning

- Teaching is focused on providing information about PID, including
  1. Identification of recurrences
  2. Meticulous perineal hygiene
- Treatment of the sexual partner for STDs is necessary.
- The nurse
  1. Provides counseling about complications of PID, including infertility, increased risk of ectopic pregnancy, and development of chronic pelvic pain
  2. Teaches contraceptive measures, including oral contraceptives and barrier methods
  3. Teaches life-style changes, including decreased sexual intercourse with multiple partners
  4. Emphasizes the importance of follow-up visits with the physician(s)

For more information on pelvic inflammatory disease, see *Medical-Surgical Nursing: A Nursing Process Approach*, **pp. 1787–1792.**

Peptic Ulcer Disease

OVERVIEW

- Peptic ulcer disease (PUD) occurs when there is a break in the continuity of the mucosa occurring in any part of the gastrointestinal tract that comes in contact with hydrochloric acid and pepsin.
- Histamine is released, resulting in acid production, vasodilation, and increased permeability.
- Types of peptic ulcers include
  1. *Gastric* ulcer, a break in the gastric mucosa extending to the muscularis mucosae and found in the junction of the fundus and the pylorus, with the majority of gastric ulcers occuring on the lesser curvature of the stomach near the pylorus and gastritis often surrounding the ulceration
  2. *Duodenal* ulcer, a chronic break in the duodenal mucosa extending through the muscularis mucosa that leaves a scar with healing; characterized by high gastric acid secretion (the most common type of peptic ulcer)
  3. *Stress* ulcer, an ulcer occurring after an acute medical crisis or trauma, with bleeding due to gastric erosion as the principal manifestation and multiple lesions occuring in the proximal portion of the stomach, beginning with the area of ischemia and evolving into erosions
- Complications of ulcers include
  1. *Intractable disease*
     a. Pain and discomfort recur.
     b. The client no longer responds to conservative management.
     c. Symptoms interfere with activities.
  2. *Hemorrhage*
     a. Ulcer bleeding varies from minimal to massive hematemesis, which usually indicates bleeding at the duodenojejunal junction.
     b. Melena is more common in duodenal ulcers.
  3. *Perforation*, with the gastroduodenal contents emptying through the anterior wall of the stomach or duodenum into the peritoneal cavity
  4. *Pyloric obstruction*
     a. The obstruction occurs at the pylorus.
     b. The cause is scarring, edema, and inflammation, causing vomiting.

483

COLLABORATIVE MANAGEMENT

Assessment

- The nurse records the client's
    1. Cigarette use
    2. Dietary intake, including alcohol, caffeine, other irritants, and patterns of eating
    3. Life-style, including perceived stress
    4. Use of over-the-counter drugs, such as corticosteroids and anti-inflammatory drugs
    5. Symptoms, including epigastric discomfort, abdominal tenderness, cramps, indigestion, nausea or vomiting and their onset, duration, location, and frequency, as well as aggravating and alleviating factors

- The nurse assesses for
    1. General appearance, including facial grimacing, restlessness, and/or moaning
    2. Presence of aching, burning, cramplike, and/or gnawing pain, possibly radiating to the back
    3. Relationship of pain to eating, with discomfort relieved by eating food or taking antacids and pain occuring after meals
    4. Early satiety, anorexia, and nausea
    5. Heartburn (common with duodenal ulcer)
    6. Vomiting

Planning and Implementation

NDx: PAIN

- The nurse
    1. Administers H_2 antagonists, as ordered, such as cimetidine (Tagamet), ranitidine (Zantac), famotidine (Pepcid), and nizatidine, to block gastric acid secretions
    2. Administers antacids (Maalox, Mylanta), as ordered, as buffering agents to decrease pain (given 2 hours after meals)
    3. Administers mucosal barrier fortifiers, such as sucralfate (Carafate), as ordered, to provide a protective coat preventing digestive action
    4. Administers anticholinergics, as ordered, to decrease vagal stimulation, reducing gastric motility and inhibiting gastric secretion
    5. Administers prostaglandin analogues, such as misoprostol (Cytotec), as ordered, to inhibit acid secretion and contribute to the mucosal barrier
    6. Teaches the client to avoid foods such as caffeine-containing coffee, tea, and cola and other foods that cause discomfort
    7. Teaches the client to avoid alcohol and tobacco
    8. Provides a bland diet with nonirritating foods

9. Instructs the client to avoid intense physical activity
10. Instructs the client to alter stressful work routines and employ coping and relaxation techniques

NDx: POTENTIAL FOR INJURY
Nonsurgical Management (Hemorrhage)
• A nasogastric (NG) tube is inserted to ascertain the presence of blood and to provide lavage.
• Selective arterial embolization may be utilized.
• Vasopressin is administered intravenously or intra-arterially to control hemorrhage.
• The nurse
  1. Administers intravenous (IV) fluids and/or blood products, as ordered, to maintain blood pressure
  2. Maintains the client on bed rest

Nonsurgical Management (Perforation)
• NG suction is used to drain gastric secretions.
• Fluid replacement is provided with IV fluids with the client given nothing by mouth (NPO).
• Antibiotics are administered to prevent infection, especially peritonitis.

Nonsurgical Management (Pyloric Obstruction)
• NG suction is employed to decompress the dilated stomach.
• Fluid replacement is provided with IV fluids while the client is NPO.

SURGICAL MANAGEMENT
• In *perforation*, surgery entails closure of the perforation after the escaped gastric contents have been evacuated.

P

• A *vagotomy* is done to eliminate stimulation of gastric cells and to decrease the responsiveness of parietal cells; there are three types of vagotomy procedures, including
  1. *Truncal,* in which each branch of the vagus nerve may be completely cut
  2. *Selective*, in which the vagus is partially cut to preserve the hepatic and celiac branches
  3. *Superselective*, in which the nerve is partially cut so as to denervate only the parietal cell mass, thus preserving innervation of both the antrum and the pyloric sphincter.
• Vagotomy and *pyloroplasty* involve cutting the right and left vagus nerves and widening the exit of the

pylorus, to prevent stasis and the resultant feeling of fullness, belching, and weight loss and to enhance gastric emptying.

- Simple *gastroenterostomy* permits neutralization of gastric acid by regurgitation into the stomach of alkaline duodenal contents; drainage of gastric contents diverts acid away from the ulcerated area to promote healing.
- *Antrectomy*, removal of the antrum of the stomach, reduces the acid-secreting portions of the stomach.
- *Subtotal gastrectomy* includes
    1. *Billroth I*, in which part of the distal portion of the stomach is removed, including the antrum, and anastamosed to the duodenum (gastrojejunostomy)
    2. *Billroth II*, which is an anastomosis of the stomach and proximal jejunum (gastrojejunostomy)
- The nurse provides routine preoperative care.
- The nurse provides postoperative care
    1. Provides routine postoperative care
    2. Monitors the patency of the NG tube and the type of drainage
    3. Never repositions or irrigates the NG tube
    4. Assesses for fluid and electrolyte imbalances
    5. Assesses for development of a *gastrojejunocolic fistula*, which arises from perforation of a recurrent ulceration at the gastrojejunal anastamosis site, by monitoring for
        a. Fecal vomiting
        b. Diarrhea
        c. Weight loss
        d. Anorexia
        e. Belching of fecal-smelling gas
    6. Assesses for development of *afferent loop syndrome*, which occurs when the duodenal loop is partially obstructed after a Billroth II resection, by monitoring for
        a. Painful contractions
        b. Vomiting
    7. Assesses for the development of *acute gastric dilation*, in the immediate postoperative period, which is manifested by
        a. Epigastric pain
        b. Tachycardia
        c. Hypotension
        d. Feelings of fullness, hiccups, and/or gagging
    8. Assists with the insertion of an NG tube, which

remains in place until postoperative edema subsides in afferent loop syndrome and gastric dilation

9. Administers vitamin B_{12}, folic acid, and iron preparations to prevent *problems of nutrition*, which develop from removal of the stomach, including deficiencies of vitamin B_{12}, folic acid, and iron; impaired calcium metabolism; and reduced absorption of calcium and vitamin D

10. Assesses for the development of the *dumping syndrome*, which occurs after gastric resection in which the pylorus is bypassed and is a postprandial problem secondary to the rapid entry of food into the bowel, manifested by

    a. Vertigo
    b. Tachycardia
    c. Syncope
    d. Sweating
    e. Pallor
    f. Palpitation
    g. Epigastric fullness
    h. Abdominal distention
    i. Diarrhea
    j. Abdominal cramping
    k. Nausea with occasional vomiting
    l. Borborygmi (intestinal rumbling noise caused by gas movement)

11. Assists in management of the dumping syndrome by

    a. Decreasing the amount of food taken by the client at one time
    b. Providing a high-protein, high-fat, low-carbohydrate diet
    c. Avoiding provision of liquids with meals
    d. Administering pectin in a dry powder form
    e. Placing the client in a recumbent or semirecumbent position while eating
    f. Positioning the client in a flat position after meals
    g. Administering sedatives and antispasmodics, as ordered, to delay gastric emptying

12. Assesses for the occurrence of *alkaline reflux gastritis*, which is the reflux of duodenal contents with bile acids, resulting in injury to the gastric mucosal barrier and manifested by

    a. Persistent pain
    b. Nausea and vomiting accentuated after meals
    c. Epigastric burning, partially relieved by vomiting

- *Delayed gastric emptying*, often present after gastric

surgery and usually resolving within 1 week, usually results from

1. Mechanical causes, such as edema at the anastamosis or adhesions obstructing the distal loop
2. Metabolic causes, such as hypokalemia, hypoproteinemia, and/or hyponatremia

• Delayed gastric emptying is resolved with NG suction and maintenance of fluid and electrolyte balance and proper nutrition.

Discharge Planning

• The nurse provides verbal and written postoperative instructions

1. Eat small, frequent meals; avoid drinking liquids with meals.
2. Do not skip meals or go for long periods without eating.
3. Avoid hot, spicy foods.
4. Eliminate caffeine and alcohol.
5. Stop smoking.
6. Avoid products containing aspirin and ibuprofen.

• The nurse teaches the client relaxation techniques to help with coping to decrease ulcer recurrence.

For more information on peptic ulcer disease, see *Medical-Surgical Nursing: A Nursing Process Approach*, **pp. 1308–1328.**

Pericarditis

OVERVIEW

• Pericarditis is an inflammation or alteration of the pericardium, the membranous sac enclosing the heart.
• The two types of pericarditis include

1. *Acute* pericarditis, which is caused by viruses, bacteria, trauma, uremia, postmyocardial infarction syndrome, postpericardiotomy syndrome, metastatic tumors, lymphomas,

radiation therapy, rheumatoid arthritis, idiopathic
   2. *Chronic constrictive* pericarditis, caused by tuberculosis, radiation therapy, trauma, and metastatic cancer, with the pericardium becoming rigid, preventing adequate ventricular filling and resulting in cardiac failure

COLLABORATIVE MANAGEMENT

- Assessment findings include
   1. Substernal precordial pain that radiates to the left neck, shoulder, and/or back; pleuritic pain aggravated by breathing, coughing, and swallowing
   2. Pericardial friction rub
   3. Acute pericarditis
      a. Elevated white blood count
      b. ST-T wave elevation on an electrocardiography
      c. Fever
   4. Chronic constrictive pericarditis
      a. Right-sided heart failure
      b. Pericardial thickening on echocardiogram and computerized tomography scan
      c. Inverted or flat T waves on ECG
      d. Atrial fibrillation
- Treatment depends on the type of pericarditis.
- For acute pericarditis, the nurse
   1. Administers analgesics or anti-inflammatory agents, as ordered
   2. Administers corticosteroid therapy, as ordered
   3. Administers antibiotics, as ordered
   4. Provides rest
- For chronic constrictive pericarditis, the nurse
   1. Administers digoxin, as ordered
   2. Administers diuretics, as ordered
- Complications of pericarditis include
   1. Pericardial effusions
   2. Pericardial tamponade

P

For more information on pericarditis, see *Medical-Surgical Nursing: A Nursing Process Approach*, **pp. 2181–2182.**

Peripheral Nerve Trauma

- Mechanisms of injury for peripheral nerve trauma include
  1. Partial or complete severance of a nerve(s)
  2. Contusion, stretching, constriction, and/or compression of a nerve(s)
  3. Ischemia
  4. Electrical, thermal, and/or radiation injury
- The most commonly affected nerves are the median, ulnar, and radial nerves of the upper extremities and the peroneal, femoral, and sciatic nerves of the legs.
- Regeneration of the damaged nerve(s) may occur.
- Nerve damage is characterized by pain, burning, and/or other abnormal sensations distal to the trauma, weakness or flaccid paralysis, and change in skin color and temperature.
- Treatment consists of immobilization of the area.
- Surgery may be performed, such as resection and suturing to reapproximate the severed nerve ends, nerve grafts, and nerve and tendon transplants.
- Nursing care is directed toward frequent skin care and assessment, management of pain, and providing psychosocial support.

For more information on peripheral nerve trauma, see *Medical-Surgical Nursing: A Nursing Process Approach,* **pp. 982–985.**

Peripheral Vascular Disease: Arterial Disease

OVERVIEW

- Peripheral vascular disease (PVD) is a group of diseases that alter the natural flow of blood through the arteries, veins, and lymphatics of the peripheral system or the extremities.
- Partial or total arterial occlusion disrupts the oxygen and nutrient supply, causing tissue death.
- The most common cause of altered flow is atherosclerosis.
- The location of the occlusion determines the location of tissue damage.
- Inflow disease is located above the superficial femoral artery; outflow disease is located below the superficial femoral artery.
- Clients with *chronic peripheral arterial disease* (PAD) seek treatment for the characteristic leg pain known as intermittent claudication.
- Four stages of PAD include
  1. Stage I: Asymptomatic
     a. No claudication is present.
     b. Bruit or aneurysm may be present.
     c. Physical examination may rarely reveal decreased pulses.
  2. Stage II: Claudication
     a. Muscle pain, cramping, or burning is exacerbated by exercise and relieved by rest.
     b. Symptoms are reproducible with exercise.
  3. Stage III: Rest pain
     a. Pain while resting commonly wakes the client at night.
     b. Pain is described as a numbness, burning, toothache-type of pain.
     c. Pain usually occurs in the distal portion of the extremity (toes, arch, forefoot, or heel) and only rarely the calf or ankle.
     d. Pain sometimes is relieved by placing the extremity in a dependent position.
  4. Stage IV: Necrosis/gangrene
     a. Ulcers and blackened tissue occur on the toes, forefoot, and heel.
     b. A distinctive gangrenous odor is present.

P

- Acute peripheral vascular disease occurs when there is an acute obstruction by a thrombus or embolus, causing severe, acute pain below the level of the obstruction.
- Risk factors for acute disease include hypertension, hyperlipidemia, diabetes mellitus, cigarette smoking, obesity, and familial predisposition.

COLLABORATIVE MANAGEMENT
Assessment
- The nurse records the client's
  1. Leg pain with exercise
  2. Relief of leg pain
  3. Discomfort in the lower back, buttocks, and/or thighs (inflow disease)
  4. Burning and/or cramping in the calves, ankles, feet, and toes (outflow disease)
  5. History of acute or chronic pain
- The nurse assesses for
  1. Ischemic changes of the extremity
     a. Loss of hair on the lower calf, ankle, and foot
     b. Dry, scaly skin
     c. Thickened toenails
     d. Color changes (ascending pallor/descending rubor)
     e. Mottled and cool or cold
     f. Delayed capillary filling
  2. Pulses present/absent
  3. Ulcer formation
     a. Arterial ulcers develop on the toes, between the toes, and/or on upper aspect of the foot. They are painful.
     b. Diabetic ulcers develop on the plantar surface of the foot, over metatarsal heads, on the heel, or on pressure areas. They may not be painful.
     c. Venous stasis ulcers occur at the ankles, with discoloration of the lower extremity at the ulcer. They cause minimal pain.

Planning and Implementation
ND$_x$: ALTERED TISSUE PERFUSION
Nonsurgical Management
- The nurse teaches methods of increasing arterial blood flow in chronic arterial disease
  1. Exercise, which promotes collateral circulation
  2. Position changes, which promote circulation and decrease swelling

3. Improvement of vasodilation by providing warmth to the affected extremity, such as wearing socks or insulated bedroom shoes; maintenance of a warm home environment; cautioning the client not to apply direct heat to the lower limbs, which may cause burns due to decreased sensitivity
4. Prevention of vasoconstriction by decreasing exposure to cold; avoiding nicotine, caffeine, and emotional stress
5. Drug therapy, including vasodilators, defibrination agents, and antiplatelet therapy
6. Control of hypertension

• *Percutaneous transluminal angioplasty* (PTA) dilates arteries that are occluded or stenosed with a balloon catheter.

• Laser-assisted angioplasty may be used to open an occluded artery.

• Mechanical rotational abrasive atherectomy is being investigated for scraping plaque while minimizing danger to the vessel wall.

• The nurse prepares the client for PTA or laser-assisted angioplasty by giving the client nothing by mouth after midnight and scrubbing the groin area with an aseptic soap, as ordered.

• Post-PTA, the nurse
1. Observes the puncture site for bleeding
2. Closely monitors vital signs
3. Checks the distal pulses on the affected limb
4. Maintains bed rest for 6 to 8 hours, as ordered, with the limb in a straight position
5. Administers anticoagulation therapy, such as heparin, for 3 days, as ordered; then administers dipyridamole for 3 to 6 months, as ordered
6. Encourages the client to take aspirin on a permanent basis, as ordered

P

Surgical Management
• An emergency surgical *embolectomy* is performed on clients who experience an acute peripheral artery occlusion by an embolus

• Clients with acute occlusion from a thrombus usually undergo an emergency bypass grafting procedure.

• Surgery for clients with chronic PAD is usually elective.

• Arterial revascularization surgery is used to increase arterial blood flow in an affected limb and includes *inflow* procedures, such as aortoiliac bypass, aortofemoral bypass, and axillofemoral bypass; and *outflow* procedures, including femoropopliteal bypass and femorotibial bypass.

- Grafting material for bypass surgeries includes the autogenous saphenous vein or a synthetic graft material, such as polytetrafluoroethylene material.
- The nurse provides routine preoperative care.
- The nurse provides postoperative care
  1. Provides routine postoperative care
  2. Monitors for the patency of the graft by checking for changes in the extremity
     a. Color
     b. Temperature
     c. Pulse intensity
     d. Pain intensity (pain changes from a throbbing pain, which occurs from increased blood flow to the affected limb, to ischemic pain, as experienced prior to surgery)
  3. Marks the site of the distal pulses, which are best palpated or auscultated with Doppler ultrasonography
  4. Monitors the client's blood pressure, notifying the physician for increases and decreases beyond desired ranges
  5. Avoids bending the knee and hip of the affected limb
  6. Utilizes aseptic wound care and proper hand washing techniques to prevent infection
  7. Monitors for signs and symptoms of infection at or around the graft and incision sites, such as hardness, tenderness, redness, and/or warmth

NDx: IMPAIRED SKIN INTEGRITY
Nonsurgical Management

- The nurse
  1. Teaches prevention of skin breakdown/ulceration
  2. Educates the client on how ulcers are formed
  3. Teaches proper foot care and protective measures
  4. Applies sterile dressings (wet-to-dry dressings for arterial ulcers)
  5. Avoids the use of tape on surrounding tissues
  6. Administers antibiotics, as ordered

Surgical Management

- *Surgical débridement* is the procedure of choice to remove eschar and promote wound healing.
- If the wound does not heal, a distal surgical *amputation* may be performed (for care of the client, see Amputation).

NDx: ACTIVITY INTOLERANCE

- The nurse
  1. Plans an exercise program to increase activity tolerance
  2. Works with the client and physician to develop a suitable pain management program

Discharge Planning

- The nurse
  1. Instructs the client on methods to increase vasodilation
  2. Reinforces the need for individualized positioning and an exercise plan
  3. Teaches the client to avoid raising the legs above the level of the heart
  4. Provides written and oral foot care instructions
     a. Keep the feet clean by washing with a mild soap in room-temperature water.
     b. Keep the feet dry.
     c. Avoid injury or extended pressure to the feet and ankles.
     d. Always wear comfortable, well-fitting shoes.
     e. Keep the toenails clean, and cut them straight across.
     f. Prevent dry, cracked skin.
     g. Prevent exposure to extreme heat or cold.
     h. Avoid heating pads.
     i. Avoid constricting garments.
  5. Provides postoperative care instructions, if necessary
  6. Provides dressing change instructions, if necessary
  7. Emphasizes the importance of follow-up visits with the physician(s)

P

For more information on peripheral arterial disease, see *Medical-Surgical Nursing: A Nursing Process Approach*, **pp. 2205–2214.**

Peripheral Vascular Disease: Venous Disease

OVERVIEW

- Peripheral vascular disease (PVD) is a group of diseases that alter the natural flow of blood through the arteries, veins, and lymphatics of the peripheral system or the extremities.

- Veins must be patent with functioning valves.

- Venous blood flow may be altered by thrombus formation and defective valves.

- A *thrombus* (blood clot) results from an endothelial injury, venous stasis, and/or hypercoagulability.

- *Thrombophlebitis* occurs when a thrombus is associated with inflammation in superficial veins.

- *Phlebothrombosis* is the presence of a thrombus without inflammation.

- *Deep venous thrombosis* (DVT) usually occurs in the deep veins of the lower extremities and presents a major risk for pulmonary embolism.

- *Venous insufficiency* occurs from prolonged venous hypertension, which stretches the veins and damages valves, resulting in venous stasis ulcers with swelling and cellulitis.

COLLABORATIVE MANAGEMENT

Assessment

- The nurse records the client's
    1. Age
    2. History of thrombophlebitis
    3. Recent surgery
    4. Recent trauma
    5. Immobilization for long periods
    6. Pregnancy
    7. Estrogen therapy
    8. Leg swelling
- The nurse assesses for
    1. Calf or groin tenderness and pain
    2. Leg swelling
    3. Pain in the calf on dorsiflexion of the foot (Homan's sign)
    4. Warmth and edema of the extremity
    5. Size comparison with the contralateral limb

6. Localized pitting edema
7. Discoloration along the ankles, extending up to the calf
8. Ulcer formation
   a. Arterial ulcers develop on the toes, between the toes, and/or on the upper aspect of the foot. They are painful.
   b. Diabetic ulcers develop on the plantar surface of the foot, over metatarsal heads, and/or on the heel and/or pressure areas. They may not be painful.
   c. Venous stasis ulcers occur at the ankles. Minimal pain is present.

Planning and Implementation

NDx: ALTERED TISSUE PERFUSION (PERIPHERAL)

- The goal of management is to prevent complications such as pulmonary emboli.
- The nurse
   1. Promotes bed rest and elevates the extremity above the level of the heart
   2. Applies intermittent or continuous warm, moist soaks
   3. Administers intravenous heparin therapy, as ordered, to reduce the formation of other clots
   4. Administers oral warfarin sodium (Coumadin), as ordered, after weaning from intravenous heparin
   5. Applies elastic stockings
   6. Teaches the client to avoid sitting or standing for long periods
- Surgical removal of a deep venous thrombosis (thrombectomy) is rarely performed.
- An inferior vena cava filter may be inserted to trap emboli before they progress to the lungs.

P

NDx: IMPAIRED SKIN INTEGRITY

- The goal of management is to heal the ulcer and prevent stasis with recurrence of ulcer formation.
- The nurse
   1. Applies oxygen-permeable polyethelene film occlusive dressings, such as Op Site, as ordered.
   2. Applies oxygen-impermeable hydrocolloid occlusive dressings, such as DuoDerm, as ordered
   3. Monitors the Unna boot dressing with zinc oxide after application by a physician
   4. Applies topical agents, as ordered, for venous ulcers, including proteolytic enzymes such as

sutilains (Travase), which digest necrotic tissue, and fibrinolysin and desoxyribonuclease (Elase), which débride necrotic tissue and fibrinous exudates
5. Administers systemic antibiotics to prevent or resolve infection

• Surgical débridement of the ulcer may be necessary to remove eschar.

Discharge Planning

• Clients recovering from venous disease are usually discharged from the hospital on a regime of warfarin.

• The nurse teaches anticoagulation instructions to the client and family

1. Avoid potential trauma.
2. Observe and report signs and symptoms of bleeding
   a. Hematuria
   b. Frank or occult blood in stool
   c. Ecchymoses
   d. Petechiae
   e. Altered level of consciousness
   f. Pain
3. Apply direct pressure to bleeding sites.
4. Seek medical assistance immediately if bleeding occurs.
5. Wear a Medic Alert bracelet or necklace and carry a card at all times.
6. Inform other health care providers, such as dentists, about the therapy.
7. Avoid other medications, unless prescribed by the same physician.
8. Avoid high-fat and vitamin-K-rich foods.
9. Have routine monitoring of prothrombin time levels.

• The nurse teaches the client to

1. Avoid standing still or sitting for long periods.
2. Avoid crossing the legs when sitting.
3. Avoid constrictive garments.
4. Wear support hose/antiembolism stockings as prescribed.
5. Follow the prescribed exercise program.
6. Follow the prescribed weight reduction plan, if needed.
7. Follow written and oral foot care instructions (see "Discharge Planning" under Peripheral Vascular Disease: Arterial Disease).

8. Keep follow-up appointments with the physician(s).

For more information on venous disease, see *Medical-Surgical Nursing: A Nursing Process Approach*, **pp. 2214–2218.**

Peritonitis

OVERVIEW

● Peritonitis is defined as an inflammation of the peritoneal cavity from contamination by bacteria or chemicals; it may be localized or generalized.

● *Primary* peritonitis results from an acute bacterial infection that is not associated with a perforated viscus or an infection from another body source that is carried to the peritoneum by the vascular system.

● *Secondary* peritonitis is caused by bacterial invasion as a result of perforation or rupture of an abdominal viscus and also results from a severe chemical reaction to pancreatic enzymes, digestive juices, bile, and/or injury to and/or perforation of the intestinal tract.

P

COLLABORATIVE MANAGEMENT
Assessment
● The nurse records the client's
   1. History of abdominal pain, which is aggravated by movement and respiratory effort and relieved by knee flexion
   2. Abdominal distention
   3. Anorexia
   4. Nausea or vomiting
   5. Elevated temperature with chills
   6. Inability to pass flatus or feces

7. Past medical history, including the date of the last menstrual period
- The nurse assesses for
    1. Pain, which may be sharp and localized or poorly localized and/or referred to either the shoulder or thoracic areas
    2. Adbominal rigidity and/or distention with rebound tenderness
    3. Absent bowel sounds
    4. Fever with tachycardia
    5. Dehydration as evidenced by dry mucous membranes, poor skin turgor, orthostatic blood pressure changes, and decreased urinary output

Planning and Implementation

NDx: Altered (Gastrointestinal) Tissue Perfusion

- The nurse
    1. Gives the client nothing by mouth (NPO)
    2. Monitors and records drainage from the nasogastric (NG) tube used for gastric and intestinal decompression
    3. Administers intravenous (IV) fluids and broad-spectrum antibiotics, as ordered
- Surgical management may be necessary to identify and repair the underlying cause of the peritonitis.
- Surgery is focused on controlling the bacterial contamination, removing foreign material from the peritoneal cavity, and draining fluid collections.
- During surgery, the peritoneum is irrigated with antibiotic solutions, and drainage catheters are inserted.

NDx: Fluid Volume Deficit

- IV fluids are given to replace fluids lost from the extracellular space to the peritoneal cavity, NG drainage losses, and NPO status.
- A saline solution with potassium supplements is given based on the client's electrolyte levels.

Discharge Planning

- The nurse provides written postoperative instructions
    1. Inspection of the incision for redness, tenderness, swelling, and drainage
    2. Care of the incision and/or dressing
    3. The need to report temperature higher than 101° F(38.2° C) to the physician
    4. Pain medication administration and monitoring
    5. Dietary limitations, if necessary

6. Activity limitations, including avoidance of heavy lifting until healing has occurred

For additional information on peritonitis, see *Medical-Surgical Nursing: A Nursing Process Approach*, **pp. 1347–1351.**

Peritonsillar Abscess

- Peritonsillar abscess is a complication of acute tonsillitis known as quinsy.
- Acute infection spreads from the tonsil to the surrounding peritonsillar tissue, forming an abscess.
- The common cause is group A *beta-hemolytic streptococcus.*
- Marked asymmetric swelling and deviation of the uvula from pus collection cause difficult swallowing, drooling, severe throat pain radiating to the ear, and voice change.
- Treatment includes
  1. Warm saline gargles or irrigations
  2. Ice collar
  3. Analgesics
  4. Antibiotics
  5. Incision and drainage of the abscess
  6. Posthealing tonsillectomy

P

For more information on peritonsillar abscesses, see *Medical-Surgical Nursing: A Nursing Process Approach*, **pp. 1249–1250, 1960.**

Pharyngitis

- Pharyngitis is an infection of the mucous membranes of the pharynx, usually preceding or occurring with acute rhinitis or sinusitis.
- Multiple causes of acute pharyngitis include bacteria, viruses, and physical and chemical causes.
- Pharyngitis is most commonly caused by a virus; the most common bacterial cause is group A *beta-hemolytic streptococcus.*
- Pharyngitis is characterized by soreness and dryness in the throat, pain, difficulty swallowing, dysphagia, and fever.
- Viral sore throats are usually accompanied by a gradual onset, rhinorrhea, headache, mild hoarseness, and low-grade fever.
- Bacterial infection is associated with an abrupt onset, dysphagia, arthralgias, myalgias, malaise, and fever.
- Viral and bacterial pharyngitis may be associated with mild to severe hyperemia, with or without enlarged erythematous tonsils and with or without exudate.
- Nasal discharge varies from thin and watery to purulent.
- Management of *viral* pharyngitis includes
    1. Rest
    2. Increased fluid intake
    3. Analgesics for pain
    4. Warm saline throat gargles
    5. Mild antiseptic throat lozenges
- Management of *bacterial* pharyngitis includes antibiotics and supportive care measures.

For more information on pharyngitis, see *Medical-Surgical Nursing: A Nursing Process Approach,* **pp. 1957–1959.**

Pheochromocytoma

OVERVIEW

• A pheochromocytoma is a catecholamine-producing tumor that arises in the chromaffin cells of the adrenal medulla.

• Most of these tumors are benign, but they may occur in a malignant form.

COLLABORATIVE MANAGEMENT

• The nurse assesses for

1. Paroxysmal hypertensive episodes, which vary in length from a few minutes to several hours
2. Palpitations
3. Severe headache
4. Profuse diaphoresis
5. Flushing
6. Apprehension or a feeling of impending doom
7. Pain in the chest or abdomen
8. Nausea and vomiting
9. Heat intolerance
10. Weight loss
11. Tremors

• Surgery is performed to remove the tumor and the affected adrenal gland.

• The nurse provides preoperative care

1. Identifies factors that contribute to hypertensive crisis
2. Provides a diet rich in calories, vitamins, and minerals
3. Ensures adequate hydration
4. Administers alpha-adrenergic blocking agents, as ordered, to decrease the risk of hypertension during surgery

• The nurse provides postoperative care

1. Provides the same care as that for an adrenalectomy (see Adrenal Hyperfunction)
2. Monitors for shock and hemorrhage

• The tumor is managed with alpha- and beta-adrenergic blocking agents if inoperable.

• Clients who are medically managed must be

P

instructed in the correct technique to monitor their
own blood pressure.

For more information on pheochromocytoma, see
*Medical-Surgical Nursing: A Nursing Process
Approach,* **pp. 1555–1557.**

Phlebitis

- Phlebitis is an inflammation of the superficial veins
caused by an irritation, commonly caused by
intravenous therapy.
- Phlebitis is manifested as a reddened, warm area
radiating up an extremity.
- The client additionally may experience pain,
soreness, and swelling of the extremity.
- Treatment involves application of warm, moist
soaks, which dilate the vein and promote circulation.

For more information on phlebitis, see *Medical-
Surgical Nursing: A Nursing Process Approach,*
p. 2227.

Pneumonia

OVERVIEW

• Pneumonia is an infection of pulmonary tissue, including the interstitial spaces, the alveoli, and the bronchioles.

• Pathogens penetrate the airway mucosa and multiply in the alveolar spaces, causing white blood cell migration into the alveoli and a thickening of the alveolar wall.

• The edema associated with inflammation stiffens the lung, decreasing compliance and vital capacity.

• The pneumonic process causes a shunt-type ventilation-perfusion defect, resulting in arterial hypoxemia.

• Pneumonia presents as diffuse patches throughout both lungs or consolidates in one lobe.

• *Community-acquired* pneumonias are caused by *Mycoplasma pneumoniae*, *Legionella pneumophila*, *Streptococcus pneumoniae*, and viruses.

• *Hospital-acquired* pneumonias are caused by *Staphylococcus aureus*, *Klebsiella pneumoniae*, *Pseudomonas aeruginosa*, and fungi.

COLLABORATIVE MANAGEMENT

Assessment

• The nurse records the client's

1. Age
2. Environmental changes
3. Cigarette and alcohol use
4. Medications
5. Drug abuse history
6. Chronic pulmonary illness
7. Recent medical history (influenza, pneumonia, viral infections)
8. Home respiratory equipment use and cleaning regime
9. Current symptomology

• The nurse assesses for

1. General appearance
2. Breathing pattern
3. Use of accessory muscles
4. Cyanosis
5. Rales, rhonchi, and wheezes on auscultation
6. Bronchial breath sounds over areas of density or consolidation

P

7. Tactile fremitus
   8. Dull percussion
   9. Character of cough
  10. Sputum production, including amount, color, and odor
  11. Fever and chills
  12. Mental status changes (especially in the elderly)
  13. Gastrointestinal symptoms

Planning and Implementation

NDx: INEFFECTIVE AIRWAY CLEARANCE

- The nurse
   1. Encourages coughing and deep breathing
   2. Encourages the use of incentive spirometry
   3. Provides chest physical therapy
   4. Increases fluid intake to liquefy secretions
   5. Changes the client's position frequently
   6. Ambulates the client and gets the client out of bed in a chair, as tolerated
   7. Performs nasotracheal suctioning if the client is unable to clear secretions
   8. Administers antibiotic therapy as determined by sputum analysis, as ordered
   9. Administers mucolytic agents and expectorants, as ordered
  10. Administers aerosolized bronchodilators such as metaproterenol sulfate (Alupent), isoetharine (Bronkosol), and terbutaline sulfate (Brethine), as ordered
  11. Provides oxygen therapy via a Venturi mask or cannula
  12. Maintains intubation with mechanical ventilation, if needed

NDx: INEFFECTIVE BREATHING PATTERN

- The nurse
   1. Monitors the rate and depth of respirations, use of accessory muscles, and pursed-lip breathing
   2. Elevates the head of the bed to facilitate breathing and lung expansion
   3. Allows the client to lean over the bedside table to facilitate breathing, if needed
   4. Encourages slow, deep breathing or diaphragmatic breathing
   5. Helps the client alleviate anxiety

NDx: ACTIVITY INTOLERANCE

- The nurse
   1. Balances rest and activity periods
   2. Increases activity gradually
   3. Continues oxygen use during activity

Discharge Planning

- The nurse provides client/family education
  1. Importance of rest
  2. Proper nutrition
  3. Adequate fluid intake
  4. Avoidance of chilling
  5. Avoiding exposure to others with respiratory infections or viruses
  6. Risk of increased susceptibility
  7. Antibiotic therapy including prescriptions, as ordered
  8. Notification of the physician for chills, fever, dyspnea, hemoptysis, increasing fatigue, or other complications
  9. Importance of follow-up visits with the physician(s)

- The influenza vaccine is highly recommended for clients older than 65 years of age and for younger people with chronic cardiac disease, severe diabetes, or impaired immune defenses.
- High-risk clients should be given the pneumococcal vaccine, which provides immunity against several strains of pneumococcus.

For more information on pneumonia, see *Medical-Surgical Nursing: A Nursing Process Approach*, **pp. 1977–1986.**

P

Pneumothorax

- Pneumothorax is an accumulation of atmospheric air in the pleural space, resulting in a rise in intrathoracic pressure and reduced vital capacity.
- Pneumothorax is caused by thoracic injury, including blunt chest trauma.

- Assessment findings include
  1. Diminished breath sounds
  2. Hyperresonance on percussion
  3. Prominence of the involved hemothorax
  4. Pleuritic chest pain
  5. Tachypnea
  6. Subcutaneous emphysema
- Interventions are aimed at rapid removal of trapped atmospheric air, including a large-bore needle insertion and chest tubes to ensure lung inflation.

For more information on pneumothorax, see *Medical-Surgical Nursing: A Nursing Process Approach*, **p. 2056.**

Poliomyelitis

- Poliomyelitis (polio) is an acute viral disease characterized by destruction of the motor cells of the anterior horn of the spinal cord, the brain stem, and the motor strip of the frontal lobe.
- Polio is transmitted through droplet infection or via the fecal or oral route and the gastrointestinal tract.
- The disease is rare in North America due to immunization during childhood.
- Polio is characterized by fever, chills, excessive perspiration, severe muscle aches and weakness, increased deep-tendon reflexes, abdominal tenderness, dysphagia, and irritability.
- Treatment is symptomatic.
- Analgesics are used to relieve pain, and respiratory status is monitored carefully.

For more information on polio, see *Medical-Surgical Nursing: A Nursing Process Approach,* **p. 905.**

Polycystic Kidney Disease

OVERVIEW

- Polycystic kidney disease (PKD) is an inherited kidney disorder of the renal parenchyma that occurs bilaterally.
- The nephron is the primary site of cyst development; cysts develop in the glomeruli and tubules, resulting in less effective glomerular filtration, tubular reabsorption, and tubular secretion.
- The kidneys become grossly enlarged; cysts become progressively larger, with diffuse distribution.

COLLABORATIVE MANAGEMENT

Assessment

- The nurse records the client's
  1. Family history of PKD
  2. Known history of PKD
  3. Current health status
  4. Age at development of clinical manifestations
  5. Family history of sudden death from a strokelike phenomenon
  6. History of constipation
  7. Changes in urine or frequency of urination
  8. History of hypertension
  9. History of headaches
- The nurse assesses for
  1. Protruding and distended abdomen
  2. Enlarged kidney on palpation
  3. Abdominal discomfort
  4. Tender tissue and flank pain
  5. Hematuria or cloudy urine
  6. Dysuria
  7. Severe headache
  8. Hypertension
  9. Edema
  10. Uremic symptoms

Planning and Implementation

NDx: PAIN

Nonsurgical Management

- The nurse
  1. Administers analgesics for comfort, as ordered, avoiding aspirin-containing products
  2. Administers antibiotics, as ordered, for the infectious process

P

3. Applies dry heat to the abdomen or flank
4. Teaches relaxation techniques

Surgical Management
- *Nephrectomy* (kidney removal) is performed when pain, infection, and/or bleeding are not controlled by medical management. (See Renal Carcinoma for care of the client undergoing a nephrectomy.)

NDx: FLUID VOLUME EXCESS
- The nurse
  1. Administers antihypertensive agents, as ordered, including vasodilators, beta-blockers, and centrally acting agents
  2. Administers mild diuretics, as ordered, to clients with renal insufficiency
  3. Administers more potent diuretics, as ordered, for renal function deterioration
  4. Monitors intake and output
  5. Records daily weights
  6. Provides a low-sodium diet initially
  7. Maintains protein restriction as renal insufficiency progresses

NDx: ANXIETY; INEFFECTIVE COPING
- The nurse
  1. Provides counseling, support, and education about health maintenance
  2. Develops a relationship that promotes trust and communication
  3. Discusses coping strategies used successfully in past
  4. Refers the client to support groups
  5. Refers the client to professional counseling services

Discharge Planning
- The nurse teaches the client/family
  1. How to measure and monitor blood pressure and body weight
  2. Dietary restrictions and fluid intake limits
  3. Desired effects and adverse effects of antihypertensive drugs and diuretics, including prescriptions
  4. Measures for preventing constipation and their rationale
  5. Need to report symptoms of uremia to the physician (nephrologist) that may indicate the need for dialysis

6. Importance of follow-up visits with the physician(s)

For more information on polycystic kidney disease, see *Medical-Surgical Nursing: A Nursing Process Approach*, **pp. 1827–1833**.

Polyneuritis/ Polyneuropathy

- Inflammatory as well as noninflammatory processes may damage cranial and peripheral nerves.
- *Polyneuritis* implies an inflammatory process, but the terms *polyneuritis* and *polyneuropathy* may be used interchangeably.
- These syndromes are characterized by muscle weakness with or without atrophy, pain, paresthesia or loss of sensation, impaired reflexes, autonomic manifestations, unsteadiness, injury without pain, or a combination of these symptoms.
- The most common type of this disorder is a symmetric polyneuropathy in which the client experiences decreased sensation, along with a feeling that the extremity is asleep and tingling, burning, tightness, or aching sensations, usually starting in the feet and progressing to the level of the knee before being noted in the hands (glove and stocking neuropathy).
- Factors associated with polyneuropathy include diabetes, renal or hepatic failure, alcoholism, vascular disease, vitamin B_1, B_6, B_{12} deficiency, and exposure to heavy metals and/or industrial solvents.
- Assessment includes
  1. Light touch and pain in the distal extremities
  2. Position sense and/or kinesthetic sensation

P

3. Sensitivity to vibration by placing a tuning fork on a bony prominence
4. Any signs of injury
5. Indications of autonomic dysfunctions such as orthostatic hypotension, abnormal sweating, and/or miosis

• Treatment consists of removal or treatment of the underlying cause and symptomatic therapy
1. Supplementing the diet with vitamins
2. Client teaching, including the importance of foot care and inspecting the extremities for injuries
3. Importance of wearing shoes at all times and purchasing well-fitting shoes
4. Teaching how to recognize potential hazards, such as exposure to extremes of environmental temperature
5. Discouraging smoking

For more information on polyneuritis and polyneuropathy, see *Medical-Surgical Nursing: A Nursing Process Approach,* **pp. 980–982.**

Polyp, Gastrointestinal

• Gastrointestinal tract polyps are small growths covered with mucosa and attached to the intestinal surface; most are benign but have the potential to become malignant.

• Adenomas require medical consultation because of their malignant potential.

• Pedunculated polyps are stalklike with a thin stem attaching them to the intestinal wall.

• Polyps are usually asymptomatic but can cause rectal bleeding, intestinal obstruction, and/or intussusception.

- Polyps can usually be removed by *polypectomy* with an electrocautery snare that fits through a colonoscope, removing the need for abdominal surgery.
- Postoperatively the nurse monitors for
  1. Abdominal distention and pain
  2. Rectal bleeding
  3. Mucopurulent rectal drainage
  4. Fever
- The nurse instructs the client to follow up with a repeated colonoscopy or sigmoidoscopy, as ordered

For more information on gastrointestinal polyps, see *Medical-Surgical Nursing: A Nursing Process Approach*, **pp. 1402–1403.**

Postmenopausal Bleeding

- Postmenopausal bleeding is vaginal bleeding occurring after a 12-month cessation of menses, after the onset of menopause.
- The three most common causes of postmenopausal bleeding are atrophic vaginitis, cervical polyps, and endometrial abnormalities, including hyperplasia, a precursor of malignancy.
- Assessment includes
  1. Menstrual and obstetrical history
  2. Family history
  3. Age at menopause
  4. Frequency and amount of bleeding
  5. Previous bleeding episodes
  6. Use of medications, especially estrogen-only replacement therapy
  7. Gastrointestinal symptoms
  8. Urinary symptoms

P

- Interventions include
  1. Dilation and curettage (D&C)
  2. Hysterectomy
  3. Combination of surgery, radiation, and chemotherapy
  4. Progesterone injections
  5. Estrogen replacement therapy

For more information on postmenopausal bleeding, see *Medical-Surgical Nursing: A Nursing Process Approach*, **pp. 1693–1694.**

Postoperative Care

OVERVIEW

- Postoperative care begins when the client is admitted to the postanesthesia care unit (PACU) (recovery room) and extends through discharge from the hospital or ambulatory care facility.
- Time spent in the PACU varies with the client's age and physical health, type of procedure, anesthesia used, and postoperative complications.

COLLABORATIVE MANAGEMENT
Assessment
- The nurse assesses for
  1. Postanesthesia score (PACU nurse)
  2. Respiratory function
     a. Patent airway
     b. Adequate respiratory exchange
     c. Breath sounds bilaterally
     d. Symmetrical movement of the chest wall
     e. Indications of diaphragmatic breathing and sternal retraction

3. Cardiovascular function
   a. Vital signs
   b. Peripheral pulses
   c. Presence of Homan's sign
   d. Edema, redness, and pain (indications of thrombophlebitis)
4. Fluid and electrolyte balance
   a. Intake and output
   b. Complete blood count
   c. Electrolytes
5. Neurologic system
   a. Level of consciousness
   b. Eye opening
   c. Ability to follow commands
   d. Motor movement
   e. Sensation/pain
   f. Orientation
6. Genitourinary system
   a. Output, color of urine
   b. Inspection, palpation, and percussion of the client's abdomen for bladder distention
7. Gastrointestinal system
   a. Auscultation for bowel sounds
   b. Palpation of the abdomen
   c. Patency of the nasogastric tube or any abdominal tubes and drains
8. Integumentary system, integrity of the wound site
9. Dressings and drains
   a. Color, amount, and consistency of drainage
   b. Integrity of Penrose drains (a single-lumen, soft latex tube inserted into or close to the surgical site)
   c. Patency and integrity of Hemovac, VacuDrain, or Jackson Pratt drains to ensure maintenance of suction
   d. Patency of all other drains or tubes
10. Pain
11. Anxiety and restlessness

Planning and Implementation

- The nurse
  1. Monitors vital signs every 4 hours or more frequently if clinically indicated (significant changes in blood pressure may indicate myocardial depression, hemorrhage, oversedation, and/or pain)

515

2. Performs a complete systems assessment every shift
3. Measures and records intake and output
4. Observes for and reports postoperative complications
   a. Urinary retention
   b. Pulmonary atelectasis, pneumonia, emboli
   c. Alterations in wound healing, infection
   d. Urinary tract infection
   e. Thrombophlebitis

NDx: IMPAIRED GAS EXCHANGE

- The nurse in the PACU
  1. Positions the client on the side or with the head turned to prevent possible aspiration
  2. Keeps the head of the bed flat until the client regains a gag reflex and to prevent hypotension as long as it is not contraindicated
  3. Raises the head of the bed to promote respiratory function, when appropriate
  4. Monitors for stridor or snoring, which are signs of upper airway obstruction from tracheal or laryngeal spasm, mucus in the airway, or occlusion of the airway from relaxation of the tongue
- The nurse (after transfer from PACU)
  1. Completes a respiratory assessment once each shift for at least 48 hours after surgery
  2. Administers oxygen, if needed
  3. Encourages the client to turn, cough, and deep breathe (splints wound as needed)
  4. Provides incentive spirometry and/or chest physiotherapy, as clinically indicated
  5. Suctions the client, as needed
  6. Monitors for complications such as atelectasis, pneumonia, pulmonary edema, and/or emboli

NDx: IMPAIRED SKIN INTEGRITY

- The nurse
  1. Observes the wound for separation
     a. Checks for *dehiscence*, the partial or complete separation of the upper layers of the wound (applies a sterile nonadherent or saline dressing and binder to the wound and notifies the surgeon immediately)
     b. Checks for *evisceration*, the total separation of the layers and extrusion of internal organs or viscera through an open wound (covers the wound with a sterile towel or nonadherent

dressing moistened with normal saline, notifies the surgeon immediately, and does not attempt to reinsert the protruding organ or viscera)

   c. Monitors vital signs and assesses for signs of shock

   d. Supports and reassures the client

   e. Prepares the client for surgery to repair the wound

2. Performs dressing changes, as ordered (with the first change usually done by the physician)

   a. Reinforces the dressing if it becomes wet from drainage

   b. Documents the color, type, amount, and odor of drainage fluid and time of observation on the client's chart

   c. Notifies the surgeon of excessive drainage; documents the time of the call and the physician's response

   d. Recognizes that wet dressings are a source of infection; obtains an order from the surgeon for dressing changes using aseptic technique

   e. Follows facility procedure for dressing changes and wound care

3. Observes the wound for infection; may give antibiotics prophylactically

NDx: Pain

- Narcotics and nonnarcotics such as meperidine hydrochloride (Demerol), morphine sulfate, codeine sulfate, butorphanol tartrate (Stadol), oxycodone hydrochloride with aspirin (Percodan), and oxycodone with acetaminophen (Tylox or Percocet) are routinely given immediately postoperatively.

- The nurse

1. Assesses the type, location, and intensity of the pain before giving the medication

2. Assesses and documents the effectiveness of the medication

3. Monitors patient-controlled analgesia (PCA), as ordered, via an intravenous or internal pump, to control pain, with the rate or dosage of infusion of a narcotic analgesic adjusted by the client on the basis of his or her pain level and physical response to the drug

4. Tapers pain medication as recovery progresses and administers nonnarcotic medication such as acetaminophen (Tylenol) and nonsteroid anti-inflammatory drugs such as ibuprofen (Motrin, Advil), as ordered

5. Positions the client based on surgical procedure and medical condition
6. Turns the client every 2 hours or more often as needed
7. Provides back rubs, relaxation techniques, and distraction to control pain

Discharge Planning

- The nurse
    1. Collaborates with the client/family to identify and correct any hazards in the home prior to discharge
    2. Identifies strategies that can be used to modify the environment to accommodate any client limitations, meal preparation, or dressing changes
    3. Teaches the care of the surgical wound and provides written instruction as needed
        a. Importance of hand washing
        b. Disposal procedure for the soiled dressing
        c. Return demonstration of wound care
    4. Reinforces diet therapy and obtains a dietary consultation if necessary; advises a high-protein, high-calorie diet to promote wound healing unless on a restricted/special diet
    5. Provides information on drug therapy
        a. Taking all medications in the correct dosage, at the right time, and by the right route
        b. What to do if a dose is missed or if complications or side effects occur
    6. Reinforces restrictions in activity and exercise
    7. Teaches the importance of follow-up visits with the physician(s)

For more information on postoperative care, see *Medical-Surgical Nursing: A Nursing Process Approach,* **pp. 473–488.**

Postpolio Syndrome

• Postpolio syndrome (PPS) is a new onset of weakness, pain, and fatigue in persons who had poliomyelitis 30 or more years previously.

• Physical and emotional stressors are contributing factors.

• Treatment is symptomatic and includes life-style modifications to preserve energy and physiologic function.

For more information on postpolio syndrome, see *Medical-Surgical Nursing: A Nursing Process Approach,* **p. 905.**

Premenstrual Syndrome

• Premenstrual syndrome (PMS) is a collection of symptoms that are cyclic in nature, occurring each month during the luteal phase of the menstrual cycle, followed by relief with menses and a symptom-free phase.

• The etiology is not well understood, but many theories have been reported in the literature.

• Clinical manifestations are highly variable and include
    1. Dermatologic: acne, urticaria, herpes
    2. Respiratory: sinusitis, asthma, rhinitis, colds
    3. Urologic: oliguria, cystitis, enuresis, urethritis
    4. Ophthamologic: conjunctivitis, styes, glaucoma
    5. Neurologic: headaches, migraine, syncope, vertigo, numbness of hands and feet, epilepsy (if susceptible)

6. Metabolic: edema, breast tenderness
7. Emotional/psychologic: depression, irritability, tension, panic attacks, changes in libido, mood swings, anxiety
8. Behavioral: lowered work performance, food cravings, alcohol and drug overindulgence, confusion, sleeplessness, lack of coordination, suicide, lethargy, child abuse, assaultive behavior
9. Other: allergies, hypoglycemia, joint pain, backache, palpitations, water retention

- Management is focused on eliminating uncomfortable symptoms and is highly individualized

1. Dietary measures such as limiting sugar, red meat, alcohol, coffee, tea, chocolate, caffeine, salt, and sodium; vitamin B_6 to relieve depression and vitamin E and magnesium to decrease breast tenderness
2. Drug therapy, which is controversial: diuretics, progesterone therapy, and tension-relief drugs, such as meprobamate, are prescribed
3. Education about PMS and its symptoms
4. Self-help groups and support groups

For more information on premenstrual syndrome, see *Medical-Surgical Nursing: A Nursing Process Approach*, **pp. 1690–1692.**

Preoperative Care

OVERVIEW

- Preoperative management is the care provided to the client before surgery.

- The primary role of the nurse is as an educator and client advocate.

- *Inpatient* refers to a client who is admitted to a hospital the day before or the same day of surgery and who requires hospitalization after surgery.

- *Outpatient* refers to the patient who goes to the surgical area (surgical center, ambulatory care center) the day of surgery and goes home on the same day (same-day surgery).
- The government has mandated and compiled a list of surgical procedures that should be performed on an outpatient basis and are reimbursed by Medicare, including cataract extraction, hernioplasty, cryosurgery, arthroscopy, and hemorrhoidectomy.

COLLABORATIVE MANAGEMENT

Assessment

- The nurse records the client's
  1. Age
  2. Allergies to medication and food
  3. Current medication (prescription and over the counter)
  4. History of medical and surgical problems
     a. Myocardial infarction within the past 6 months
     b. Congestive heart failure
     c. Dysrhythmias
     d. Pneumonia
     e. Pulmonary disease such as chronic obstructive pulmonary disease
  5. Previous surgical experiences
  6. Previous experience with anesthesia
  7. Tobacco, alcohol, and drug use
  8. Family medical history and problems with anesthetics that may indicate possible intraoperative needs and reactions to anesthesia, such as malignant hyperthermia
  9. Self-care capabilities, support system, and home environment (particularly important to obtain for clients having outpatient surgery)

P

- Preoperative assessment is done to determine baseline data, hidden medical problems, potential complications related to the administration of anesthesia, and potential complications of surgery.
- The nurse assesses the client's
  1. Vital signs
  2. Cardiovascular system
     a. Palpates peripheral pulses; observes for indications of arteriosclerosis
     b. Auscultates the heart for rate, regularity, and abnormalities
     c. Records blood pressure to determine hypertension, increased diastolic pressure

3. Respiratory system
   a. Observes for
      (1) Posture, fingers (for clubbing)
      (2) Rate, rhythm, depth of respirations
      (3) Lung expansion
   b. Auscultates the lungs to determine the quality and presence of adventitious sounds and congestion
4. Renal system
   a. Observes for
      (1) Frequency of urination
      (2) Dysuria
      (3) Anuria
      (4) Appearance and odor of urine
   b. Obtains a urinalysis to determine the presence of glucose, protein, blood, and bacteria
   c. Recalls that scopolamine, morphine, meperidine, and barbiturates may cause confusion, disorientation, apprehension, and restlessness when administered to clients with decreased renal function
5. Neurologic system
   a. Level of consciousness
   b. Orientation
   c. Ability to follow commands and communicate
   d. Gait, ability to ambulate
6. Musculoskeletal system (for the following because they may have an impact on positioning)
   a. Arthritis
   b. Osteoporosis
   c. Skeletal deformities
   d. Length of client's neck and shape of client's thoracic cavity, which may interfere with respiratory and cardiac function
7. Nutritional status
   a. Recognizes that malnutrition and obesity can cause poor wound healing and increase surgical risk
   b. Assesses for indicators of fluid and electrolyte imbalance and malnutrition
      (1) Brittle nails
      (2) Wasting muscles
      (3) Dry, flaky skin
      (4) Dull, sparse, dry hair
      (5) Decreased skin turgor
      (6) Postural hypotension
      (7) Decreased serum albumin
      (8) Abnormal electrolytes

8. Psychosocial status
    a. Anxiety and fear
    b. Coping mechanisms

Planning and Implementation

NDx: KNOWLEDGE DEFICIT

• Informed consent for the surgical procedure is obtained by the physician; the nurse may witness the client's signature.

• Consent implies that the client has been provided with information necessary to understand the

1. Nature of and reasons for surgery
2. Available options and risks associated with each option
3. Risks of surgical procedure and potential outcomes
4. Risks associated with the administration of anesthesia

• The nurse

1. Notifies the physician of any indications that the client did not understand the information given concerning the procedure or is not adequately informed
2. Clarifies facts presented by the physician
3. Dispels myths about surgery
4. Ensures that special permits that may be needed are obtained by the physician

• The client is allowed *nothing-by-mouth* (NPO) for 6 to 8 hours before surgery; it is customary to make the client NPO after midnight.

• The nurse

1. Emphasizes the consequences of not adhering to NPO
    a. Surgery may be cancelled.
    b. There is an increased risk of aspiration during surgery.
2. Consults the physician concerning the administration of medications such as corticosteroids and those used for hypertension, cardiac disease, glaucoma, and epilepsy

• *Bowel preparation* is usually done for clients having major abdominal, pelvic, perineal or perianal surgery or diagnostic procedures such as a colonoscopy.

• *Skin preparation* varies depending on the procedure and facility/physician preference.

• Skin preparation may include a shower or washing the involved area with special soap, providone-iodine (Betadine), or hexachlorophene.

P

- Shaving is generally not done until immediately before the start of the surgical procedure or not at all.
- The nurse prepares the client for the possibility of tubes, drains, and intravenous lines postoperatively
    1. Foley catheter, nasogastric tube
    2. Drains that promote the evacuation of fluid from the surgical wound
    3. Intravenous line, which is usually started on all clients
- The nurse teaches the client and family postoperative *exercises* preoperatively to reduce apprehension and to increase postoperative cooperation and participation.
    1. Ensures client mastery by observing correct performance on return demonstration
    2. Encourages the client to practice frequently
        a. Diaphragmatic breathing
        b. Incentive spirometry
        c. Coughing and deep breathing
        d. Splinting the wound
        e. Turning and leg exercises
- The nurse informs the family about the client's care and allows them to participate in the client's care if they desire to do so.
- The nurse informs the family of the scheduled time of surgery and of any change
    1. Reminds the family that 45 to 60 minutes of preparation time is often needed before surgery actually starts; frequently the physician does not include this time in their estimates of how long surgery will take
    2. Informs the family where they should wait during the surgery
    3. Reinforces to the family that it will be several hours before they will be able to see the client due to recovery room time and time required to admit the client to the unit after surgery
- Preoperative teaching reduces stress and anxiety associated with surgery.
- The nurse encourages the client to verbalize feelings freely without fear of ridicule or judgment.
- The nurse provides an environment conducive to sleep and offers the client a sedative if one is ordered.

CLIENT TRANSFER TO THE SURGICAL SUITE

- The nurse reviews the chart for
    1. Operative permit and other special permits
    2. Results of all laboratory, radiographic, and diagnostic tests

3. Abnormal results that are documented and reported to the physician
4. Height and weight
5. Current vital signs
6. Special needs flagged (e.g., client refusal to allow blood transfusion)

- Client preparation includes
  1. Hospital gown
  2. Antiembolism stockings or Ace bandages, if ordered
  3. Security of all client valuables (if rings cannot be removed cover with tape and note on preoperative checklist)
  4. Identification band, allergy band
  5. Removal of dentures, including partial plates; hair pins and clips of any type; wigs and toupees; prosthetic devices; all jewelry such as earrings and watches
  6. Checking facility policy regarding removal of hearing aids and fingernail polish
  7. Instructing the client to void

- After the medication is given, the client should remain in bed with the side rails up.

- Common preoperative medications
  1. Sedatives and hypnotics (e.g., pentobarbital sodium, secobarbital sodium, and chloral hydrate)
  2. Tranquilizers (e.g., chlorpromazine hydrochloride, hydroxyzine hydrochloride, diazepam, and promethazine hydrochloride)
  3. Narcotics (e.g., meperidine hydrochloride, morphine sulfate, and hydromorphine hydrochloride)
  4. Anticholinergics (e.g., atropine sulfate, glycopyrrolate and scopolamine)

P

For more information on preoperative care, see *Medical-Surgical Nursing: A Nursing Process Approach,* **pp. 427–453.**

Priapism

- Priapism is an uncontrolled and long-maintained erection without sexual desire, which causes the penis to become large, hard, and painful.
- Priapism occurs from neural, vascular, or pharmacologic causes.
- Common causes are thrombosis of the veins of the corpus cavernosa, leukemia, sickle cell anemia, diabetes, and malignancies.
- Priapism is also associated with psychotropic medications, antidepressants, and antihypertensives.
- Priapism is considered a urologic emergency because penile circulation may be compromised, and the client may not be able to void with an erect penis.
- Conservative treatment measures include
  1. Prostatic massage
  2. Sedation
  3. Bed rest
  4. Warm enemas to cause venous dilation and increase outflow of trapped blood
- Urinary catheterization is required.
- Aspiration of the corpora cavernosa with a large-bore needle or surgical intervention may be required.
- Priapism should be resolved within the first 24 to 30 hours to prevent penile ischemia, gangrene, fibrosis, and impotence.

For more information on priapism, see *Medical-Surgical Nursing: A Nursing Process Approach*, **p. 1768.**

Progressive Systemic Sclerosis

OVERVIEW

- Progressive systemic sclerosis (PSS), also referred to as systemic *scleroderma*, is a chronic connective tissue disease characterized by inflammation, fibrosis, and sclerosis and is similar to lupus erythematosus.
- PSS is manifested by arthralgia; stiffness; painless, symmetric, pitting edema of the hands and fingers, which may progress to include the entire upper and/or lower extremities and face; and taut and shiny skin that is free from wrinkles.
- In PSS, inflammation is replaced by tightening, hardening, and thickening of skin tissue; the skin loses its elasticity, and range of motion is markedly decreased.
- Joint contractures may develop, and the client is unable to perform activities of daily living.
- Major organ involvement is manifested in
    1. Gastrointestinal tract: hiatal hernia, esophageal reflux, dysphagia, reflux of gastric contents that can cause esophagitis, partial bowel obstruction, and malabsorption
    2. Cardiovascular system: Raynaud's phenomenon, digit necrosis, vasculitis, myocardial fibrosis, dysrhythmias, and chest pain

COLLABORATIVE MANAGEMENT

P

- Treatment of PSS is directed toward forcing the disease into remission and slowing its progress and includes
    1. Drugs such as steroids and immunosuppressants in large doses
    2. Local skin measures such as using mild soap, lotion, and gentle cleaning
    3. Bed cradle and footboard
    4. Constant room temperature
    5. Small, frequent meals, minimizing foods that stimulate gastric secretion (spicy foods, caffeine, alcohol) and having the client sit up for 1 to 2 hours after meals (if there is esophageal involvement)

- Refer to Rheumatoid Arthritis for care of joint pain.

For more information on progressive systemic sclerosis, see *Medical-Surgical Nursing: A Nursing Process Approach,* **pp. 704–706.**

Prostatic Cancer

OVERVIEW

- Prostatic cancer is the most common cancer among American men and the third leading cause of cancer deaths.
- Although its etiology is unclear, two factors influence its development
  1. Intact hypothalmic-pituitary-testicular pathway
  2. Advancing age
- An increase in dietary fat is thought to promote development of the tumor.
- Several viruses are found more frequently in cancerous prostatic tissue.
- Ninety-five percent of cancers of the prostate are adenocarcinomas arising from the epithelial cells of the prostate and are usually located in the posterior lobe or outer portion of the gland.
- A prostatic tumor is a slow-growing malignancy with a predictable metastatic pattern to the prostatic and perivesicular lymph nodes, pelvic lymph nodes, bone marrow, and bones of the pelvis, sacrum, and lumbar spine.

COLLABORATIVE MANAGEMENT

- Clinical manifestations include
  1. Symptoms related to bladder neck obstruction
     a. Difficulty in initiating urination

     b. Recurrent bladder infections

     c. Urinary retention

  2. Bone pain (advanced disease)

- Assessment includes

  1. Digital rectal examination by the physician for a stony hard prostate gland with irregularities or indurations

  2. Biopsy of prostatic tissue

- Management includes

  1. Surgical intervention—prostatectomy with pelvic lymphadenectomy

  2. Interstitial radiation therapy or radioactive seed implantation for localized disease (see Cancer)

  3. Androgen deprivation by simple orchiectomy or hormone therapy with estrogens such as diethylstilbesterol (DES) or a gonadotropin-releasing hormone agonist or androgen-blocking agent such as flutamide

- Client/family education includes a discussion about quality-of-life issues, including sexuality, body image, and the impact of a cancer diagnosis on life.

For more information on prostatic cancer, see *Medical-Surgical Nursing: A Nursing Process Approach*, **pp. 1750–1754.**

P

Prostatitis

- Prostatitis is an inflammatory condition of the prostate.
- The most common cause is a bacterial prostatitis, which can occur after a viral illness or results from a sudden decrease in sexual activity.
- Bacterial prostatitis is usually associated with urethritis or an infection of the lower urinary tract.

- Common causative organisms include *Escherichia coli, Enterobacter, Proteus,* and group D streptococci.
- *Acute* bacterial prostatitis is manifested by
  1. Fever and chills
  2. Dysuria
  3. Urethral discharge
  4. Boggy, tender prostate
  5. Decreased sexual function
  6. Urinary tract infections
- *Chronic* prostatitis is manifested by
  1. Backache
  2. Perineal pain
  3. Mild dysuria
  4. Urinary frequency
  5. Hematuria
  6. An irregularly enlarged, firm, and slightly tender prostate
  7. Decreased sexual functions
  8. Urinary tract infections
- Complications include epididymitis and cystitis.
- Treatment includes antimicrobials such as carbenicillin indanyl sodium (Geocillin) and comfort measures such as sitz baths, stool softeners, and analgesia.
- Client education includes measures that will drain the prostate, including intercourse, masturbation, and prostatic massage.

For more information on prostatitis, see *Medical-Surgical Nursing: A Nursing Process Approach,* **p. 1769.**

Psoriasis

OVERVIEW

- Psoriasis is a lifelong scaling skin disorder with underlying dermal inflammation characterized by exacerbations and remissions.
- Lesions occur anywhere on the body and may be limited to one or two localized plaques or involve large epidermal areas.

- Abnormal proliferation of epidermal cells in the outer skin areas results in cell shedding every 4 to 5 days.
- *Psoriasis vulgaris* is the most common type and is characterized by
    1. Thick erythematous papules or plaques surmounted by silvery-white scales
    2. Sharply defined borders between lesions and normal skin lesions distributed symmetrically, with the common sites of the scalp, elbows, trunk, knees, sacrum, and extensor surfaces of the limbs
    3. Associated nail involvement
- *Guttate psoriasis* appears as isolated droplet-shaped papules, primarily scattered over the trunk, sparing the palms and the soles.
- *Exfoliative psoriasis* (erythrodermic psoriasis) is characterized by generalized erythema and scaling without obvious lesions.
- *Pustular psoriasis* is a rare, fatal manifestation, with generalized erythema and scaling occurring with pustules and secondary infection of the lesions.

COLLABORATIVE MANAGEMENT
Assessment
- The nurse records the client's
    1. Precipitating factors, including skin trauma, upper respiratory infections, surgeries, past and current medications, and stress
    2. Family history of psoriasis
    3. Age at onset
    4. Description of progression and patterns of recurrences
    5. Gradual or sudden onset of episode
    6. Description of lesion location
    7. Associated symptoms such as fever and pruritis
    8. Previous treatment modalities
- The nurse assesses for
    1. Character and distribution of skin lesions
    2. Character of lesions responding to treatment
    3. Signs of dehydration
    4. Hypothermia or hyperthermia
    5. Skin tenderness

Planning and Implementation
NDx: IMPAIRED SKIN INTEGRITY
- The nurse
    1. Applies topical steroids, as ordered, to skin lesions, followed by warm, moist dressings to increase absorption

P

531

2. Applies tar preparations, as ordered, which contain crude coal tar and derivations and are available in solution, ointment, lotion, gel, and shampoo

• Ultraviolet light therapy decreases epidermal growth rate.

• Systemic treatment with a cytostatic agent is given for severe, debilitating psoriasis.

NDx: PAIN

• The nurse
  1. Administers antihistamine therapy, as ordered
  2. Maintains skin hydration and lubrication

NDx: INEFFECTIVE INDIVIDUAL COPING

• The nurse
  1. Identifies precipitating stressors and alleviates if possible
  2. Teaches relaxation techniques
  3. Promotes physical exercise
  4. Refers the client to professional counseling, if necessary

NDx: BODY IMAGE DISTURBANCE

• The nurse
  1. Promotes contact with other clients with psoriasis
  2. Facilitates group discussions to promote socialization
  3. Uses touch to promote acceptance

Discharge Planning

• The nurse
  1. Identifies precipitating factors
  2. Explains the rationale of the treatment plan and the importance of compliance
  3. Teaches the proper application and side effects of the therapeutic agents
  4. Emphasizes the control of symptoms by the identification of precipitators and complying with treatment
  5. Emphasizes the importance of follow-up visits with the physician(s)

For more information on psoriasis, see *Medical-Surgical Nursing: A Nursing Process Approach*, **pp. 1186–1197.**

Ptosis

- Ptosis is the drooping of, or the inability to use, the upper eyelid.
- Types of ptosis include
  1. Neurogenic, resulting from interference with the third cranial nerve
  2. Myogenic, relating to altered myoneural impulse function
  3. Mechanical, caused by abnormal weight of the eyelids from edema, inflammation, or a tumor
  4. Traumatic, caused by an injury to the third cranial nerve or the levator muscle
- Treatment is palliative; surgery may be indicated if visual acuity or appearance is adversely affected.
- Nursing management after surgery consists of assessing the eye for drainage and infection, cool compresses, ophthalmic antibiotic or an antibiotic-steroid combination ointment, teaching the client the procedure to instill the ointment, and notifying the physician if dryness or burning of the eye occurs.

P

For more information on ptosis, see *Medical-Surgical Nursing: A Nursing Process Approach,* **pp. 1013–1014.**

Pulmonary Contusion

- Pulmonary contusion is characterized by interstitial hemorrhage associated with intra-alveolar hemorrhage, resulting in decreased pulmonary compliance.
- Respiratory failure develops over time following

blunt chest trauma from rapid deceleration injuries during motor vehicle accidents.

- Manifestations include
  1. Hypoxemia
  2. Dyspnea
  3. Irritated bronchial mucosa
  4. Increased bronchial secretions
  5. Hemoptysis
  6. Decreased breath sounds, rales, and wheezes

- Treatment is aimed at maintenance of ventilation and oxygenation; the distressed client requires mechanical ventilation with positive end-expiratory pressure. The major complication is adult respiratory distress syndrome (ARDS).

For more information on pulmonary contusion, see *Medical-Surgical Nursing: A Nursing Process Approach*, **p. 2057.**

Pulmonary Embolism

OVERVIEW

- Pulmonary embolism occurs when a thrombus that forms in a deep vein detaches and travels to the right side of the heart and then lodges in a branch of the pulmonary artery.

- Physiologic responses include platelet accumulation, triggering the release of potent vasoconstrictors and causing widespread pulmonary vasoconstriction, which impairs ventilation and perfusion.

- Clients prone to pulmonary embolism are those at risk for deep vein thrombosis (DVT), including prolonged immobilization, surgery, obesity, pregnancy, congestive heart failure, advanced age, and prior history of thromboembolism.

COLLABORATIVE MANAGEMENT

- Nursing interventions are aimed at preventing venous stasis and include range-of-motion exercises, early ambulation, antiembolism or pneumatic compression stockings, and preventing pressure under the popliteal space.
- Subcutaneous heparin injections are given to prevent hypercoagulability.
- The nurse assesses for
  1. Dyspnea accompanied by anginal and pleuritic pain exacerbated by inspiration
  2. Cough
  3. Blood-tinged sputum
  4. Rales on auscultation
  5. Tachycardia
  6. Shallow respirations
  7. Low-grade fever
  8. Distended neck veins
  9. Cyanosis
  10. Dysrhythmias
  11. Positive Homans' sign
- Interventions include
  1. Oxygen
  2. Intubation and mechanical ventilation for severe hypoxemia
  3. Anticoagulation with intravenous heparin (bolus followed by continuous infusion) during the acute phase; warfarin (Coumadin) orally when the heparin drip is discontinued, with prothrombin time and partial thromboplastin time monitored closely)
  4. Surgical embolectomy
  5. Surgical vein ligation
  6. Insertion of an umbrella filter

P

For more information on pulmonary embolism, see *Medical-Surgical Nursing: A Nursing Process Approach*, **pp. 2059–2060.**

Pulmonary Sarcoidosis

- Pulmonary sarcoidosis is a chronic interstitial or fibrotic lung disease associated with an intense cellular immune response in the alveolar structures.

- The hallmark of sarcoidosis is noncaseating granuloma of the alveolar structures composed of lymphocytes, macrophages, epithelioid cells, and giant cells.

- Interstitial fibrosis results in a loss of lung compliance and functional ability to exchange gases.

- Cor pulmonale (right-sided congestive heart failure) develops due to the heart's inability to pump against the noncompliant, fibrotic lung.

- The disease affects Black persons 10 times more frequently than Caucasians and develops between the ages of 20 and 40 years.

- Indications for treatment vary.

- If the client is asymptomatic, with no abnormalities in pulmonary function tests, there is no treatment.

- For reduced pulmonary function, steroids are administered.

For more information on pulmonary sarcoidosis, see *Medical-Surgical Nursing: A Nursing Process Approach*, **pp. 2040–2041.**

Rabies

- Rabies is a severe and often fatal neurologic disease caused by a virus transmitted by a bite from a rabid mammal.

- All animal and human bites or potentially

contaminated cuts are thoroughly cleansed with detergent and running water for 5 minutes, followed by the application of a topical antiseptic.

- Deep wounds require exploration to remove foreign objects.
- Occlusive dressings are avoided since moist wounds can promote the growth of viral organisms.
- The rabies virus is killed by exposure and drying.

For more information on rabies, see *Medical-Surgical Nursing: A Nursing Process Approach*, **pp. 1209–1210.**

Raynaud's Phenomenon/ Raynaud's Disease

- Raynaud's is caused by vasospasm of the arterioles and arteries of the upper and lower extremities.
- Cutaneous vessels are constricted, causing blanching of the extremities, followed by cyanosis.
- When the vasospasm is relieved, the tissue becomes reddened or hyperemic.
- *Raynaud's phenomenon* usually occurs unilaterally in individuals older than 30 years and occurs in both sexes.
- *Raynaud's disease* occurs bilaterally between the ages of 17 and 50 years and is more common in females.
- Clinical manifestations include
  1. Color changes in the extremity or digits from blanched, to reddened, to cyanotic
  2. Numbness of the extremity or digits
  3. Coldness of the extremity or digits
  4. Pain

R

5. Swelling
6. Ulcerations
7. Aggravation of symptoms by cold or stress
8. Gangrene of digits in severe cases

- Interventions include
    1. Drug therapy to prevent vasoconstriction
    2. Lumbar sympathectomy to relieve symptoms in the feet
    3. Sympathetic ganglionectomy to relieve symptoms in the upper extremities

- Client education emphasizes methods to minimize vasoconstriction
    1. Decrease exposure to cold
    2. Decrease stress
    3. Wear warm clothes, socks, and/or gloves
    4. Keep the home at a comfortable, warm temperature

For more information on Raynaud's phenomenon/ Raynaud's disease, see *Medical-Surgical Nursing: A Nursing Process Approach,* **pp. 2226–2227.**

Rectocele

- A rectocele is a protrusion of the rectum through a weakened vaginal wall.
- A rectocele may develop as a result of the pressure of a baby's head during a difficult delivery, a traumatic forceps delivery, or a congenital defect of the pelvic support tissues.
- Assessment findings include
    1. Constipation
    2. Hemorrhoids
    3. Fecal impaction

4. Feelings of vaginal or rectal fullness
5. Bulge of the posterior vaginal wall during pelvic examination

- Management is focused on promoting bowel elimination
  1. High-fiber diet
  2. Stool softeners
  3. Laxatives
- The surgical intervention is a posterior colporrhaphy or posterior repair.
- Care is similar to other rectal surgeries.
- If both a cystocele and rectocele are repaired, the client has an anterior and posterior (A&P) repair.

For more information on rectocele, see *Medical-Surgical Nursing: A Nursing Process Approach*, **pp. 1706–1707.**

Refractive Error

R

- Refractive errors result from problems in the ability of the eye to focus images on the retina.
- Types of refractive errors include
  1. *Myopia*, also referred to as nearsightedness; when distant objects appear blurred
  2. *Hyperopia*, also referred to as farsightedness; when close objects appear blurred
  3. *Presbyopia*, when the lens is unable to alter its shape to focus the eye for close work
  4. *Astigmatism*, a refractive defect that prevents focusing of sharp, distinct images
  5. *Aphakia*, the absence of the crystalline lens
- Treatment of refractive errors includes
  1. Eyeglasses

2. Contact lenses (complications of contact lenses include corneal edema, corneal abrasions, and giant papillary cell conjunctivitis)
3. Surgery
   a. *Radical keratotomy* to treat mild to moderate myopia is done if the client is unable to tolerate glasses or contact lenses. Complications include over- or undercorrection of the refractive error, corneal scars, and failure to achieve adequate correction.
   b. *Epikeratophakia* is the surgical grafting of donor corneal tissue onto the client's own cornea to alter its refractive ability.

For more information on refractive errors, see *Medical-Surgical Nursing: A Nursing Process Approach,* **pp. 1060–1064.**

Rehabilitation

OVERVIEW

- Chronic disease is characterized by
  1. Duration longer than 6 months
  2. Residual disability
  3. Nonreversible pathologic alterations as the cause
  4. The need for special training of the client in rehabilitation
  5. The expectation that a long period of supervision, observation, or care will be required

- *Rehabilitation* is the process of learning to live with disability. Impairment is an abnormality of a body structure or structures or an alteration in a system function resulting from any cause.

- *Disability* is the consequence of an impairment; a *handicap* is the disadvantage experienced by an individual as a result of impairments and disabilities.

- Settings for rehabilitation include
  1. Freestanding rehabilitation hospitals
  2. Rehabilitation units within acute care hospitals or within skilled nursing or long-term-care facilities
  3. Outpatient hospital rehabilitation centers
  4. Transitional living centers, a step between a rehabilitation center and an independent living center (ILC), with the goal of preparing the client to live at home or in the ILC
  5. ILCs, in which the client shares an apartment or home with other disabled clients and with supervision and support available
  6. Vocational rehabilitation
- Rehabilitation team members typically include the
  1. Nurse
  2. Occupational therapist (OT)
  3. Orthotist
  4. Physicians
     a. Psychiatrist
     b. Internal medicine
     c. Orthopedic surgeon
     d. Neurologist, neurosurgeon
     e. Urologist
     f. Other medical specialists
  5. Physical therapist (PT)
  6. Psychologist
  7. Recreational therapist
  8. Respiratory therapist
  9. Speech language pathologist (SLP)
  10. Social worker and/or case manager
  11. Vocational counselor

COLLABORATIVE MANAGEMENT

Assessment

- The nurse records the client's health history with a rehabilitation focus

R

  1. History of existing condition
  2. Occupation
  3. Educational background
  4. Home situation
     a. Architectural features
     b. Proximity of shopping centers, transportation
     c. Availability of support for help in the home such as cooking and cleaning
  5. Daily schedule and activities of daily living (ADL)
  6. Bowel and bladder routine and habits
  7. Sexuality patterns
  8. Sleep habits, bedtime routine

- The nurse assesses for
  1. Cardiovascular system
     a. Routine cardiovascular assessment
     b. Alteration in cardiac status such as hyper- or hypotension, chest pain, and diuresis
     c. Manifestations of activity intolerance
     d. Knowledge of the cardiovascular problem, risk factors, and compliance with medication and the rehabilitation regimen
  2. Respiratory system
     a. Routine respiratory assessment
     b. Level of activity the client can perform without becoming short of breath
  3. Gastrointestinal (GI) system
     a. Routine GI assessment
     b. Oral intake and pattern for eating
     c. Indications of anorexia, dysphagia, nausea, vomiting, and/or discomfort related to and/or interfering with oral intake
     d. Height, weight, hemoglobin and hematocrit levels, and serum albumin and blood glucose concentrations
     e. Changes in the client's normal elimination patterns
  4. Urinary system
     a. Routine urologic assessment
     b. Baseline urinary patterns
        (1) Output
        (2) Number of times the client usually voids and at what time of day
        (3) Problems with incontinence or retention
     c. Usual fluid intake patterns and volume, including the type of fluids ingested and the time of fluid consumption
  5. Neurologic system
     a. Routine neurologic assessment
     b. Functional aspects of cognition, pain, comfort, sensation, strength, and dexterity
     c. Preexisting problems, general physical condition, and communication abilities
     d. Sensory/perceptual deficits
  6. Musculoskeletal system
     a. Routine musculoskeletal assessment
     b. Impact of deficits on the client's home, work, and/or school environment
  7. Integumentary system
     a. Routine integumentary assessment

    b. Actual and potential interruptions in skin integrity

    c. Use of the facility assessment tool to predict the risk of skin breakdown

    d. Client's understanding of the cause and treatment of skin breakdown

8. Functional assessment, with various tools used to measure objectively the level at which a person is performing in any of a variety of areas

    a. Physical health

    b. Quality of self-maintenance

    c. Quality of role activity

    d. Intellectual status

    e. Attitude toward the world and toward self

    f. Emotional status

9. Psychological assessment

    a. Changes in body image, self-esteem, role performance, anger, and anxiety

    b. Defense mechanisms

    c. Availability of support systems such as family and significant others

10. Vocational assessment (information on the client's current occupation, work history)

Planning and Implementation

NDx: IMPAIRED PHYSICAL MOBILITY

- The nurse

1. Assesses for and intervenes to prevent complications of immobility

    a. Contractures

        (1) Provides active-assist or passive range-of-motion (ROM) exercises at least daily

        (2) Provides foot support while in bed

    b. Constipation/decreased GI motility

        (1) Assists the client to increase his or her activity level

        (2) Provides a high-fiber diet

    c. Decreased cardiac output (performs ROM exercises)

    d. Increased venous stasis/thrombus formation/embolism

        (1) Applies antiembolism stockings

        (2) Avoids leg massage

        (3) Performs ROM exercises

        (4) Monitors vital signs

    e. Disorientation

        (1) Helps the client maintain a normal sleep-wake cycle

R

(2) Orients the client as needed

(3) Controls sensory stimulation to the client

f. Postural hypotension (avoids sudden position changes)

g. Renal calculi

    (1) Decreases dietary calcium

    (2) Increases fluids

    (3) Maintains acidic urine through diet or drugs

h. Pneumonia

    (1) Turns, coughs, and deep breathes the client at least every 2 hours

    (2) Teaches respiratory exercises

i. Pressure ulcers

    (1) Repositions the client frequently (at least every 2 hours)

    (2) Applies pressure-relief devices as appropriate

2. Performs ROM exercises

a. Exercises all joints

b. Completes full range movement of each joint at least 5 or more times

c. Performs exercises at least 3 times daily

d. Does not move the joint beyond the point at which the client expresses pain or the nurse perceives stiffness or difficulty

3. Utilizes and teaches correct transfer techniques

a. Bed to wheelchair or chair

    (1) Places the chair at an angle to the bed on the client's strong side

    (2) Locks the wheelchair brakes or secures the chair position

    (3) Assists the client to stand and move his or her strong hand to the armrest

    (4) Keeps the client's body weight forward and pivots

    (5) Assists the client in sitting when the client's legs touch the chair edge

b. Wheelchair to chair or bed

    (1) Places the chair with the client's strong side next to the bed

    (2) Locks or secures the wheelchair brakes

    (3) Assists the client to stand and moves the client's strong hand to the armrest

    (4) Keeps the client's body weight forward and pivots

    (5) Assists the client in sitting and then

reclining when the client's legs touch the bed edge

c. Use of a sliding board
  (1) Places the chair or wheelchair as close to the bed as possible
  (2) Removes the armrest from the chair (if removable) or wheelchair
  (3) Powders the sliding board
  (4) Places the sliding board under the client's buttocks
  (5) Instructs the client to reach toward his or her side
  (6) Assists the client in sliding gently to the bed or chair

4. Assists the client in gait training
  a. Walker assisted
    (1) Applies a gait belt around the client's waist
    (2) Assists the client to a standing position
    (3) Assists the client in placing both hands on the walker
    (4) Ensures that the client is well balanced
    (5) Assists the client repeatedly to perform the following sequence
      —Lift the walker
      —Move the walker 2 ft forward and set it down on all legs
      —While resting on the walker, take small steps
      —Check balance

  b. Cane assisted
    (1) Applies a gait belt around the client's waist
    (2) Assists the client to a standing position
    (3) Assists the client in placing his or her strong hand on the cane
    (4) Ensures that the client is well balanced
    (5) Assists the client repeatedly to perform the following sequence:
      —Move the cane forward
      —Move the weaker leg one step forward
      —Move the stronger leg one step forward
      —Check balance

NDx: TOTAL SELF-CARE DEFICIT

- The nurse
  1. Encourages the client to perform ADL within his or her abilities
  2. Follows the care plan initiated by physical and occupational therapy

3. Reinforces the correct use of assistive devices
4. Encourages the client to eat a balanced diet

NDx: POTENTIAL FOR IMPAIRED SKIN INTEGRITY

- The nurse
  1. Assesses the client for risk level
  2. Repositions the client every 2 hours or more and assesses the skin with each positioning
  3. Encourages the client to eat a balanced diet
  4. Provides frequent skin care
  5. Obtains mechanical devices as appropriate
     a. Water bed
     b. Foam mattress
     c. Air mattress
     d. Alternating-pressure mattress
     e. Air-fluidized device (e.g., Clinitron bed)

NDx: CONSTIPATION; BOWEL INCONTINENCE; DIARRHEA

- The nurse designs a bowel program
  1. Plans and implements the program based on the cause
     a. *Upper motor neuron* disease may result in a reflex bowel pattern with defecation occurring suddenly without warning.
        (1) Initiates a bowel training program
        (2) Provides a high-fiber diet
        (3) Administers suppositories, as ordered
        (4) Maintains a consistent toileting schedule
     b. *Lower motor neuron* disease may result in a flaccid bowel pattern with defecation occurring infrequently and in small amounts.
        (1) Initiates a bowel program
        (2) Provides a high-fiber diet
        (3) Administers suppositories, as ordered
        (4) Maintains a consistent toileting schedule
        (5) Performs manual disimpaction as needed
     c. *Uninhibited bowel pattern* may result in frequent defecation, urgency, and complaints of constipation.
        (1) Maintains a consistent toileting schedule
        (2) Provides a high-fiber diet
        (3) Administers stool softeners, as ordered
  2. Modifies the bowel program if complications occur, such as constipation, diarrhea, or flatulence

NDx: ALTERED PATTERNS OF URINARY ELIMINATION; REFLEX INCONTINENCE; TOTAL INCONTINENCE; URINARY RETENTION

- *Reflex* bladder results in urinary frequency and urgency.
- *Flaccid* bladder results in dribbling, overflow, and incontinence.
- *Uninhibited bladder* results in frequency, urgency, and voiding in small amounts.
- The nurse
  1. Initiates a bladder training program as appropriate
     a. Intermittent catheterization/residual urine determination
     b. Consistent scheduling of toileting routines
     c. Facilitating or triggering techniques to stimulate voiding
     d. Valsalva's and Credé's maneuvers
  2. Administers drug therapy, as ordered
     a. Cholinergics: bethanechol chloride (Urecholine)
     b. Antispasmodics: oxybutynin chloride (Ditropan), flavoxate hydrochloride (Urispas)
     c. Anticholinergics: propantheline bromide (Pro-Banthine)
     d. Skeletal muscle relaxants: dantrolene (Dantrium), baclofen (Lioresal)
  3. Provides and teaches diet therapy
     a. Encourages fluids to 3000 mL per day unless contraindicated
     b. Encourages fluids that promote an acidic urine such as tomato juice, cranberry juice, and bouillon
     c. Avoids excessive milk and citrus juices, which promote alkaline urine
  4. Intervenes to prevent complications
     a. Autonomic hyperreflexia or dysreflexia
     b. Bladder overdistention
     c. Increased urinary residual volume

Discharge Planning

- The nurse
  1. Assists the client/family to identify and correct hazards in the home prior to discharge
  2. Ensures that the client can correctly use all adaptive-assistive devices ordered for home use
  3. Provides a detailed plan of care at the time of

R

discharge for the client to be transferred to a long-term-care facility or rehabilitation center
4. Assesses for support systems to help the client to cope with disability
- The nurse teaches the client
    1. Use of orthotic and ambulatory aids (with the PT)
    2. Prescribed exercise regimen (client mastery is ensured by observing correct performance on return demonstration)
    3. Skills for ADL (with the OT)
    4. Bladder and bowel training
    5. Prevention of immobility complications

For more information on rehabilitation, see *Medical Surgical Nursing: A Nursing Process Approach*, **pp. 504–522.**

Renal Abscess

- A renal abscess is a collection of fluid and cells resulting from an inflammatory response to bacteria in the renal parenchyma, renal fascia, or the flank.
- An abscess is suspected when fever and symptoms are unresponsive to antibiotic therapy.
- Symptoms include
    1. Fever
    2. Flank pain
    3. General malaise
    4. Local edema
- Treatment includes
    1. Broad-spectrum antibiotics
    2. Drainage by surgical incision or needle aspiration

For more information on renal abscess, see *Medical-Surgical Nursing: A Nursing Process Approach*, **p. 1843.**

Renal Artery Stenosis

- Renal artery stenosis involves pathologic processes affecting the renal arteries, resulting in severe narrowing of the lumen and reducing blood flow to the renal parenchyma.
- Uncorrected stenosis leads to ischemia and atrophy of renal tissue.
- Renal artery stenosis is suspected when a sudden onset of hypertension occurs.
- Atherosclerotic changes in the renal artery are associated with corresponding disease of the aorta and other major vessels.
- Fibromuscular changes of the vessel wall occur throughout the length of the renal artery between the aortic junction and branching into the renal segmental arteries.
- The location of the defect, the overall condition of the client, and the size of the atrophied kidney influence the decision for therapeutic intervention.
- Treatment includes
    1. Antihypertensive drugs
    2. Percutaneous transluminal balloon angioplasty
    3. Renal artery bypass surgery

For more information on renal artery stenosis, see *Medical-Surgical Nursing: A Nursing Process Approach*, **p. 1856.**

R

Renal Failure, Acute

OVERVIEW

- Acute renal failure (ARF) is the rapid deterioration of renal function associated with an accumulation of nitrogenous wastes in the body (azotemia) not due to extrarenal factors.

- The three types of acute renal failure include
  1. *Prerenal failure*
     a. Failure results from decreased blood flow to the kidneys, leading to ischemia in the nephrons.
     b. Prolonged hypoperfusion can lead to tubular necrosis and ARF.
     c. Conditions that cause decreased cardiac output and ultimately hypoperfusion to the kidneys include shock, congestive heart failure, pulmonary embolism, anaphylaxis, pericardial tamponade, and sepsis.
  2. *Intrarenal failure*
     a. Failure results from actual tissue damage to the kidney caused by inflammatory or immunologic processes.
     b. The cause is exposure to nephrotoxins, acute glomerulonephritis, vasculitis, hepatorenal syndrome, and acute tubular necrosis (ATN).
  3. *Postrenal failure*
     a. Failure results from an obstruction of the urinary collecting system or the bladder.
     b. The causes may be urethral or bladder cancer, renal calculi, atonic bladder, prostatic hyperplasia or cancer, or cervical cancer.
- The four phases of ARF include
  1. *Onset* phase: begins with the precipitating event and continues until oliguria is observed; lasts hours to several days; clinical manifestations are rising blood urea nitrogen (BUN) and creatinine levels and urinary output of less than 400 mL/24 hours
  2. *Diuretic* or high-output phase: urine output up to 10 L/day; usually occurs 2 to 6 weeks after onset and continues until the BUN ceases to rise
  3. *Recovery* phase: begins when the BUN level starts to fall and lasts until the BUN reaches normal levels; normal renal tubular function is reestablished
  4. *Convalescence* phase: returns to normal activities but functions at a lower energy level

COLLABORATIVE MANAGEMENT

Assessment

- The nurse records the client's
  1. Exposure to nephrotoxins
  2. Recent surgery or trauma

3. Transfusions
4. Known renal disease
5. History of diabetes mellitus, systemic lupus erythematosus, and chronic malignant hypertension
6. History of acute illnesses, including influenza, colds, gastroenteritis, and sore throat
7. History of intravascular volume depletion
8. History of urinary obstructive disease

- The nurse assesses for

  1. Cardiovascular manifestations

     a. Chest pain
     b. Tachycardia
     c. Hypotension
     d. Decreased cardiac output
     e. Decreased central venous pressure
     f. Peripheral edema
     g. Cardiac irritability

  2. Respiratory symptoms

     a. Shortness of breath
     b. Pulmonary edema
     c. Friction rub

  3. Neurologic manifestations

     a. Lethargy
     b. Somnolence
     c. Tremors
     d. Headache
     e. Mental confusion
     f. Muscle cramps
     g. Generalized weakness
     h. Seizures
     i. Flaccid paralysis
     j. Coma

  4. Gastrointestinal (GI) manifestations

     a. Nausea
     b. Vomiting
     c. GI bleeding
     d. Constipation
     e. Diarrhea
     f. Flank pain

  5. Genitourinary manifestations

     a. Decreased urinary output
     b. Hematuria
     c. Changes in urine stream
     d. Difficulty starting urination
     e. Dysuria
     f. Urgency
     g. Incontinence

R

6. Integumentary manifestations
   a. Ecchymoses
   b. Yellow pallor

Planning and Implementation

NDx: FLUID VOLUME DEFICIT

• The client with ARF receives multiple medications, as does the client with chronic renal failure (see Renal Failure, Chronic).

• Fluid challenges and diuretics are frequently used to promote renal perfusion.

• A low-dose dopamine infusion may be used to promote renal perfusion.

• Hypercatabolism results in the breakdown of muscle for protein, which leads to increased azotemia; clients require increased calories. Total parenteral nutrition (TPN) with intralipid infusion may be required to reduce catabolism.

• Indications for hemodialysis or peritoneal dialysis in ARF are symptoms of uremia, persistent hyperkalemia, persistent acidosis, severe fluid overload, severe hyponatremia, pericarditis, toxins, and the need for prophylaxis. (See Renal Failure, Chronic for a discussion of dialysis.)

• Continuous arteriovenous *hemofiltration* (CAVH), an alternative to dialysis, may be used to treat hypervolemia and toxic solute accumulation.

• Also known as ultrafiltration, CAVH necessitates the insertion of a vascular access device, which is then connected to a low-flow filter system, driven by the client's own blood pressure and gravity; blood circulates at a much slower rate, which avoids hypotension and extreme fluid shifts.

• The nurse
   1. Monitors the client's status, assessing for hypotension
   2. Monitors the hemofiltration circuit
   3. Observes the amount and color of the filtered drainage (ultrafiltrate)
   4. Monitors for signs of infection at the venous access site
   5. Monitors laboratory values
   6. Records intake and output accurately

Discharge Planning

• Discharge planning and client/family education are centered around the specific pathophysiology and precipitating factors of the disease, clinical manifestations of progressive renal failure, and treatment measures.

• The needs of the client vary depending on the status of the disease on discharge. Refer to "Discharge Planning" under Renal Failure, Chronic.

For more information on acute renal failure, see *Medical-Surgical Nursing: A Nursing Process Approach*, **pp. 1917–1925.**

Renal Failure, Chronic

OVERVIEW

• Chronic renal failure (CRF) is a condition in which the kidney ceases to remove metabolic wastes and excessive water from the blood.
• The progression toward CRF occurs in three stages

1. *Stage I*, or *diminished renal reserve*
   a. There is a reduction in renal functioning without accumulation of metabolic wastes.
   b. The unaffected kidney may compensate.
2. *Stage II*, or *renal insufficiency*
   a. Metabolic wastes begin to accumulate in the blood because the unaffected nephrons no longer compensate.
   b. The degree of insufficiency is determined by the decreasing glomerular filtration rate and is classified as mild, moderate, or severe.
3. *Stage III*, or *end-stage renal disease* (ESRD)
   a. ESRD occurs when excessive amounts of metabolic wastes accumulate in the blood.
   b. The kidneys are unable to maintain homeostasis and require dialysis.

• Pathologic alterations include disruptions in the glomerular filtration rate (GFR), abnormalities of urine production and water excretion, electrolyte imbalance, and metabolic anomalies.

R

- Metabolic alterations include disturbances in blood urea nitrogen (BUN) and creatinine excretion.
- *Urea* is the primary product of protein metabolism and is normally excreted by the kidney; BUN varies with dietary intake of protein.
- *Creatinine* is derived from creatine and phosphocreatine; the normal rate of excretion depends on muscle mass, physical activity, and diet.
- *Azotemia* is the increased accumulation of BUN and creatinine in the blood; it is a classic indicator of renal failure.
- Variations in sodium excretion occur depending on the stage of CRF.
- *Hyponatremia,* or sodium depletion, in early CRF is due to obligatory loss.
- *Hypernatremia* occurs when the kidney's ability to excrete sodium decreases as urine production decreases.
- *Hyperkalemia* results from an increase in potassium load, including ingestion of potassium in medications, failure to restrict potassium in the diet, blood transfusions, and excess bleeding.
- Other pathologic occurrences include numerous metabolic disturbances such as changes in pH (metabolic acidosis), calcium (hypercalcemia) and phosphorus (hypophosphetemia) imbalances, and vitamin D insufficiency.
- Renal *osteodystrophy* caused by hypocalcemia and phosphorus retention results in skeletal demineralization manifested by bone pain, pseudofractures, sclerosis of the spine, skull demineralization, osteomalacia, reabsorption of bone, and loss of tooth lamina.
- Cardiovascular alterations include anemia, hypertension, congestive heart failure, and pericarditis.

COLLABORATIVE MANAGEMENT

Assessment

- The nurse records the client's
    1. Age and sex
    2. Height and weight
    3. Current and past medical conditions
    4. Medications, prescription and over the counter
    5. Family history of renal disease
    6. Dietary and nutritional habits
    7. Change in food tastes
    8. History of gastrointestinal (GI) problems such as

nausea, vomiting, anorexia, diarrhea, and/or constipation
9. Current energy level
10. Recent injuries and/or bleeding
11. Weakness
12. Shortness of breath
13. Detailed urinary elimination

- The nurse assesses for

  1. Cardiovascular abnormalities

     a. Hypertension
     b. Anemia
     c. Abnormal bleeding
     d. Peripheral edema
     e. Congestive heart failure
     f. Pulmonary edema

  2. Respiratory manifestations

     a. Breath that smells like urine
     b. Deep sighing or yawning
     c. Shortness of breath
     d. Hyperventilation
     e. Kussmaul's respirations
     f. Uremic lung or hilar pneumonitis

  3. Neurologic manifestations

     a. Weakness and lassitude
     b. Extreme drowsiness
     c. Shortened attention span
     d. Peripheral neuropathies (numb, weakened extremities)
     e. Headaches
     f. Muscle twitching
     g. Convulsions
     h. Coma

  4. GI disruptions

     a. Anorexia
     b. Nausea
     c. Vomiting
     d. Unpleasant or metallic taste
     e. Constipation
     f. Diarrhea
     g. GI bleeding

  5. Genitourinary findings

     a. Change in urinary frequency
     b. Hematuria
     c. Change in urine appearance
     d. Proteinuria

  6. Integumentary or dermatologic manifestations

     a. Pale, yellow skin

b. Uremic frost (urea crystals on the face and eyebrows)
c. Severe itching (pruritis)
d. Dry skin
e. Purpura
f. Ecchymoses

Planning and Implementation

NDx: Fluid Volume Excess

Nonsurgical Management

• The nurse administers and monitors the complex drug therapy, as ordered
  1. Cardiotonics, such as digoxin
  2. Vitamins and minerals, including folic acid, ferrous sulfate, and calcium gluconate
  3. Phosphate binders, such as aluminum hydroxide gel (Amphojel, Alternagel, Alu-Cap) and aluminum carbonate gel (Basaljel), to decrease serum phosphorus
  4. Stool softeners and laxatives, such as docusate sodium (Colace) and bisacodyl (Dulcolax)
  5. Antihypertensives, such as hydralazine hydrochloride (Apresoline), methyldopa (Aldomet), metoprolol tartrate (Lopressor), prazosin (Minipress), propranolol (Inderal), and clonidine hydrochloride (Catapres)
  6. Diuretics
     a. Osmotic diuretics act on the proximal convoluted tubule, such as mannitol and urea.
     b. Thiazide and thiazide-like diuretics act on the cortical diluting site of the ascending limb of the loop of Henle, such as chlorothiazide (Diuril), hydrochlorothiazide (HydroDiuril), chlorthalidone (Hygroton), and metolazone (Zaroxolyn).
     c. Loop diuretics act on the ascending limb of the loop of Henle, such as furosemide (Lasix), bumetanide (Bumex), and ethacrynic acid (Edecrin).
     d. Potassium-sparing diuretics act on the distal convoluted tubule, such as spironolactone (Aldactone) and triamterene (Dyazide).

• *Hemodialysis* is used to remove the body's excessive fluid and waste products via vascular accesses, such as external arteriovenous (AV) shunts, internal access or AV fistula, or temporary external vascular access such as subclavian or femoral vein catheters.

• Hemodialysis is based on the principle of diffusion, in which the client's blood is circulated through a semipermeable membrane that acts as an artificial kidney.

- Nurses are specially trained to perform hemodialysis.
- After hemodialysis, the nurse
  1. Closely monitors for side effects
     a. Hypotension
     b. Headache
     c. Nausea
     d. Malaise
     e. Vomiting
     f. Dizziness
     g. Muscle cramps
  2. Obtains the client's weight and vital signs
  3. Avoids invasive procedures for 4 to 6 hours, due to heparinization of the dialysate
  4. Monitors for signs of bleeding
  5. Monitors laboratory results
- *Peritoneal dialysis* (PD), an alternative and slower dialysis method, is accomplished by the surgical insertion of a silicone rubber catheter (Tenckhoff's catheter) into the abdominal cavity to instill dialysis solution into the abdominal cavity.
- The PD process occurs via a transfer of fluid and solutes from the bloodstream through the peritoneum.
- There are three types of PD: intermittent, continuous ambulatory, and continuous cycling.
- The nurse
  1. Implements and monitors PD therapy and instills, dwells, and drains the solution, as ordered
  2. Maintains PD flow data and monitors for negative or positive fluid balances
  3. Obtains baseline and daily weights
  4. Monitors laboratory results to measure the effectiveness of the treatment
  5. Maintains accurate intake and output records

Surgical Management

- *Renal transplantation* is appropriate for select clients.
- After a suitable donor kidney is found, the client undergoes a *nephrectomy*, removal of the diseased kidney, with reimplantation of the donor organ.
- Postoperative care of the renal transplant recipient is similar to other abdominal surgeries.
- The nurse additionally
  1. Monitors for the return of renal functioning by assessing hourly urine output for oliguria or diuresis

2. Administers immunosuppressants, as ordered
3. Monitors for signs of organ rejection

    a. Hyperacute rejection, which occurs within 48 hours after surgery

        (1) Increased temperature
        (2) Increased blood pressure
        (3) Pain at the transplant site

    b. Acute rejection, which occurs within 1 week to 2 years after the transplant (most commonly in the first 2 weeks)

        (1) Oliguria or anuria
        (2) Increased temperature
        (3) Increased blood pressure
        (4) Enlarged, tender kidney
        (5) Lethargy
        (6) Changes in urinalysis and blood chemistry values

    c. Chronic rejection, which occurs gradually during a period of months to years

        (1) Gradual increase in BUN and serum creatinine levels
        (2) Fluid retention
        (3) Changes in serum electrolyte levels

NDx: Altered Nutrition: Less Than Body Requirements

- Dietary principles are based on the regulation of protein intake, limitation of fluid intake, restriction of potassium, sodium, and phosphorus intake, administration of vitamin and mineral supplements, and providing adequate calories.
- The nurse

    1. Limits the client's protein intake

        a. Chronic uremia: 0.55 g/kg of body weight per day
        b. Hemodialysis: 1.0 to 1.3 g/kg of body weight per day
        c. Peritoneal dialysis: 0.8 to 1.5 g/kg of body weight per day

    2. Closely monitors the client's fluid intake

        a. Chronic uremia: 1500 to 3000 mL/day
        b. Hemodialysis: 700 mL/day plus amount of urinary output
        c. Peritoneal dialysis: restricts fluid based on fluid weight gain and blood pressure

    3. Monitors sodium intake and restricts sodium intake to

        a. Chronic uremia: 1 to 3 g/day

    b. Hemodialysis: 1 to 2 g/day
    c. Peritoneal dialysis: restricted based on the
       fluid weight gain and blood pressure
  4. Monitors potassium intake and serum
    potassium levels
    a. Chronic uremia: 70 mEq/day
    b. Hemodialysis: 70 mEq/day
    c. Peritoneal dialysis: usually not restricted
  5. Monitors phosphorus intake and limits to 700 to
    800 mg/day
  6. Administers vitamin and mineral supplements,
    as ordered
  7. Collaborates with the dietitian/nutritionist
  8. Assists the client in adapting the diet to food
    preferences, ethnic background, and the budget
  9. Teaches the client to minimize caloric intake
    within the dietary restrictions
 10. Emphasizes the importance of complying with
    the dietary restrictions

Discharge Planning

• The nurse provides in-depth, clear, concise verbal
and written instructions about diet, drug therapy, renal
pathology, and renal failure.
• The nurse
  1. Teaches hemodialysis principles and care of the
    vascular access, as appropriate
  2. Stresses the necessity to comply with the
    treatment schedule
  3. Provides and reinforces in-depth education for
    clients with home dialysis
  4. Teaches peritoneal dialysis principles, as
    appropriate, validates the client's performance of
    the procedure, and explains the care of the
    peritoneal catheter

• Renal transplantation clients and family have
specialized educational needs, including
immunosuppressant drug information and side effects,
clinical manifestations of transplant rejection and
infection, and changes in diet and activity level.
• The nurse emphasizes the importance of follow-up
visits with the physician(s)

For more information on chronic renal failure, see
*Medical-Surgical Nursing: A Nursing Process
Approach*, **pp. 1884–1917.**

Renal Trauma

OVERVIEW
- Renal trauma is injury to one or both kidneys.
- The injuries include
  1. *Minor* injuries: contusion, small lacerations, and disruption of the integrity of the parenchyma and the calyx
  2. *Major* injuries: lacerations to the cortex, medulla, or one of the segmental branches of the renal artery or vein; likely to follow penetrating abdominal, flank, or back wounds
  3. Pedicle injuries: a laceration or disruption of the renal artery and/or vein, resulting in rapid and extensive hemorrhage.

COLLABORATIVE MANAGEMENT
Assessment
- The nurse records the client's
  1. History of events surrounding the trauma
  2. History of renal or urologic disease
  3. Previous surgical intervention
  4. History of diabetes or hypertension
- The nurse assesses for
  1. Abdominal and/or flank pain
  2. Presence of flank asymmetry
  3. Presence of flank bruising
  4. Penetrating injuries of the lower thorax or back
  5. Abdominal ecchymoses
  6. Abdominal distention
  7. Penetrating abdominal wounds

Planning and Implementation
NDx: ALTERED (RENAL) TISSUE PERFUSION
Nonsurgical Management
- The nurse
  1. Administers low-dose dopamine, as ordered, to ensure renal perfusion
  2. Administers fluids, such as crystalloids and red blood cells, to restore circulatory blood volume; plasma volume expanders may also be given

Surgical Management
- Depending on the extent of the injury, *nephrectomy* (the surgical removal of the kidney) may be required.

• For major vascular tearing, the kidney may be surgically removed, repaired through revascularization techniques, and then surgically reimplanted.

• Postoperative care is similar to any other client undergoing abdominal surgery. (See Colorectal Cancer).

• The nurse monitors for signs of hematuria and oliguria.

Discharge Planning

• The nurse
   1. Instructs the client to observe the pattern and frequency of urination and to note the color, clarity, and amount of urine produced
   2. Instructs the client to seek medical attention for feelings of bladder distention, inadequate bladder emptying, and signs of infection
   3. Describes the signs and symptoms of urinary infection, including chills, fever, lethargy, and/or cloudy, foul-smelling urine

For more information on renal trauma, see *Medical-Surgical Nursing: A Nursing Process Approach*, **pp. 1877–1880.**

Renal Tuberculosis

R

• Renal tuberculosis, or granulomatous nephritis, occurs when the kidney is invaded by *Mycobacterium tuberculosis*, usually by the blood-borne route.

• Normal renal parenchyma is replaced by scar tissue or a granuloma.

• Symptoms include
   1. Urinary frequency
   2. Dysuria
   3. Hypertension
   4. Hematuria

5. Proteinuria
6. Renal colic
- Treatment includes
  1. Chemotherapy
  2. Surgical excision of diseased tissue

For more information on renal tuberculosis, see *Medical-Surgical Nursing: A Nursing Process Approach*, **p. 1843.**

Respiratory Acidosis

OVERVIEW

- An alteration in some area of respiratory function results in an inadequate exchange of oxygen and carbon dioxide.

- Respiratory acidosis is characterized by a low pH, elevated carbon dioxide partial pressure (PCO_2), and decreased oxygen tension (PO_2).

- Changes in bicarbonate, serum potassium, serum chloride, and anion gap levels vary with the duration of the acidosis and the degree of renal compensation.

- Common causes include
  1. Respiratory depression
     a. Chemical depression
     b. Drugs/narcotics
     c. Poisons
     d. Trauma
     e. Hypoxia, ischemia
     f. Spinal cord injury
     g. Guillain-Barré syndrome
     h. Myasthenia gravis
  2. Inadequate chest expansion
     a. Skeletal deformities and trauma
        (1) Scoliosis
        (2) Osteoporosis
     b. Muscular dystrophy
     c. Obesity

  d. Pleural effusion
  e. Thoracic tumor
  f. Ascites
 3. Airway obstruction
  a. Bronchiolitis
  b. Asthma
  c. Bronchitis
 4. Alveolar-capillary block
  a. Thrombus or embolus formation
  b. Vascular occlusive disease
  c. Pneumonia
  d. Pulmonary edema
  e. Atelectasis
  f. Emphysema

COLLABORATIVE MANAGEMENT

Assessment

- The nurse records the client's
  1. Age
  2. Prescribed and over-the-counter medications, especially those containing aspirin or alcohol
  3. Current and past medical history
     a. Respiratory problems
     b. Renal failure
     c. Diabetes mellitus
     d. Pancreatitis
     e. Persistent diarrhea
     f. Fever
  4. Diet history
  5. Behavior or personality changes
- The nurse assesses for
  1. Central nervous system changes
     a. Lethargy, confusion, stupor
     b. Reduced attention span
  2. Neuromuscular changes
     a. Hyporeflexia
     b. Skeletal muscle weakness
     c. Flaccid paralysis
  3. Cardiac changes
     a. Delayed electrical conduction
        (1) Bradycardia
        (2) Tall T waves
        (3) Widened QRS complex
        (4) Prolonged PR interval
     b. Hypotension
     c. Thready peripheral pulses

R

4. Respiratory changes
   a. Diminished respiratory efforts
   b. Shallow respirations; rate may vary from rapid to absent
5. Integumentary changes (pale to cyanotic skin)

Planning and Implementation
NDx: INEFFECTIVE BREATHING PATTERN
- The nurse
  1. Performs a respiratory assessment every 4 hours or more often as indicated by the client's clinical condition
     a. Rate and depth of respirations
     b. Auscultation of breath sounds
     c. Ease with which the client moves air in and out of the lungs
     d. Presence of retractions
  2. Administers drugs to improve gas exchange, as ordered
     a. Aminophylline (Amoline, Lixaminol, Somophyllin)
     b. Theophylline (Bronkodyl, Theo-Dur)
     c. Ephedrine, fenoterol (Berotec)
     d. Isoproterenol (Aerolone, Isuprel)
     e. Metaproterenol (Alupent)
     f. Terbutaline (Brethaire, Brethine, Bricanyl)
  3. Administers nebulized oxygen cautiously, particularly if the client has chronic obstructive pulmonary disease (COPD) and carbon dioxide narcosis
  4. Places the client in the Fowler's or semi-Fowler's position
  5. Implements chest physiotherapy, as ordered, to all lung fields
  6. Teaches deep-breathing exercises
  7. Examines nail beds and mucous membranes for color

NDx: ACTIVITY INTOLERANCE
- The nurse
  1. Encourages the client to ingest enough calories to meet at least basal energy requirements
     a. Plan small, frequent meals that have a high protein and carbohydrate content, unless contraindicated.
     b. Plan foods that are easy to eat and require less energy to consume.

2. Plans activities and procedures to allow the client frequent rest periods
3. Reschedules bath, activities, and tests that are not absolutely necessary, if possible

NDx: ALTERED THOUGHT PROCESSES

- The nurse
    1. Assesses the client's mental status every 4 hours
        a. Level of consciousness
        b. Orientation
        c. Past and recent memory
        d. Ability to concentrate and other cognitive functions
    2. Maintains a safe environment
    3. Orients the client to time and place at every interaction
    4. Places large calendars and clocks where they can easily be seen by the client
    5. Ensures that the client wears/uses required assistive devices (hearing aid, glasses)
    6. Reduces environmental stimuli
    7. Ambulates the client with assistance
    8. Keeps the bed in a low position and the side rails up at all times
    9. Places the call light within easy reach
    10. Assesses the need for a vest or jacket restraint; strictly adheres to facility policy regarding the use of restraints

Discharge Planning

- The nurse
    1. Ensures that the client/family know how to use all assistive-adaptive devices correctly prior to discharge
    2. Provides drug information, as needed
    3. Instructs the client/family on the use of oxygen, if ordered
        a. Application and amount
        b. Safety measures for the home
        c. Importance of notifying the power company and local fire and police of the presence of oxygen in the home
    4. Reviews the symptoms of respiratory acidosis
    5. Discusses how to schedule and pace activities
        a. Strenuous activities should be performed in the morning.
        b. Naps or rest periods should be scheduled throughout the day.

   c. Objects needed frequently should be within easy reach.

- Also see Chronic Obstructive Pulmonary Disease.

For more information on respiratory acidosis, see *Medical-Surgical Nursing: A Nursing Process Approach*, **pp. 340–350.**

Respiratory Alkalosis

OVERVIEW

- Respiratory alkalosis results from the excessive loss of carbon dioxide through hyperventilation, direct stimulation of the central chemoreceptors, or stimulation of the peripheral chemoreceptors.
- Common causes include
  1. Hyperventilation
  2. Anxiety and fear
  3. Improperly set ventilators
  4. Compensation for metabolic acidosis
  5. Drugs
     a. Salicylates
     b. Catecholamines
     c. Progesterone
  6. Hypoxemia
  7. Asphyxiation
  8. High altitudes
  9. Shock
  10. Pneumonia
  11. Asthma
  12. Pulmonary emboli

COLLABORATIVE MANAGEMENT
Assessment

- The nurse records the client's
  1. Age
  2. Use of prescribed and over-the-counter medications
     a. Antacids

    b. Diuretics

    c. Antihypertensive agents

    d. Products containing aspirin or other salicylates

  3. Current and past medical history

    a. Nausea and vomiting

    b. Fever

    c. Severe pain

    d. Excessive licorice ingestion

    e. Problems with respirations

  4. Urinary output, including the frequency and quantity

  5. Actual fluid intake over the previous 24 hours

  6. Recent weight loss

  7. Disturbance in sleep pattern or insomnia

- The nurse assesses for

  1. Central nervous system changes

    a. Memory changes

    b. Changes in the ability to concentrate

    c. Anxiety, irritability

    d. Tetany, seizures

    e. Positive Chvostek's sign

    f. Positive Trousseau's sign

    g. Paresthesia

  2. Neuromuscular changes

    a. Hyperreflexia

    b. Muscle cramping and twitching

    c. Skeletal muscle weakness

  3. Cardiac changes

    a. Increased heart rate

    b. Normal or low blood pressure

    c. Increased digitalis toxicity

  4. Respiratory changes (increased rate and depth of ventilation)

Planning and Implementation

- Respiratory alkalosis is managed by treating the underlying cause of the alkalosis.

For more information on respiratory alkalosis, see *Medical-Surgical Nursing: A Nursing Process Approach,* **pp. 352–355.**

Retinal Hole/Tear/ Detachment

OVERVIEW

- A *retinal hole* is a break in the integrity of the peripheral sensory retina and is frequently associated with trauma and aging.
- A *retinal tear* is a more jagged and irregularly shaped break in the retina that occurs as a result of traction on the retina.
- *Retinal detachment* is the separation of the sensory retina from the pigmented epithelium.
- Rhegmatogenous detachments occur after the development of a hole or tear in the retina creates an opening for the vitreous to filter into the subretinal space.
- Traction detachments are created when the retina is pulled away from the epithelium by bands of fibrous tissue in the vitreous humor.
- Exudative detachments are caused by fluid accumulation in the subretinal space as a result of an inflammatory process.

COLLABORATIVE MANAGEMENT

Assessment

- The nurse assesses for
  1. Risk factors, including aphakia, increased age, vitreoretinal degeneration, and myopia
  2. Previous ocular and medical history
  3. Visual changes
- The nurse records the client's description of
  1. Time symptoms first developed
  2. Length of time since the onset of symptoms
  3. Severity of symptoms
  4. Aggravating or relieving factors
  5. Anxiety and fear
- Indirect ophthalmoscopic examination reveals gray bulges or folds in the retina that quiver with movement; a hole or tear may be seen.

Planning and Implementation

NDx: SENSORY/PERCEPTUAL ALTERATIONS (VISUAL)

- Repair of retinal holes or tears is done by surgery.
- Treatment is directed toward sealing the break by

creating an inflammatory response that will bind the retina and choroid together around the break.

- Treatment includes
  1. *Cryotherapy hair:* A supercooled metal probe is placed on the conjunctiva over the area that corresponds to the retinal break.
  2. *Photocoagulation:* A laser light is focused on the pigmented epithelium. The epithelium absorbs the light and converts it to heat.
  3. *Diathermy hair:* A high-frequency current applied to the sclera directly over the site of the break causes a burn that creates a local inflammatory response and results in the sealing of the retinal break.

- For repair of *retinal detachments*, the treatment is directed toward placing the retina in contact with the underlying structures.

- The *scleral buckling* procedure is most often performed.

- During the scleral buckling procedure, the ophthalmologist repairs wrinkles or folds in the retina so that the retina can assume its normal smooth position.

- The nurse provides preoperative care
  1. Provides routine preoperative care
  2. Maintains activity restrictions
  3. Maintains the eye patch over the affected eye to reduce eye movement
  4. Administers topical medications, as ordered, to inhibit accommodation and constriction, such as phenylephrine hydrochloride (Neo-synephrine, tropicamide (Mydriacyl), and cyclopentolate hydrochloride (Cyclogel)

- The nurse provides postoperative care
  1. Provides routine postoperative care
  2. Reports any drainage to the physician immediately
  3. Does not remove the initial eye patch and shield without a specific order
  4. Positions the client, as ordered, to allow gas that may have been used to promote reattachment to float against the retina
     a. The client lies on the abdomen with the head turned so that he or she lies with the unaffected eye down.
     b. The client sits on the side of the bed with his or her head on a bedside stand.
  5. Withholds food and fluids until the client is fully

569

awake and nausea has passed; administers
antiemetics as ordered

6. Administers analgesics, as ordered, such as
meperidine (Demerol), acetaminophen
(Tylenol), and/or codeine

7. Instructs the client to avoid activities that will
increase intraocular pressure, such as sneezing,
straining at stool, and bending over from the
waist

8. Administers antibiotic-steroid drops, as ordered,
which are given to prevent infection

9. Administers cycloplegic agents, as ordered,
which dilate the pupil and rest the muscles used
for accommodation

10. Enforces activity restrictions, including
avoidance of reading, writing, and performing
close work such as needlepoint

Discharge Planning

- The nurse

1. Assists with the identification and correction of
hazards in the home prior to discharge

2. Reviews signs and symptoms of complications
and what to do should they develop

3. Emphasizes the importance of follow-up visits
with the physician(s)

4. Reminds the client to wear protective eyewear
during the day and the eye shield at night

5. Provides verbal and written drug information, as
needed, for the client/family

For more information on retinal holes, tears, and
detachment, see *Medical-Surgical Nursing: A Nursing
Process Approach,* **pp. 1055–1060.**

Rheumatoid Arthritis

OVERVIEW

- Rheumatoid arthritis (RA) is a chronic, progressive,
systemic, inflammatory process that affects primarily
synovial joints.
- RA is considered to be a probable autoimmune
disease.

- Other areas of the body can be affected; vasculitis can cause malfunction and eventual failure of an organ or system.

COLLABORATIVE MANAGEMENT
Assessment
- The nurse assesses the joints for
    1. Inflammation, tenderness, and stiffness; bilateral and symmetric joint involvement
    2. Deformities
    3. Moderate to severe pain and morning stiffness (more than 30 minutes)
    4. Softness/spongy feeling because of synovitis and effusions
    5. Muscle atrophy
    6. Decreased range of motion (ROM)
- The nurse assesses for systemic involvement
    1. Low-grade fever
    2. Fatigue
    3. Weakness
    4. Anorexia, weight loss
    5. Paresthesia
    6. Osteoporosis
    7. Anemia
    8. Vasculitis
    9. Peripheral neuropathy
    10. Pericarditis
    11. Fibrotic lung disease
    12. Renal disease
    13. Sjögren's syndrome
    14. Subcutaneous nodules
    15. Respiratory compromise, including pleurisy, pneumonitis, diffuse interstitial fibrosis, and pulmonary hypertension
    16. Ocular involvement, such as iritis and/or scleritis
    17. Body image disturbance, poor self-esteem

Planning and Implementation
CHRONIC PAIN
- The nurse administers drug therapy, as ordered
    1. Salicylates
        a. The initial dose is 12 to 18 tablets each day in 4 divided doses, until a therapeutic serum salicylate level of 20 to 25 mg/100mL is achieved.
        b. When symptoms are relieved, the dosage is adjusted to a maintenance level of 15 to 20 mg/100mL.

c. Toxicity is manifested by tinnitus; other side effects include nausea, vomiting, and ulcers.
d. The drug is given with meals or a snack.
e. The drug may interfere with the clotting ability; observation is needed for abnormal bleeding and bruising.

2. Nonsteroidal anti-inflammatory agents

   a. These drugs may be used in combination with salicylates if pain and inflammation are not decreased within 6 to 12 weeks.
   b. They may cause retention of fluids and sodium; observation is needed for hypertension, changes in renal function, and fluid retention.

3. Gold therapy

   a. This therapy is used in combination with salicylates and nonsteroidal anti-inflamatory agents.
   b. It may induce remission as well as decrease pain and inflammation.
   c. Weekly injections of 25 to 50 mg of gold or sodium thiomalate (Myochrysine) are administered until improvement is seen or a cumulative total dosage of 1000 mg is administered.
   d. Weekly injections are tapered slowly to once a month if they are effective; if remission is not seen after a total of 1000 mg has been given, the drug is discontinued.
   e. Toxic effects include rash, blood dyscrasias, and renal involvement.
   f. Oral gold preparation such as auranofin (Ridaura) may be used in place of injections; side effects include nausea, vomiting, and diarrhea.

4. Steroids

   a. Prednisone (Deltasone) is given when commonly used agents are ineffective.
   b. Complications include diabetes mellitus, infection, hypertension, osteoporosis, and glaucoma.
   c. The client is observed for cushingoid changes such as moon-face and acne.

5. Antineoplastic agents

   a. Antineoplastic agents are used in clients with life-threatening RA.
   b. Agents include cyclophosphamide (Cytoxan), azathioprine (Imuran), and methotrexate.

- Other analgesics include acetaminophen (Tylenol, Datril), propoxyphene (Darvon), and propoxyphene with acetaminophen (Darvocet-N 100).

NDx: IMPAIRED PHYSICAL MOBILITY

- The nurse reinforces the exercise program developed by physical therapy
  1. Encourages consistency
  2. Teaches the client to stop if pain increases with exercise
  3. Teaches that the number of repetitions are decreased when inflammation is severe
  4. Teaches that exercises should be active rather than passive
- Of special importance is the need for higher-level toilet seats, chairs, and wheelchairs to facilitate mobility.

NDx: TOTAL SELF-CARE DEFICIT

- The nurse
  1. Collaborates with the occupational therapist to obtain needed assistive-adaptive devices
  2. Teaches the client alternative strategies to activities of daily living, such as using the palm of the hand to squeeze toothpaste onto the toothbrush; collaborates with the dietary department to have the tray set up so the client can easily manipulate items

NDx: FATIGUE; ACTIVITY INTOLERANCE

- The nurse identifies factors that contribute to fatigue
  1. Anemia
     a. Anemia is treated with iron, folic acid, and/or vitamin supplements.
     b. The client is assessed for drug-related blood loss, such as that caused by salicylate therapy, by testing the stool for occult blood.
  2. Muscle atrophy: daily exercise program
  3. Inadequate rest: quiet environment, warm beverage before bed
- The nurse teaches the principles of energy conservation
  1. Pacing activities
  2. Setting priorities
  3. Allowing rest periods
  4. Obtaining assistance when possible, delegating activities to the family

- The nurse
  1. Determines the client's reaction to changes
  2. Communicates acceptance of the client by establishing a trusting relationship
  3. Encourages the client to verbalize feelings
  4. Encourages the client to wear street clothes, his or her own night clothes or bathrobe
  5. Assists with grooming, such as shaving and makeup
  6. Emphasizes the client's strengths
  7. Treats the client with patience and understanding, as the client often appears to be manipulative and demanding

Discharge Planning

- The nurse
  1. Identifies and corrects hazards in the home prior to discharge
  2. Ensures that the client can correctly use all adaptive-assistive devices ordered for home use
  3. Provides a detailed plan of care at the time of discharge for clients to be transferred to a rehabilitation or long-term-care facility
  4. Provides drug information
     a. Taking all medications in the correct dosage, at the right time, and by the right route
     b. What to do if a dose is missed or if complications or side effects occur
  5. Reviews energy conservation measures
  6. Reviews the prescribed exercise program
  7. Teaches joint protection measures
  8. Emphasizes the importance of follow-up visits with the physician(s) and other therapists

For more information on rheumatoid arthritis, see *Medical-Surgical Nursing: A Nursing Process Approach,* **pp. 691–700.**

Rhinitis

- Rhinitis is an inflammation of the nasal cavities; it is the most common disorder affecting the nose and accessory nasal sinuses.

- *Acute rhinitis* is caused by allergens or virus; the offending substance causes release of vasoactive mediators, which induce vasodilation and increased capillary permeability with resultant edema and swelling of the nasal mucosa.

- Symptoms of acute rhinitis include headache, nasal irritation, sneezing, nasal congestion, rhinorrhea, and itchy, watery eyes.

- *Allergic rhinitis* (hay fever) is initiated by sensitivity reactions to allergens and occurs as acute seasonal episodes.

- *Chronic rhinitis* presents intermittently or continuously when exposed to allergens such as dust, animal dander, wool, and foods.

- *Rhinitis medicamentosa* occurs after excessive use of nosedrops or sprays as a rebound effect causing nasal congestion.

- *Acute viral rhinitis* (the common cold) is caused by one of over 30 viruses and spreads via droplet nuclei from sneezing and coughing.

- The common cold is usually self-limiting; complications include otitis media, sinusitis, and bronchitis.

- Pneumonia occurs in the elderly or in immunosuppressed individuals.

- Symptomatic relief measures include

    1. Antihistamines and decongestants
    2. Antipyretics for fever
    3. Proper rest
    4. Adequate fluid intake

- The client at risk should avoid individuals who are susceptible to infections.

- Thorough hand washing is important to avoid spread of the infection.

- Antibiotic therapy is given for secondary bacterial infections.

R

- Allergy testing and hyposensitization are commonly used in allergic rhinitis.

For more information on rhinitis, see *Medical-Surgical Nursing: A Nursing Process Approach*, **pp. 1953–1954.**

Rib Fracture

- Rib fractures result from direct blunt chest trauma; ribs five through nine are most often injured.
- Rib fractures cause a potential for intrathoracic injury, such as pneumothorax or pulmonary contusion.
- Pain with movement and defensive chest splinting result in impaired ventilation and inadequate clearance of secretions.
- Ribs usually unite spontaneously.
- Pain management is provided to maintain adequate ventilatory status; an intercostal nerve block may be required for severe pain.

For more information on rib fracture, see *Medical-Surgical Nursing: A Nursing Process Approach*, **p. 2055.**

Scabies

- Scabies is a contagious skin disease characterized by epidermal curved or linear ridges and follicular papules associated with severe pruritis.
- Hypersensitivity reactions result in excoriated erythematous papules, pustules, and crusted lesions on the elbows, nipples, lower abdomen, buttocks, thighs, and axillary folds.
- Scabies are transmitted by close and prolonged contact with an infested companion or bedding.
- Scabies mites are carried by pets and occur endemically among schoolchildren, institutional elderly clients, and clients of lower socioeconomic status.
- Treatment consists of chemical disinfection with scabicides such as lindane (Kwell) or topical sulfur preparations.
- Clothes and personal items are laundered in hot water.

For more information on scabies, see *Medical-Surgical Nursing: A Nursing Process Approach*, **pp. 1209, 1792.**

S

Scoliosis

- Scoliosis is a C- or S-shaped lateral curvature of the vertebral spine.
- Scoliosis is generally diagnosed and treated in adolescence.

- Deviations of more than 50 degrees can compromise cardiopulmonary function.
- Treatment for the adult involves a surgical fusion and the insertion of instrumentation.
    1. The *Harrington* rod system uses a compression rod on the convex side of the spine and a distraction rod on the concave side.
    2. *Dwyer* cable instrumentation requires an anterolateral surgical approach and involves entrance into the thoracic area with subsequent chest tube insertion.
    3. The *Luque* rod system requires no cast postoperatively; however, it is a longer surgical procedure, and blood loss is greater.
    4. The Cotrel-Dubousset (C-D) system is a three-dimensional segmental instrumentation using noninvasive hooks to prevent neurologic complications; the client is not immobilized by a brace or cast.
- The client may or may not have a partial body cast after surgery.
- The client may be placed on a Stryker or Foster frame postoperatively.
- Nursing management is directed toward preventing complications of immobility, such as skin breakdown, atelectasis, and deep-vein thrombosis.

For more information on scoliosis, see *Medical-Surgical Nursing: A Nursing Process Approach,* **pp. 774–775.**

Sensory Deprivation

OVERVIEW

- Sensory deprivation is described as the reduction in variety and intensity of sensory input, with or without a change in the structure or pattern of stimulation.

- Subtypes of sensory deprivation include
  1. Absolute reduction: absence of stimuli in the external environment
  2. Reception deprivation: receptor organs are impaired and either partial or complete loss of sensation occurs
  3. Perceptual deprivation: individual cannot recognize and interpret stimuli from the external environment
  4. Technological deprivation: client is in a highly technological environment in which the nurse focuses on the machines rather than the individual
  5. Confinement deprivation: individual is separated from significant others and familiar objects
  6. Immobility deprivation: client has decreased physical movement and activity

COLLABORATIVE MANAGEMENT

Assessment
- The nurse assesses for
  1. Cognitive changes, such as poor concentration, altered sequencing of thoughts or unusual ideas to bizarre thinking, impaired memory, and disorientation
  2. Emotional changes, such as anxiety, depression, crying, fear, mood swings, irritability, annoyance over trivial matters, and anger
  3. Perceptual changes, such as visual and auditory distortions, alterations in color and perceived movement of stable objects, and preoccupation with internal sensations and somatic complaints
  4. Physical changes, such as drowsiness, excessive yawning and sleep, and alterations in dexterity and hand-eye coordination movements

Planning and Implementation
NDx: SENSORY/PERCEPTUAL ALTERATIONS
- The nurse
  1. Identifies factors that contribute to sensory deprivation
  2. Increases the level of intensity of stimulation and increases the variety of patterns of incoming stimuli
  3. Tries to create an environment that resembles familiar surroundings and restores meaningful stimuli
     a. Places pictures on the walls of the hospital room

S

    b. Displays personal cards and pictures on the bedside table

    c. Encourages family members to bring inexpensive personal items in from home

    d. Allows the client to wear nightgown/pajamas from home when possible

    e. Uses radio and television appropriately

    f. Has clocks and calendars easily visible

    g. Ensures that the client uses needed assistive devices such as hearing aids, eyeglasses, or contact lenses

    h. Encourages participation in self-care activities

    i. Talks with the client, explains tests and procedures

Discharge Planning

- The nurse

    1. Identifies areas in the home that may contribute to sensory deprivation

    2. Assesses the need for a community health nurse or home health aide

For more information on sensory deprivation, see *Medical-Surgical Nursing: A Nursing Process Approach*, **pp. 148–153.**

Sensory Overload

OVERVIEW

- Sensory overload results from an increase in environmental stimuli—when there is multisensory bombardment of stimuli or when there is an increase in the pattern and intensity of stimuli so that the input is meaningless.

- Behavioral manifestations of sensory overload can have a health-threatening effect on the individual.

COLLABORATIVE MANAGEMENT
Assessment
- There are no clear differences between behaviors observed in sensory deprivation and those observed in sensory overload.
- The distinguishing feature of overload is that the client cannot use sleep as an escape mechanism.
- The nurse assesses for
  1. Cognitive changes, such as poor concentration, altered sequencing of thoughts or unusual ideas to bizarre thinking, impaired memory, and disorientation
  2. Emotional changes, such as anxiety, depression, crying, fear, mood swings, irritability, annoyance over trivial matters, and anger
  3. Perceptual changes, such as visual and auditory distortions, alterations in color and perceived movement of stable objects, and preoccupation with internal sensations and somatic complaints
  4. Physical changes, such as drowsiness and alterations in dexterity and hand-eye coordination

Planning and Implementation
NDx: SENSORY/PERCEPTUAL ALTERATIONS
- The nurse
  1. Reduces the intensity of incoming stimuli and increases the meaningfulness of the stimuli
  2. Provides a consistent, predictable pattern of stimulation
  3. Keeps the noise level to a minimum
  4. Encourages the health care team to refrain from conversations at the client's bedside
  5. Maintains a normal sleep-wake cycle by dimming the lights at night and drawing curtains around the client's bed
  6. Explains all procedures, diagnostic tests, and equipment
  7. Remains calm, uses an unhurried approach, and speaks in a low, modulated voice when interacting with the client
  8. Schedules the same nurse to care for the client, when possible
  9. Develops a routine for care and activities
  10. Orients the client to reality as often as necessary
  11. Limits the use of radio and television, visitors, and telephone calls

S

Discharge Planning

• Family or significant others should assess the home for stimuli that are potential sources of difficulties for the client.

For more information on sensory overload, see *Medical-Surgical Nursing: A Nursing Process Approach,* **pp. 150–154.**

Sexuality

OVERVIEW

• Sexual health includes one's freedom from physical and psychological impairment; the awareness of open and positive attitudes toward sexual functioning; accurate knowledge of sexuality; and congruency among gender assignment, identity, and role.

• *Homosexuality* is defined as erotic attraction to persons of the same sex.

• *Bisexuality* refers to a preference for intimate relationships with members of both sexes.

• An individual who is *transsexual* is completely dissatisfied with his or her gender assignment and is convinced that he or she is trapped with the wrong body; sex reassignment surgery may be performed.

• A *transvestite* wears clothes associated with the opposite sex for the sake of sexual arousal, but there is no conflict about his or her gender; cross-dressing occurs more frequently in men than women.

• *Pedophilia* is a sexual preference for children and is considered to be a psychiatric disorder.

COLLABORATIVE MANAGEMENT
Assessment

• The nurse records the client's
  1. Injury or disease of the genitourinary system

2. Contraceptive use
3. Development of secondary sexual characteristics
4. Unwanted or traumatic sexual events such as rape
5. Changes of sexual functioning related to drug or alcohol use
6. Changes in sexual functioning since the current illness, injury, and/or surgery
7. Current physical condition causing the body image change
8. Changes in usual activities and roles
9. Changes in beliefs and practices about sexual functioning that have occurred as a result of illness

- The nurse assesses for
  1. Changes in external genitalia and breasts (e.g., thickening or discharge from genitalia or breasts)
  2. Dyspareunia (painful intercourse)
  3. Inhibited sexual desire: loss of interest in sexual activity or decline in libido
  4. Vaginismus: muscles of the outer third of the vaginal barrel contract powerfully and prevent insertion of a tampon or other object
  5. Orgasmic dysfunction: the inability to achieve orgasm (primary dysfunction) or to achieve orgasm with intercourse or at an appropriate time during intercourse (secondary dysfunction)
  6. Erectile dysfunction: the inability to attain or maintain an erection of the penis of sufficient firmness to permit penetration
  7. Ejaculatory dysfunction, premature: ejaculation after penetration but sooner than either partner desires
  8. Retrograde ejaculation, or dry orgasm: semen discharged into the urinary bladder
  9. Sexual aversion: irrational fear or phobic reaction to the thought of sexual activity or to the actual activity
  10. Psychologic and social factors related to past and present functioning

Planning and Implementation

NDx: SEXUAL DYSFUNCTION: DYSPAREUNIA

- In females, dyspareunia may be related to
  1. An intact hymen; the nurse refers the client to a gynecologist.
  2. Scarring from an episiotomy; the nurse refers the client to a gynecologist.
  3. Infections of the vagina or vulva; the nurse
     a. Explains methods to decrease risk of infection
     b. Administers antibiotics, as ordered

583

    c. Teaches the client to avoid sexual intercourse until the infection is resolved

    d. Encourages the client to rest and to increase fluid intake

4. Insufficient vaginal lubrication; the nurse instructs the client to use a water-soluble lubricant before sexual activity or intercourse.

5. Irritation from chemical products such as contraceptives, douches; the nurse

    a. Instructs the client to avoid excessive use of these products or to stop their use completely

    b. Encourages the use of products without scents

6. Pathologic conditions of the uterus, cervix, ovaries, and fallopian tubes; the nurse refers the client to a gynecologist.

7. Psychogenic factors; the nurse refers the client to a competent therapist.

- In males, dyspareunia may be related to:

1. Inflammation or infection of the penis, prostate, urinary bladder, urethra, or testes; the nurse refers the client to a urologist.

2. Exposure to vaginal contraceptive cream, jelly, foam, or irritation from an intrauterine device; the nurse

    a. Refers the client to a urologist

    b. Provides information and alternatives to the client and his sexual partner

3. Psychosocial factors; the nurse refers the client to a competent therapist.

NDx: SEXUAL DYSFUNCTION: INHIBITED SEXUAL DESIRE

- In females, inhibited sexual desire may be related to

1. Hormonal replacement therapy; the nurse

    a. Refers the client to a gynecologist

    b. Provides support for women coping with menopause

2. Oral contraceptives; the nurse

    a. Refers the client to a gynecologist

    b. Describes alternatives to oral contraceptives

3. Eating disorders; the nurse

    a. Refers the client to a competent therapist

    b. Provides information on a balanced diet

4. Drug use or abuse; the nurse refers the client to a competent therapist.

5. Chronic illness; the nurse assists the client to seek medical management.

6. Psychosocial factors; the nurse
    a. Refers the client to a competent therapist
    b. Utilizes therapeutic communication to discuss specific factors causing the problem.
- In men, inhibited sexual desire may be related to antihypertensive drugs, drug use or abuse, chronic illness, or psychosocial factors; the nurse assists the client to seek medical management.

NDx: Sexual Dysfunction: Sexual Aversion

- The nurse
  1. Refers the client to a competent therapist
  2. Allows the client to verbalize feelings and beliefs

NDx: Sexual Dysfunction: Vaginismus

- The nurse
  1. Helps to identify and relieve underlying psychogenic factors, such as rape trauma syndrome, conflicts surrounding homosexual experimentation, or strong religious teachings
     a. Gives the client permission to express anxiety and conflict
     b. Refers the client to a competent therapist
  2. Helps to identify and relieve underlying physical factors such as sexual activity too soon after childbirth, abnormality of the hymen, or atrophy of the vagina
     a. Refers the client to a gynecologist
     b. Encourages the client to explore alternatives to vaginal intercourse during the healing process
     c. Explains the relationship between physical factors and involuntary muscular response

NDx: Sexual Dysfunction: Orgasmic Dysfunction

- Orgasmic dysfunction is the most common sexual complaint of adult women related to
  1. Adhesions of the clitoris
  2. Lack of strength in the pubococcygeal muscles
  3. Diminished contractions of the uterus
  4. Psychogenic factors
- The nurse
  1. Refers the client to a gynecologist
  2. Instructs the client in the performance of Kegel's exercises
  3. Gives the client permission to talk about the problem
  4. Provides information about the relationship

between stressors and the physical response of orgasm

NDx: SEXUAL DYSFUNCTION: ERECTILE DYSFUNCTION

- Erectile dysfunction may be related to
    1. Spinal cord injury
    2. Diabetes mellitus
    3. Alcoholism
    4. Neurologic disease
    5. Infections of the genitourinary system
    6. Drug use or abuse
    7. Psychogenic factors
- The nurse
    1. Refers the client to a urologist or competent therapist, as appropriate
    2. Instructs the client and his partner in "sensate focus" technique

NDx: SEXUAL DYSFUNCTION: EJACULATORY DYSFUNCTION

- The nurse
    1. Educates the client and his partner about the relationship between emotions and the sexual response cycle
    2. Teaches systematic relaxation exercises
    3. Refers the client to a urologist and/or competent therapist

Discharge Planning

- The nurse teaches the importance of follow-up visits with the physician(s) and other therapists.

For more information on human sexuality, see *Medical-Surgical Nursing: A Nursing Process Approach,* **pp. 173–195.**

Shock

OVERVIEW

• Shock is a pathological condition rather than a disease process.

• Shock is characterized by generalized abnormal cellular metabolism, which occurs as a direct result of inadequate delivery of oxygen to body tissues or inadequate usage of oxygen by body tissue.

• The classification of shock includes four types

1. *Hypovolemic* shock

   a. There is a loss of circulating fluid volume from the central vascular space to the extent that mean arterial pressure (MAP) decreases and the body's total need for tissue oxygenation is not adequately met.

   b. The causes include hemorrhage, dehydration, or shifting of fluid from the central vascular space to the interstitial space.

2. *Cardiogenic* shock

   a. The pumping ability of the heart is impaired either directly or indirectly.

   b. The result is inadequate cardiac output.

      (1) Direct pump failure can result from myocardial infarction (MI), cardiac arrest, serious dysrhythmias, valvular pathological changes, and myocardial degeneration associated with inadequate myocardial circulation, systemic infection, and exposure to chemical toxins.

      (2) Indirect pump failure can result from cardiac tamponade, electrolyte imbalances (especially hyperkalemia and hypocalcemia), administration of drugs that decrease the rate and vigor of cardiac contractility, and injuries to the cardioregulatory areas of the brain.

3. *Vasogenic* shock

   a. There is a loss of sympathetic tone, vasodilation, pooling of blood in the venous and capillary beds, and increased vascular permeability, which all contribute to decreased MAP.

   b. The origin of this set of reactions is neural (neurogenic shock) or chemical (anaphylaxis).

S

4. *Septic* shock
    a. This type is commonly associated with bacteremia caused by gram-negative bacteria (*Pseudomonas aeruginosa, Escherichia coli,* and *Klebsiella pneumoniae*), *staphylococcus,* and *streptococcus.*
    b. Predisposing conditions include malnutrition, immunosuppression, the presence of large, open wounds, mucous membrane fissures in prolonged contact with bloody or drainage-soaked packing, gastrointestinal (GI) ischemia, and loss of GI integrity.

COLLABORATIVE MANAGEMENT

Assessment

- The nurse records the client's
    1. Risk factors for shock
    2. Age
    3. History of recent illness, trauma, and/or procedures and/or chronic conditions that may lead to shock
    4. Current medications
    5. Allergies
    6. Intake and output for the previous 24 hours
    7. Height and weight

- The nurse assesses for general clinical manifestations of shock

    1. Cardiovascular changes
        a. Decreased cardiac output
        b. Increased pulse rate
        c. Thready pulse
        d. Decreased blood pressure (it is important to consider the client's baseline blood pressure when shock is suspected)
        e. Narrowed pulse pressure
        f. Postural hypotension
        g. Low central venous pressure
        h. Flat neck and hand veins in dependent positions
        i. Slow capillary refill in the nail beds
        j. Diminished peripheral pulses; as shock progresses, possible absence of superficial peripheral pulses
    2. Respiratory changes
        a. Increased respiratory rate
        b. Shallow respirations
        c. Decreased arterial carbon dioxide partial pressure and oxygen tension

    d. Cyanosis, especially around the lips and nail beds

    e. Indications of adult respiratory distress syndrome (ARDS)

3. Neuromuscular changes

    a. Anxiety and restlessness

    b. Decreased level of consciousness

    c. Generalized muscle weakness

    d. Diminished or absent deep-tendon reflexes

    e. Sluggish pupillary response to light

    f. Changes in behavior or personality

4. Renal changes

    a. Decreased urinary output

    b. Increased specific gravity

    c. Sugar and acetone present in the urine

5. Integumentary changes

    a. Color changes: first evident in mucous membranes and in the skin around the mouth; as shock progresses, color changes noted in the extremities

    b. Cool to cold

    c. Moist and clammy

    d. Pale to mottled to cyanotic

    e. Mouth dry, pastelike coating present

6. Gastrointestinal changes

    a. Decreased motility

    b. Diminished or absent bowel sounds

    c. Nausea and vomiting

    d. Constipation

    e. Increased thirst

• If *hypovolemic* shock is suspected, the nurse assesses for the following in addition to the general clinical manifestations

1. Poor skin turgor

2. Edema; the skin is stretched and shiny in appearance; pits may be formed in response to light pressure

• If *cardiogenic* shock is suspected, the nurse assesses for the following in addition to the general clinical manifestations

1. Elevated central venous pressure

2. Distended neck and hand veins

3. Edema

4. Pulmonary edema

5. Labored respirations, especially in the supine position

6. Crackles and wheezes on auscultation

• If *vasogenic* shock is suspected, the nurse assesses for

warm and pink skin in addition to the general clinical manifestations.

• If *septic* shock is suspected, the nurse assesses for the following in addition to the general clinical manifestations

1. Rapid onset and progression
2. Skin that is warm and pink with some edema present
3. Upper and lower airway obstruction
4. Audible stridor and wheezes
5. Loss of consciousness, which occurs quickly

Planning and Implementation

EMERGENCY CARE

• The nurse provides emergency care for the client in hypovolemic shock

1. Assesses the client for evidence of injury or apparent bleeding
2. Covers any wounds with a clean cloth/dressing and applies pressure to a wound if bleeding appears to be originating from an artery
3. Inserts an intravenous (IV) line and infuses Ringer's lactate or normal saline, as ordered
4. Applies military antishock trousers (MAST), if indicated

• The nurse provides emergency care for the client in cardiogenic shock

1. Determines the presence, severity, and location of chest pain
2. Loosens any restrictive or tight clothing
3. Places the client in a semi-Fowler's position
4. Observes for nausea and vomiting, which frequently occurs during an MI
5. Administers IV morphine to relieve pain as ordered; lidocaine may be given for dysrhythmias

• The nurse provides emergency care for the client in vasogenic shock

1. Assesses the client for neurologic deficits that may indicate head or spinal cord injury
2. Questions the client for events leading to the onset of illness, especially regarding any known allergens or recent infection
3. Obtains information about any medications or chemical substances ingested by the client recently, as well as any surgical or dental procedures
4. Monitors respiratory status frequently; observes for airway obstruction
5. Treats anaphylactic reactions with epinephrine as ordered

NDx: Decreased Cardiac Output

- The nurse administers drug therapy, as ordered
  1. Vasoconstricting agents, such as dopamine (Dopastat, Intropin, Revimine), epinephrine (Adrenalin), mephentermine (Wyamine), metaraminol (Aramine), methoxamine (Vasoxyl), norepinephrine (Levophed), phenylephrine (Neo-Synephrine), and vasopressin (Pitressin)
  2. Agents enhancing myocardial contractility, such as dobutamine (Dobutrex), dopamine amrinone (Inocor), epinephrine, isoproterenol (Isuprel), digoxin (Lanoxin, Purodigin), and deslanoside (Cedilanid-D)
  3. Agents enhancing myocardial perfusion (most beneficial for cardiogenic shock; not given to clients with a head injury), such as nitroglycerin (Ang-O-Span, Klavikordal, Nitrostat, Trates, Tridil), nitroprusside (Nipride, Nitropress), erythrityl tetranitrate (Cardilate), isosorbide dinitrate (Coronex, Iso-Bid, Isonate, Sorbitrate), and pentaerythritol tetranitrate (Duotrate, Pentol, Vaso-80)
- The nurse
  1. Provides oxygen via a face mask or nasal cannula, as needed
  2. Monitors intubation as necessary
  3. Maintains the client on strict bed rest
  4. Monitors vital signs and neurologic signs at least every hour, or more often if clinically indicated
- Clients in an intensive care unit receive sophisticated hemodynamic monitoring such as frequent measurement of cardiac output and pulmonary artery pressures.

NDx: Fluid Volume Deficit

- The nurse
  1. Administers colloid fluid replacement such as whole blood, packed red blood cells, and/or plasma to treat hypovolemic shock due to hemorrhage
     a. Monitors for a transfusion reaction
     b. Adheres strictly to facility policy and procedure for the administration of blood products
  2. Administers fluids as ordered, such as Ringer's lactate and normal saline
  3. Records strict measurement of intake and output
  4. Weighs the client daily
  5. Monitors vital signs frequently; monitors hemodynamic parameters such as pulmonary

capillary wedge pressures and central venous pressure

6. Administers antibiotics as ordered, which should be started within 30 minutes of receiving the order

NDx: IMPAIRED GAS EXCHANGE

- The nurse
  1. Performs a respiratory assessment every 2 to 4 hours; is alert for signs and symptoms of ARDS
  2. Monitors arterial blood gases
  3. Provides oxygen as indicated
  4. Assesses for cyanosis

NDx: ALTERED THOUGHT PROCESSES

- The nurse
  1. Performs neurologic checks every hour or more often, if clinically indicated
  2. Maintains a safe environment by keeping the bed in a low position and the side rails up at all times; reorients the client as needed
  3. Explains all procedures and treatments
  4. Maintains a quiet and distraction-free environment

Discharge Planning

- The nurse provides drug information, including
  1. Taking all medications in the correct dosage, at the right time, and by the right route
  2. What to do if a dose is missed or if complications or side effects occur
- The nurse
  1. Obtains a dietary consultation to help the client select personal food preferences that meet prescribed dietary requirements (e.g., low salt, low fat)
  2. Provides the telephone numbers of health care resource persons
  3. Emphasizes the importance of follow-up visits with the physician(s)

For more information on shock, see *Medical-Surgical Nursing: A Nursing Process Approach*, **pp. 402–423.**

Sinusitis

- Sinusitis is an inflammation of the mucous membranes of one or more sinuses.

- In *acute sinusitis* there is an obstruction of sinus secretion flow, which becomes infected.

- Acute sinusitis occurs with acute allergic rhinitis or from a deviated nasal septum, polyps, tumors, chronically inhaled air pollutants, or cocaine abuse.

- In *chronic sinusitis*, the mucous membranes are permanently thickened from prolonged or repeated inflammation or infection.

- Infections are caused by *Streptococcus pneumoniae*, *Haemophilus influenzae*, and *Bacteroides* species developing in the maxillary and frontal sinuses.

- Clinical manifestations include nasal swelling and congestion, headache, facial pressure and pain, low-grade fever, and purulent or bloody nasal drainage.

- Treatment measures include
    1. Broad-spectrum antibiotics
    2. Analgesics for pain and fever
    3. Decongestants
    4. Antral puncture and lavage
    5. Surgical opening of sinus cavities

S

For more information on sinusitis, see *Medical-Surgical Nursing: A Nursing Process Approach*, **p. 1954.**

Sjögren's Syndrome

- Sjögren's syndrome is a disorder in which inflammatory cells and immune complexes obstruct secretory ducts and glands.
- The disorder is manifested by dry eyes (sicca syndrome), dry mouth (xerostomia), dry vagina, swelling of the parotid and lacrimal areas, fever, fatigue, and associated connective tissue disease.
- Treatment includes steroids; meticulous mouth, eye, and perineal care; and use of artificial tears and saliva.

For more information on Sjögren's syndrome, see *Medical-Surgical Nursing: A Nursing Process Approach,* **p. 709.**

Skin Cancer

OVERVIEW

- Sunlight overexposure is the major cause of cutaneous malignancy.
- The most common skin cancers include
  1. *Actinic* or solar keratoses: premalignant lesions involving the keratinocytes of the epidermis that are common in chronic sun-damaged skin and may progress to squamous cell carcinoma
  2. *Squamous cell carcinoma*: malignant neoplasms of the epidermis, characterized by local invasion and potential for metastasis; predisposed by sun exposure and chronic epithelial damage from repeated injury or irritation

3. *Basal cell carcinomas*: lesions that arise in the basal cell layer of the epidermis, resulting primarily from ultraviolet light radiation exposure, genetic predisposition, and chronic irritation
4. *Melanomas*: highly metastatic pigmented malignant lesions originating in the melanin-producing cells of the epidermis

• Risk factors include genetic predisposition and precursor lesions that resemble unusual moles.

COLLABORATIVE MANAGEMENT
Assessment
• The nurse records the client's
1. Risk factors
2. Age and race
3. Family history of skin cancer
4. Past surgical removal of skin growths
5. Changes in size, color, or sensation of any mole, birthmark, wart, or scar
6. Sunlight exposure
7. Exposure to chemical carcinogens
8. Skin lesions subjected to repeated irritation
• The nurse assesses for
1. Skin lesions in sun-exposed areas and the entire skin surface
2. Unusual appearance of moles, warts, birthmarks, and scars
3. Associated symptoms such as tenderness and/or itching

Planning and Implementation
NDx: IMPAIRED SKIN INTEGRITY
Nonsurgical Management
• Topical chemotherapy with 5-fluorouracil cream is used for multiple actinic keratoses.
• Radiation therapy is limited to elderly clients with large, deeply invasive basal cell tumors who are poor surgical risks.

Surgical Management
• *Cryosurgery* with liquid nitrogen is performed on isolated lesions.
• Procedures used for small lesions with well-defined borders include *curettage,* to scrape away the cancerous tissue, followed by *electrodesiccation*, which involves placement of an electric probe on the wound surface to destroy the malignant tissue remnants by thermal and electrical energy.

S

- *Wide scalpel incision* is necessary for large or poorly defined cancers.

Discharge Planning
- The nurse
  1. Teaches wound care to minimize the potential for infection, including wound cleaning and dressings
  2. Discusses preventive measures, such as avoiding overexposure to sunlight and routine skin inspection

For more information on skin cancer, see *Medical-Surgical Nursing: A Nursing Process Approach*, **pp. 1197–1202.**

Skin Infection

OVERVIEW

- The majority of *cutaneous bacterial* infections are caused by *Staphylococcus* or *Streptococcus.*

- *Folliculitis* is a superficial staphylococcal infection involving the upper portion of the hair follicle and is associated with mild discomfort.

- *Furuncles* (boils) are caused by *Staphylococcus*, but the infection occurs deeper in the hair follicle.

- *Cellulitis* is a generalized nonfollicular infection with either *Staphylococcus* or *Streptococcus*, involving deeper connective tissue.

- *Viral* skin infections include *herpes simplex* virus (HSV) infections (type I virus, or classic cold sores; and type II virus, or genital herpes), and *herpes zoster* (shingles).

- Many *fungal* infections may affect the skin.

- Superficial fungal (dermatophyte) infections, or tinea, include
  1. Tinea pedis (athlete's foot)
  2. Tinea manus (hands)
  3. Tinea cruris (groin)
  4. Tinea corporis (ringworm)
  5. Tinea capitis (scalp)
  6. Tinea barbae (beard)

- *Candidiasis* is an opportunistic yeast infection of the skin and mucous membranes.

COLLABORATIVE MANAGEMENT
Assessment
- The nurse records the client's
  1. Recent history of skin trauma
  2. Past or current history of staphylococcal or streptococcccal infections
  3. Lesions appearing on the lips, oral cavity, and/or genitals
  4. Past history of similar lesions
  5. Prodromal symptoms of burning, tingling, and/or pain
  6. Previous exposure to chicken pox
  7. History of shingles
  8. Anatomic location of dermatophyte infection
  9. Social and environmental factors
  10. History of recent antibiotics or immunosuppressive drugs
  11. Medical history, including diabetes or cancer
  12. Nutritional deficiencies
- The nurse assesses for clinical manifestations of common skin infections such as
  1. Redness
  2. Warmth
  3. Edema
  4. Tenderness
  5. Pain
  6. Itching
  7. Stinging
  8. Localized areas of inflammation
  9. Blisters
  10. Pustules
  11. Papules
  12. Vesicles
  13. Scaling
  14. Single or multiple lesions

Planning and Implementation
NDx: Impaired Skin Integrity

Nonsurgical Management
- The nurse
  1. Teaches the client to bathe daily with antibacterial soap for bacterial infection
  2. Applies warm compresses to furuncles or cellulitis
  3. Applies astringent compresses such as Burow's solution to viral lesions

4. Allows the skin to dry between treatments
5. Provides optimal client positioning to promote air circulation
6. Teaches the client to avoid tight garments
7. Uses proper hand washing to prevent cross-contamination
8. Maintains strict isolation for resistant *Staphylococcus*
9. Teaches the client to avoid sexual contact when recurrent herpes lesions are present
10. Teaches the client/family to avoid sharing contaminated personal items of clients with dermatophyte infections
11. Applies antibacterial ointment such as neomycin, gentamicin, chloramphenicol, and providone-iodine and cream such as silver sulfadiazine, as ordered
12. Applies antifungal ointment and cream, such as clotrimazole, nystatin, ciclopirox, miconazole, econazole, tolnaftate, haloprogin, and undecylenic acid, as ordered, which are the treatment of choice for dermotophyte and yeast infections
13. Applies antifungal powder, such as nystatin and tolnaftate, as ordered
14. Administers antifungal oral preparation, such as nystatin and clotrimazole, as ordered
15. Administers anti-inflammatory steroid preparations, as ordered, ranging from low to potent fluorinated agents
16. Applies an antiviral ointment, such as acyclovir, as ordered, which is the treatment of choice for viral infections

Surgical Management

• Incision and drainage of *furuncles* is the primary surgical procedure that is done for skin infections.

Discharge Planning

• The nurse teaches the client/family
1. Underlying skin infection causes and treatments
2. Prevention of the spread of infection at home
3. Importance of follow-up visits with the physician(s)

For more information on skin infection, see *Medical-Surgical Nursing: A Nursing Process Approach*, **pp. 1172–1182.**

Spermatocele

- A spermatocele is a sperm-containing cystic mass that develops on the epididymis alongside the testicle.
- Spermatoceles normally remain small and asymptomatic and require no intervention.
- If necessary, a spermatocelectomy is performed by a small scrotal incision.

For more information on spermatocele, see *Medical-Surgical Nursing: A Nursing Process Approach*, **p. 1766.**

Spinal Cord Injury

OVERVIEW

- An injury to the vertebral column and spinal cord may be caused by motor vehicle accidents, falls, sports such as diving and football, and/or penetrating trauma.
- As a result, a loss or decrease in motor function, sensation, reflex activity, and bowel and bladder function may occur.
- The extent of the injury can be classified as
  1. *Complete*, where the spinal cord is transected and total motor and sensory loss occurs
  2. *Incomplete*, where some function remains and specific syndromes may occur if the cervical spinal cord is injured
     a. Anterior cord is characterized by loss of motor function below the level of the injury; sensations of touch, position, and vibration remain.
     b. Posterior cord is characterized by intact motor function and changes in sensation.
     c. Brown-Séquard is characterized by loss of

599

motor function, proprioception, vibration, and deep touch on the same side as the injury and loss of pain and temperature on the opposite side.

d. Central cord is characterized by loss of motor function that is more pronounced in the upper extremities than the lower extremities.

COLLABORATIVE MANAGEMENT

Assessment

- The nurse records the client's
  1. Description of how the injury occurred and the probable mechanism of injury
  2. Position of the client immediately after the injury
  3. Symptoms that occurred after the injury and what changes have occurred since
  4. Any problems encountered during the extrication and transport of the client
  5. Past medical history, with particular attention to a history of arthritis of the spine, congenital deformities, osteoarthritis or osteomyelitis, cancer, previous back and spinal cord injury, and respiratory problems
- The nurse assesses for
  1. Adequate airway and breathing pattern, respiratory compromise
  2. Indication of hemorrhage or bleeding around the fracture sites or in the abdomen
  3. Decreased or absent motor strength; the ability to shrug the shoulders, flex and extend the arms, elevate the arms and legs off the bed, extend the wrist, wiggle the toes, flex and extend the feet and legs
  4. Muscle wasting, spasticity, contractures, decreased muscle tone
  5. Decreased or absent sensation
  6. Cardiovascular dysfunction, such as bradycardia, hypotension, and cardiac dysrhythmias
  7. Change in thermoregulatory capacity, with the client's body tending to assume the temperature of the environment
  8. Indications of autonomic dysreflexia characterized by severe headache, hypertension, bradycardia, nasal stuffiness, and flushing
  9. Paralytic ileus manifested by decreased or absent bowel sounds and distended abdomen
  10. Heterotrophic ossification manifested by swelling, redness, warmth, and decreased range of motion (ROM) of the involved extremity

11. Coping strategies used in the past
12. Body image and self-esteem disturbances

Planning and Implementation

NDx: Altered (Spinal Cord) Tissue Perfusion
Nonsurgical Management

- The most commonly used devices for cervical injuries are cervical tongs (Gardner-Wells, Crutchfield-Vinke) and the halo fixation device to immobilize the spine.
- Traction is added, with the amount of weight to be used prescribed by the physician.
- Weights should hang free at all times; the nurse never releases the traction.
- The nurse monitors insertion sites for infection and cleans pins per hospital policy.
- The nurse administers drug therapy, as ordered
    1. Corticosteroid agent such as dexamethasone (Decadron), used for its anti-inflammatory effects
    2. Dextran, a plasma expander, used to increase capillary blood flow with the spinal cord and to prevent or treat hypotension
    3. Atropine sulfate, used to treat bradycardia
    4. Dantrolene (Dantrium) or baclofen (Lioresal), used to treat spasticity

Surgical Management

- *Decompression laminectomy* is performed to relieve compression from a hematoma, to remove bone fragments, or to remove a penetrating object such as a bullet.
- *Spinal fusion* or insertion of metal or steel rods to stabilize the vertebral column may be indicated.
- The nurse provides routine preoperative care.
- The nurse provides postoperative care
    1. Provides routine postoperative care
    2. Records vital signs and neurologic checks every hour and then every 4 to 6 hours depending on the client's condition
    3. Helps the client logroll from side to side
    4. Checks the surgical site for drainage and signs of infection

NDx: Ineffective Airway Clearance; Ineffective Breathing Pattern; Impaired Gas Exchange

- The nurse
    1. Performs a respiratory assessment at the beginning of each shift
    2. Turns the client at least every 2 hours

3. Encourages the client to cough and deep breathe every 1 to 2 hours
4. Teaches the client to use an incentive spirometer every 2 hours while awake
5. Performs tracheal suctioning if needed

NDx: Impaired Physical Mobility

- The nurse
  1. Repositions the client every 2 hours while in bed and every 30 minutes while in a chair
  2. Inspects the skin every shift for signs of pressure sores or reddened areas
  3. Performs ROM to all extremities at least once per shift
  4. Collaborates with physical and occupational therapy to determine positioning and exercise programs; determines the need for splints and a plan to prevent foot drop
  5. Assesses for signs of deep-vein thrombosis, measures the calf and thigh each day
  6. Applies thigh-high antiembolism stockings

NDx: Altered Patterns of Urinary Elimination; Bowel Incontinence

- The nurse establishes an individualized bowel program
  1. Schedules a consistent time for evacuation
  2. Encourages fluids unless contraindicated
  3. Provides a high-fiber diet
  4. Assesses the need for a suppository or stool softener
  5. Places the client on a bedside commode or bedpan at the time determined to be the client's normal time to have a bowel movement; allows for privacy
  6. Teaches the client to use the Valsalva maneuver, or to massage the abdomen from right to left to stimulate bowel evacuation
- The nurse establishes an individualized bladder program
  1. Begins an intermittent catheterization program as soon as possible
  2. Encourages fluids unless contraindicated to 2000 mL to 2500 mL; restricts fluids after 7 PM each evening
  3. Catheterizes the client every 4 hours and more frequently if the urinary output is greater than 500 mL
  4. Recognizes that over time, intervals between catheterization are increased and adjusted to the client's fluid intake and sleep times

5. Teaches the client with upper motor injury that he or she may be able to stimulate voiding by stroking the inner thigh, performing the Valsalva maneuver, or tightening the abdominal muscles
6. Catheterizes for residual urine after the client voids to ascertain the effectiveness of the above maneuvers

NDx: SELF-CARE DEFICIT

- The nurse
  1. Assesses the client's ability to perform activities of daily living (ADLs) to establish abilities and limitations
  2. Encourages the client to perform activities as independently as possible, provides assistance as needed
  3. Plans activities to follow the administration of medication to maximize independence and successful attempts at self-care
  4. Documents and monitors the client's response to or tolerance of activity
  5. Collaborates with physical and occupational therapy to identify the need for assistive-adaptive devices

NDx: IMPAIRED ADJUSTMENT

- The nurse
  1. Invites the client to ask questions and answers honestly and openly
  2. Refers questions about prognosis and potential for complete recovery to the physician because the timing and extent of recovery vary greatly
  3. Explores coping strategies with the client
  4. Redirects socially unacceptable behavior
  5. Allows the client to direct his or her care and routine as much as possible
  6. Involves the client/family in care planning and setting goals

Discharge Planning

- The nurse
  1. Identifies and suggests corrections for hazards in the home
  2. Ensures that the client can correctly use all assistive-adaptive devices ordered for home use
  3. Ensures that assistive-adaptive equipment is installed in the home prior to discharge
  4. Provides a detailed plan of care at the time of discharge for clients to be transferred to a rehabilitation facility (rehabilitation can be lengthy; see Rehabilitation)

- The nurse teaches the client/family in collaboration with other health team members
    1. Training in ADL
    2. Structured exercise program
    3. Correct use of adaptive-assistive equipment
    4. Transfer skills
    5. Diet
    6. Bowel and bladder program
    7. Drug information as needed

For more information on spinal cord injury, see *Medical-Surgical Nursing: A Nursing Process Approach,* **pp. 937–947.**

Stye

- An *external* stye (hordeolum) is an infection of the glands of Moll or Zeis near the exit of the eyelashes from the eyelid, manifested by a localized red, swollen, tender area on the skin surface side of the margin.
- An *internal* stye is caused by an infection of the sebaceous meibomian glands and is characterized by a small, beady, edematous area on the skin side of the eyelid or on the conjunctival side of the eyelid-eyelash margin.
- Treatment includes
    1. Warm compresses, with thorough hand washing before and after applying the compresses
    2. Antibacterial ointment
    3. Instructing the client to remove ointment from the eye before driving or operating machinery

4. Instructing the client to avoid rubbing the eye or wearing eye makeup

For more information on stye, see *Medical-Surgical Nursing: A Nursing Process Approach,* **pp. 1014, 1024.**

Subclavian Steal Syndrome

- Subclavian steal syndrome occurs in the upper extremities from a subclavian artery occlusion and results in altered blood flow and ischemia in the arm.
- The disorder occurs at any age but is more common with risk factors for atherosclerosis.
- Clinical manifestations include
  1. Paresthesias
  2. Syncope
  3. Dizziness
  4. Headaches
  5. Pain and discomfort
  6. Difference in blood pressure between arms
  7. Subclavian bruit on the occluded side
  8. Subclavian pulse decreased on the occluded side
  9. Discoloration of the affected arm
- Surgical intervention involves one of three procedures: endarterectomy of the subclavian artery, carotid-subclavian bypass, or dilation of the subclavian artery.
- Nursing interventions include
  1. Frequent brachial and radial pulse checks

S

2. Observation for ischemic changes of the extremity
3. Oservation for edema and redness

For more information on subclavian steal syndrome, see *Medical-Surgical Nursing: A Nursing Process Approach*, **p. 2226.**

Syndrome of Inappropriate Antidiuretic Hormone

OVERVIEW

- Syndrome of inappropriate antidiuretic hormone (SIADH) occurs when ADH (vasopressin) is secreted in the presence of low plasma osmolality because feedback mechanisms that regulate ADH do not function properly.
- Water is retained, which results in dilutional hyponatremia and expansion of extracellular fluid volume.
- SIADH is associated with
  1. Oat cell carcinoma of the lung
  2. Carcinoma of the pancreas, duodenum, and genitourinary tract
  3. Ewing's sarcoma
  4. Hodgkin's and non-Hodgkin's lymphoma
  5. Viral and bacterial pneumonia, lung abscess, active tuberculosis, pneumothorax, chronic obstructive pulmonary disease
  6. Central nervous system disorders such as trauma, cerebral vascular accident, infections, tumors, porphyria
  7. Drugs such as exogenous ADH, chlorpropamide, vincristine, cyclophosphamide, carbamazepine, general anesthetic agents, and tricyclic antibiotics

COLLABORATIVE MANAGEMENT
Assessment
- The nurse records the client's
  1. Past medical history
  2. Weight, especially a history of weight gain
- The nurse assesses for
  1. Gastrointestinal disturbances such as loss of appetite, nausea, and vomiting
  2. Edema of the extremities
  3. Water and sodium retention
  4. Seizure activity
  5. Decreased or sluggish deep-tendon reflexes
  6. Vital sign changes (tachycardia, hypothermia)
  7. Irritability, anxiety

Planning and Implementation
NDx: FLUID VOLUME EXCESS
- The nurse
  1. Restricts fluid intake, as ordered (may be as low as 500 to 600 mL/day)
  2. Weighs the client daily
  3. Carefully measures intake and output
  4. Provides frequent mouth care
  5. Suggests hard candy to relieve dryness of the mouth

- The nurse administers diuretics as ordered, particularly if congestive heart failure results from fluid overload

NDx: ALTERED THOUGHT PROCESSES
- The nurse
  1. Monitors neurologic status
  2. Promotes a safe environment

Discharge Planning
- The nurse teaches the client
  1. To restrict fluids if SIADH is not completely resolved
  2. To use the same scale for daily weights
  3. To avoid over-the-counter medications such as aspirin or nonsteroidal anti-inflammatory drugs, which may contribute to hyponatremia

S

For more information on syndrome of inappropriate antidiuretic hormone, see *Medical-Surgical Nursing: A Nursing Process Approach,* **pp. 1540–1544.**

Syphilis

OVERVIEW

- Syphilis is a classic sexually transmitted disease.
- The primary population affected is young adults in their early 20s.
- The causative organism is *Treponema pallidum*, a spirochete with a slender, spiral shape.
- In *primary* syphilis, the chancre is the first lesion developing at the site of inoculation or entry of the organism.
- During the highly infectious stage, the chancre begins as a small papule; within 3 to 7 days, it breaks down into its characteristic appearance—a painless, indurated, smooth, weeping lesion.
- Without treatment, the chancre disappears within 6 weeks; however, the organism disseminates throughout the bloodstream.
- *Secondary* syphilis, which develops from 6 weeks to 6 months after the onset of primary syphilis, becomes a systemic disease because spirochetes circulate throughout the bloodstream.
- Symptoms of secondary syphilis include malaise, low-grade fever, headache, muscular aches and pains, and sore throat.
- A generalized rash usually evolves from papules, to squamous papules, to pustules.
- *Latent* syphilis is a later stage of the disease.
- *Early latent* syphilis occurs during the first year after infection, and infectious lesions can recur.
- *Late latent* syphilis is a disease of more than one year's duration after infection; it is noninfectious except to the fetus of a pregnant woman.
- *Late* syphilis develops after a highly variable period—from 4 to 20 years in untreated cases.
- Manifestations of late syphilis include benign lesions of the skin, mucous membranes, and bones, aortitis and aneurysms, and neurosyphilis.

COLLABORATIVE MANAGEMENT

- Assessment includes
  1. Sexual history
     a. Type and frequency of sexual activity
     b. Number of contacts
     c. Past history of sexually transmitted diseases

    d. Potential sites of infection

    e. Sexual preferences

2. Chief complaint
3. Inspection of the external genitalia for chancre lesion
4. Positive Venereal Disease Research Laboratory (VDRL) and fluorescent treponemal antibody absorption tests

- Management includes antibiotic therapy with penicillin.
- Client education includes

1. Treatment and side effects
2. Complications of untreated syphilis
3. Follow-up care
4. Treatment for sexual partners
5. Disease reported to the health department
6. Contagiousness of the disease

For more information on syphilis, see *Medical-Surgical Nursing: A Nursing Process Approach*, **pp. 1775–1778.**

Tension Pneumothorax

S

- Tension pneumothorax is a complication of blunt chest trauma or mechanical ventilation with positive end-expiratory pressure and occurs as a result of an air leak into the lung or chest wall.
- Air forced into the thoracic cavity causes complete collapse of the affected lung.
- Air entering the pleural space during expiration does not exit during inspiration; therefore, the air accumulates under pressure, compressing the mediastinal vessels and interfering with venous return.

- Assessment findings include
    1. Tracheal deviation to the unaffected side
    2. Respiratory distress
    3. Unilateral absence of breath sounds
    4. Distended neck veins
    5. Cyanosis
    6. Hypertympanic sound over the affected hemothorax

- Initial treatment includes emergency insertion of a large-bore needle into the second intercostal space in the midclavicular line on the affected side to relieve pressure.

- Chest tube placement into the fourth intercostal space of the midaxillary line follows; underwater seal drainage is maintained until the lung is fully expanded.

For more information on tension pneumothorax, see *Medical-Surgical Nursing: A Nursing Process Approach*, **p. 2056.**

Testicular Cancer

OVERVIEW

- Testicular cancer is the third leading cause of cancer deaths in young men.
- Primary testicular cancers fall into two groups
    1. *Germinal* tumors, arising from the sperm-producing germ cells, which include seminoma and nonseminoma tumors (embryonal, teratoma, and choriocarcinoma)
    2. *Nongerminal* tumors, arising from other structures in the testicles, including interstitial cell tumors and androblastoma

COLLABORATIVE MANAGEMENT
Assessment
- The nurse records the client's
    1. Age and race

2. History or presence of undescended testes
3. Family history of testicular cancer
- The nurse assesses for
  1. Palpable lymphadenopathy
  2. Abdominal masses
  3. Gynecomastia

Planning and Implementation

NDx: KNOWLEDGE DEFICIT

Nonsurgical Management

- Combination chemotherapy is dramatically effective in treating nonseminomatous testicular cancer, especially cisplatin (Platinol) in combination with other agents.
- External beam radiation therapy may be used.

Surgical Management

- *Unilateral orchiectomy* (removal of the testis) is done for diagnosis and primary surgical management.
- *Radical retroperitoneal lymph node dissection* is used to stage the disease and to reduce tumor volume so that chemotherapy or radiation therapy is more effective.
- The nurse provides preoperative care
  1. Provides routine preoperative care
  2. Prepares the client for an extensive surgical procedure and a large incision if retroperitoneal lymph node dissection is to be performed.
- The nurse provides postoperative care
  1. Provides routine postoperative care
  2. Assesses for signs of shock after prolonged anesthesia and excess blood loss
  3. Assesses the wound for potential complications
  4. Monitors fluid and electrolyte balance
  5. Maintains accurate intake and output records

NDx: SEXUAL DYSFUNCTION

- Infertility is related to oligospermia and azoospermia.
- The nurse provides important client education about reproduction, fertility, and sexuality in the pretreatment stage, including discussion of options.
- Sperm storage for adequate sperm counts prior to undergoing treatment may be suggested.
- Other options include donor insemination, adoption, or not fathering children.

Discharge Planning

- The nurse provides postoperative instructions
  1. Notify the physician of chills, fever, increasing

T

tenderness or pain around the incision, drainage, or dehiscence of the incision.
2. Resume normal activities except lifting objects heavier than 20 lb or stair climbing.
3. Perform monthly testicular self-examination on the remaining testis.
4. Follow instructions for radiation and/or chemotherapy.
5. Follow-up with visits to the physician(s) for at least 3 years.

For more information on testicular cancer, see *Medical-Surgical Nursing: A Nursing Process Approach*, **pp. 1756–1765.**

Tetanus

- Tetanus, also know as lockjaw, is caused by *Clostridium tetani* and is easily prevented through immunization.
- Tetanus is characterized by tonic rigidity, opisthotonos, cramps, muscle spasms, stiffness, and facial expression known as risus sardonicus.
- Treatment includes intramuscular antitoxin, human tetanus immune globulin, or hyperimmune equine or bovine serum.
- Sedation, antianxiety agents, and muscle relaxants to decrease muscle spasms and increase the client's comfort are provided.
- Propranolol (Inderal) is given to treat cardiac irregularities, and the client receives aggressive respiratory support.

For more information on tetanus, see *Medical-Surgical Nursing: A Nursing Process Approach*, **pp. 905–906.**

Thoracic Outlet Syndrome

- Thoracic outlet syndrome is a compression of the subclavian artery at the thoracic outlet by anatomic structures, such as a rib or muscle.
- Damage of the arterial wall produces thrombosis or embolization to distal arteries of the arm.
- The common sites of compression of the thoracic outlet are the interscalene triangle; between the coracoid process of the scapula and the pectoralis minor tendon; and, most common, the costoclavicular space.
- Clinical manifestations include
    1. Neck, shoulder, and arm pain
    2. Numbness of the extremity
    3. Moderate edema of the extremity
    4. Increasing pain and numbness when the arm is held over the head or out to the side
- Conservative treatment includes
    1. Physical therapy
    2. Exercise
    3. Avoidance of aggravating positions
- Surgical treatment involves resection of the anatomic structures compressing the artery.

For more information on thoracic outlet syndrome, see *Medical-Surgical Nursing: A Nursing Process Approach*, **p. 2226.**

Thyroid Cancer

OVERVIEW

- There are four types of thyroid cancer
    1. *Papillary* carcinoma
        a. This type is a slow-growing tumor found more frequently in women.

    b. If it is localized to the thyroid gland, the prognosis is good.

2. *Follicular* carcinoma

    a. Follicular carcinoma invades blood vessels and metastasizes to bone and lung tissue.

    b. It can adhere to the trachea, neck muscles, great vessels, and skin, resulting in dysphagia and dyspnea.

    c. The prognosis is fair if metastasis is minimal at the time of diagnosis.

3. *Medullary* carcinoma

    a. Medullary carcinoma involves metastasis that occurs via regional lymph nodes and invades surrounding structures.

    b. It may occur as part of multiple endocrine neoplasia type II, a familial endocrine disorder.

    c. Excessive secretion of calcitonin, adrenocorticotropic hormone, prostaglandins, and serotonin may occur.

4. *Anaplastic* carcinoma

    a. Anaplastic carcinoma is a rapidly growing, extremely aggressive tumor.

    b. It directly invades adjacent structures, causing stridor, hoarseness, and dysphagia.

    c. Its prognosis is poor.

COLLABORATIVE MANAGEMENT

- The treatment for papillary, follicular, and medullary carcinoma includes

1. Partial or total *thyroidectomy* with a modified radical neck dissection if regional lymph nodes are involved

2. Postoperative suppressive doses of thyroid hormone for 3 months, followed by a radioactive iodine (RAI) uptake study; if there is RAI uptake, clients are treated with ablative amounts of RAI

3. If recurrent thyroid cancer does not respond to RAI, a course of chemotherapy

- The treatment for anaplastic carcinoma is palliative surgery, radiation, or chemotherapy. For nursing care, see Cancer, General and Hyperthyroidism.

For more information on thyroid cancer, see *Medical-Surgical Nursing: A Nursing Process Approach,* **p. 1575.**

Thyroiditis

OVERVIEW

- Thyroiditis is the inflammation of the thyroid gland.
- There are three types of thyroiditis.
  1. *Acute* suppurative thyroiditis, caused by bacterial invasion of the thyroid gland and manifested by neck tenderness, pain, fever, malaise, and dysphagia
  2. *Subacute* granulomatous thyroiditis, which results from a viral infection of the thyroid gland and is manifested by fever, chills, dysphagia, and muscle and joint pain; on palpation the gland feels hard
  3. *Chronic* thyroiditis (Hashimoto's disease), believed to be an autoimmune disease, which is manifested by dysphagia, painless enlargement of the thyroid gland, low serum thyroid levels, and increased thyroid-stimulating hormone secretion, which causes a euthyroid state for some time, followed by the development of hypothyroidism

COLLABORATIVE MANAGEMENT

- Acute suppurative thyroiditis is treated symptomatically and with antibiotics.
- Subacute granulomatous thyroiditis is treated with rest, fluids, and acetylsalicylic acid (aspirin); severe cases may be treated with corticosteroids.
- Chronic thyroiditis is usually treated with thyroid hormone; a subtotal thyroidectomy may be necessary. See "Surgical Management" under Hyperthyroidism.

For more information on thyroiditis, see *Medical-Surgical Nursing: A Nursing Process Approach,* **pp. 1574–1575.**

Tonsillitis

- Tonsillitis is an inflammation of the tonsils and lymphatic tissue of the oropharynx.
- Tonsillitis is a contagious airborne or food-borne infection.
- The acute form lasts 7 to 10 days and is caused by a bacterial organism, usually *Streptococcus*, and viruses.
- Acute symptoms begin with the sudden onset of a mild to severe sore throat, fever, muscle aches, chills, dysphagia, ear pain, headache, anorexia, and malaise.
- The tonsils are swollen and red with pus and covered with white or yellow exudate.
- The uvula may be edematous and inflamed, and the cervical lymph nodes are tender and enlarged.
- Treatment includes
  1. Systemic antibiotics for 7 to 10 days
  2. Warm saline gargles
  3. Analgesics
  4. Antipyretics
  5. Antiseptic anesthetic lozenges
  6. Tonsillectomy and adenoidectomy (T&A)
- Tonsillectomy and adenoidectomy are indicated for
  1. Recurrent acute infections or chronic infections unresponsive to antibiotic therapy
  2. Peritonsillar abscess
  3. Malignant tonsils
  4. Hypertrophy of tonsils and adenoids, causing airway obstruction
  5. Diphtheria carriage
- The chronic form of tonsillitis results from unresolved acute infections or recurrent infections.

For more information on tonsillitis, see *Medical-Surgical Nursing: A Nursing Process Approach*, **pp. 1959–1962.**

Toxic Shock Syndrome

- The pathophysiology of toxic shock syndrome (TSS) is not fully understood.

- Certain strains of *Staphylococcus aureus* produce a toxin associated with TSS.

- Menstrual-related TSS theories focus on tampon use and conclude that toxins readily cross the vaginal mucosa.

- Highly absorbent tampons rub the vaginal walls and cause ulceration, which allows transport of the toxins; prolonged or continued tampon use can cause chronic vaginal ulcerations through which *S. aureus* is absorbed; and plastic tampon inserters can cause ulceration.

- Diaphragms, cervical caps, and vaginal contraceptives have also been implicated.

- Physical findings include
  1. Fever (temperature greater than 102° F)
  2. Diffuse rash
  3. Peeling of the skin
  4. Hypotension
  5. Influenza-type symptoms, including sore throat, vomiting, diarrhea, and generalized rash

- Primary treatment includes
  1. Fluid replacement due to dehydration
  2. Antibiotics (oxacillin, nafcillin, and cephalosporin)
  3. Administration of platelets, if needed
  4. Corticosteroids for skin changes
  5. Vaginal irrigations with a vaginal disinfectant

- Client education is focused on prevention, including instructions on proper tampon, vaginal sponge, and diaphragm use.

T

For more information on toxic shock syndrome, see *Medical-Surgical Nursing: A Nursing Process Approach*, **pp. 1702–1703.**

Tracheobronchial Trauma

- Most tears of the tracheobronchial tree are the result of severe blunt trauma, primarily involving the mainstem bronchi.
- Injuries to the cervical trachea occur at the junction of the trachea and cricoid cartilage.
- Clients with laceration of the trachea develop massive air leaks, which produce pneumomediastinum (air in the mediastinum) and extensive subcutaneous emphysema.
- Upper airway obstruction may occur, producing severe respiratory distress and inspiratory stridor.
- Most cervical tears are managed by cricothyroidotomy or tracheostomy below the level of the injury.
- The nurse
    1. Assesses for respiratory distress
    2. Administers oxygen, as ordered
    3. Maintains mechanical ventilation, if required
    4. Assesses for subcutaneous emphysema
    5. Auscultates the lungs to assess for further complications
    6. Provides care to the tracheostomy, if needed

For more information on tracheobronchial trauma, see *Medical-Surgical Nursing: A Nursing Process Approach*, **p. 2057.**

Trachoma

- Trachoma is a chronic, bilateral scarring form of conjunctivitis caused by *Chlamydia trachomatis.*
- Trachoma is the leading cause of blindness in the world and is manifested by tearing, photophobia,

edema of the eyelids, conjunctival edema, profuse drainage, eyelid scars, and turns inward, leading to corneal abrasion.

- Treatment includes oral tetracycline (Achromycin) or erythromycin (E-Mycin, E.E.S.), which may also be used as a topical ointment.
- The client is taught to
  1. Control the fly population
  2. Use warm water to clean the face and eye
  3. Not to share washcloths for bathing and to launder them separately in hot water
  4. Wash the hands before and after touching the eyes
  5. Use warm, moist compresses if eye drainage is present
  6. Avoid crowded, public areas until the infection is cleared

For more information on trachoma, see *Medical-Surgical Nursing: A Nursing Process Approach,* **p. 1028.**

Tuberculosis, Pulmonary

OVERVIEW

- Pulmonary tuberculosis (TB) is a highly communicable disease typically caused by *Mycobacterium tuberculosis.*
- The tubercle bacillus is transmitted via aerosolization to a susceptible site in the lung's bronchi or alveoli and freely multiplies.
- Granulomatous inflammation is surrounded by collagen, fibroblasts, and lymphocytes; areas of caseation localize and undergo reabsorption, hyaline degeneration, and fibrosis.
- Calcification and liquefaction occur.

T

• The initial infection is seen most often in the middle or lower lobes, with the upper lobes as the most common sites of reinfection.

COLLABORATIVE MANAGEMENT

Assessment
• The nurse records the client's
  1. Past exposure to TB
  2. Country of origin
  3. Travel to foreign countries
  4. Prior TB tests
  5. History of bacille Calmette-Guérin vaccine
• The nurse assesses for
  1. Progressive fatigue
  2. Lethargy
  3. Anorexia, nausea
  4. Weight loss
  5. Irregular menses
  6. Low-grade fever
  7. Night sweats
  8. Cough with mucoid, blood-streaked, mucopurulent sputum
  9. Chest tightness
  10. Dull, aching chest pain
  11. Dullness with chest percussion
  12. Bronchial breath sounds and/or rales
  13. Increased transmission of spoken or whispered sounds
  14. Localized wheezing

Planning and Implementation
NDx: POTENTIAL FOR INJURY
• The nurse reviews the multiple-drug regime required to prevent spread of the disease
  1. Isoniazid (INH)
  2. Rifampin (Rifadin)
  3. Ethambutol (Myambutol) and streptomycin in the initial 2 to 8 weeks
• The nurse
  1. Teaches the client to cover the mouth and nose when coughing or sneezing
  2. Collects sputum for examination every 2 to 4 weeks until negative culture results are obtained
  3. Teaches the client to avoid excess exposure to silicone or dust
  4. Wears a mask (respiratory precautions) when in contact with the client who is hospitalized
  5. Practices thorough hand washing

- The nurse
  1. Teaches the client to take chemotherapeutic drugs at bedtime to minimize the effects of nausea
  2. Administers antinausea drugs, as ordered
  3. Teaches the client to increase the intake of foods rich in iron, protein, and vitamin C

Discharge Planning

- The nurse teaches the client/family
  1. Adherence to the prescribed drug regimen for 9 to 12 months
  2. Side effects of medications and ways to minimize them to ensure compliance
  3. Need to resume usual activities gradually
  4. Maintenance of proper nutrition
  5. Identification of individuals who have been exposed to the client to determine infection with TB
  6. Importance of follow-up visits with the physician(s)

For more information on pulmonary tuberculosis, see *Medical-Surgical Nursing: A Nursing Process Approach*, **pp. 2041–2045.**

Ulcerative Colitis

OVERVIEW

- Ulcerative colitis is a chronic inflammatory process of the bowel with unknown cause that results in poor absorption of vital nutrients.
- Classified as an inflammatory bowel disease, it is characterized by diffuse inflammation of the intestinal mucosa, resulting in loss of surface epithelium, causing ulceration and abscess formation.

T
U

• Ulcerative colitis typically begins in the rectum and proceeds in a uniform, continuous manner proximally toward the cecum.

• *Acute* ulcerative colitis results in vascular congestion, hemorrhage, edema, and ulceration of the bowel mucosa.

• *Chronic* ulcerative colitis causes muscular hypertrophy, fat deposits, and fibrous tissue with bowel thickening, shortening, and narrowing.

• Complications of the disease include abscess formation, bowel stenosis, bowel perforation with peritonitis, fissures, and fistula formation.

COLLABORATIVE MANAGEMENT
Assessment
• The nurse records the client's
  1. Family history of inflammatory bowel disease
  2. Previous and current therapy for illnesses
  3. Diet history, including usual patterns and intolerances to milk products and greasy, fried, or spicy foods
  4. History of liquid, bloody stools
  5. Anorexia
  6. Fatigue
• The nurse assesses for
  1. The presence or absence of bowel sounds
  2. Increased or localized abdominal tenderness or cramping
  3. Bowel elimination patterns, noting color, consistency, and character of stools and the presence or absence of blood
  4. The relationship between the occurrence of diarrhea and the timing of meals, pain, emotional distress, and activity

Planning and Implementation
NDx: Diarrhea
Nonsurgical Management
• Management of ulcerative colitis is aimed at resting the bowel to permit inflammation to resolve.

• The prescribed diet depends on the severity of the disease and if surgery is done
  1. Nothing by mouth, with intravenous fluids and electrolytes; diet resumes with clear liquids and is gradually increased to low-residue foods, as tolerated
  2. Low-roughage diet, limiting high-residue foods and avoiding foods such as whole wheat grains,

nuts, raw fruits, and vegetables; thorough chewing of solid foods is stressed
3. Elemental formulas, which are absorbed in the upper bowel, thereby minimizing stimulation while providing fluid and nutrients
4. Parenteral nutrition with hyperosmolar dextrose and amino acid solutions
- The nurse
  1. Teaches the client to avoid caffeinated beverages, alcohol, and pepper
  2. Encourages the client to stop smoking
  3. Adminsters antidiarrheal agents, as ordered, to manage symptoms, including diphenoxylate hydrochloride and atropine sulfate (Lomotil), loperamide (Imodium), and camphorated tincture of opium (paregoric)
  4. Administers antimicrobial agents, as ordered, to prevent secondary infections, including sulfonamides
  5. Administers corticosteroids, as ordered, to reduce inflammation, including prednisone or intravenous adrenocorticotropic hormone
  6. Administers immunosuppressants, as ordered, including azathioprine (Imuran), in combination with steriods
  7. Restricts the client's activity to reduce intestinal activity, promoting comfort and intestinal healing

Surgical Management
- The need for surgery is based on the client's response to medical interventions.
- Surgical procedures include
  1. *Total proctocolectomy with permanent ileostomy*, which involves removal of the colon, rectum, and anus with anal closure; the end of the terminal ileum forms the stoma, which is located in the right lower quadrant
  2. *Kock ileostomy (pouch)*, which involves an intra-abdominal pouch or reservoir constructed from the terminal ileum; the pouch is connected to the stoma with a nipplelike valve constructed from an intusscepted portion of the ileum; the stoma is flush with the skin
  3. *Ileoanal reservior*, which is a two-stage procedure involving the excision of the rectal mucosa, abdominal colectomy, construction of the reservoir or pouch to the anal canal, and a temporary loop ileostomy; over 3 to 4 months, the capacity of the reservoir is increased by a series of fluid instillations, after which the loop ileostomy is closed

U

- The nurse provides extensive preoperative teaching
  1. Provides routine preoperative instructions
  2. Provides instructions on care of the ostomy
     a. Empty the ileostomy pouch when it is 1/3 to 1/2 full
     b. Change the pouch during inactive times, such as before meals, retiring at night, on waking in the morning, or 2 to 4 hours past meals
     c. Change the entire pouch system every 3 to 7 days
     d. Use a pectin-based skin barrier to protect the skin from contact with the ostomy contents
     e. Use skin care products if the skin continues to have contact with the ostomy contents
     f. Monitor the skin for irritation and redness
- The nurse provides routine postoperative care.
- Specific nursing care interventions are determined by the procedure performed, including ostomy or perineal wound care.
- The nurse consults the enterostomal therapist, as needed.

NDx: PAIN
- The nurse
  1. Assesses the client for changes in complaints and responses to pain that may indicate disease complications
  2. Assesses for pain, including its character, pattern of occurrence such as before or after meals, during the night, and before or after bowel movements, and duration
  3. Administers antidiarrheal drugs, as ordered, to control diarrhea
  4. Administers anticholinergics, as ordered, prior to meals to provide relief of pain caused by cramping
  5. Provides measures to relieve irritated skin caused by frequent contact with diarrheal stool
     a. Cleansing with mild soap and water after each stool
     b. Providing frequent sitz baths
     c. Applying a thin coat of mineral oil, petroleum jelly, vitamin A and D ointment, or other skin protective care product
     d. Applying medicated wipes such as witch hazel or Tucks

Discharge Planning
- The nurse teaches the client
  1. Information on the nature of the disease,

624

including acute episodes, remissions, and symptom management

2. Postoperative continuing care
   a. Incision and wound management
   b. Inspection of the incision for redness, tenderness, swelling, and drainage
   c. Inspection of the stoma for unusual swelling or color changes, reporting abnormalities to the physician
3. Self-care of the ileostomy or Kock pouch, including when to empty the pouch and change the pouch system
4. Pain medication administration according to the physician's order
5. Activity limitations, including avoidance of heavy lifting
6. Reporting a marked increase or decrease in ileostomy drainage to the physician

For more information on ulcerative colitis, see *Medical-Surgical Nursing: A Nursing Process Approach*, **pp. 1351–1362.**

Upper Airway Obstruction

OVERVIEW

- Upper airway obstruction is a life-threatening emergency, defined as any interruption in airflow through the nose or mouth into the lungs.
- The obstruction may be caused by laryngeal edema, peritonsillar abscess, laryngeal carcinoma, tumor growth, cerebral vascular accident, thickened secretions, tongue occlusion, smoke inhalation injury, tracheal and laryngeal trauma, foreign body aspiration, and anaphylaxis.
- Assessment includes increasing anxiety, sternal retractions, seesawing chest, abdominal movements, air hunger, and the universal distress sign for airway obstruction (hands to the neck).

U

- Management depends on the cause, including
  1. Hyperextension of the neck
  2. Suctioning of oral secretions
  3. Heimlich maneuver for a foreign body
  4. Cricothyroidotomy as an emergency procedure
  5. Endotracheal intubation
  6. Tracheostomy

For more information on upper airway obstruction, see *Medical-Surgical Nursing: A Nursing Process Approach*, **pp. 1974–1975.**

Urethritis

- Urethritis is inflammation of the urethra.
- Urethritis in the *male* client presents as
  1. Burning on urination
  2. Difficult urination
  3. Discharge from the urethral meatus
- Urethritis in the *female* client presents as
  1. Bacterial cystitis (mimics)
  2. Painful urination
  3. Difficulty with urination
  4. Lower abdomen discomfort
  5. Pyuria
- The most common cause in males is gonorrhea.
- Nonspecific urethritis may be caused by *Ureaplasma, Chlamydia,* or *Trichomonas vaginalis.*

For more information on urethritis, see *Medical-Surgical Nursing: A Nursing Process Approach*, **p. 1839.**

Urolithiasis

OVERVIEW

• Urolithiasis is the presence of stones or urologic calculi in the urinary tract; the exact mechanism of formation is not known.

• A supersaturation of urinary filtrate with a particular element is believed to be the primary factor contributing to calculi formation.

• Other factors include the acidity or alkalinity of the urine, urinary stasis, and other substances, such as pyrophosphate, magnesium, and citrate.

• Calculi may be formed from calcium, phosphate, oxalate, uric acid, struvite, and cystine crystals, with the majority of stones containing calcium as one component.

COLLABORATIVE MANAGEMENT

Assessment

• The nurse records the client's
   1. History of previous renal stones
   2. Family history of renal stones
   3. Diet history
   4. Previous interventions to eliminate stones
• The nurse assesses for
   1. Presence, location, and duration of pain
   2. Nausea and vomiting
   3. Chills and fever
   4. Changes in the pattern of urination
   5. Flank pain
   6. Ureteral spasm or colic
   7. Color, amount, clarity, and odor of urine
   8. Bladder distention
   9. Diaphoresis
   10. Pale, ashen skin

Planning and Implementation

NDx: PAIN

Nonsurgical Management

• The nurse administers drug therapy, as ordered
   1. Narcotic agents such as morphine sulfate
   2. Spasmolytic agents such as oxybutynin chloride (Ditropan) and propantheline bromide (Pro-Banthine)

U

Surgical Management

- Stone removal procedures include

   1. *Cystoscopy*: insertion of an endoscope through the urethra to visualize stones and to extract stones with a basket
   2. *Percutaneous nephrostomy*: use of an endoscope to visualize the stone with a special attachment to extract the stone (via a small flank incision)
   3. *Percutaneous ultrasonic lithostripsy*: use of sound waves directed by a probe inserted via cystoscopy or nephrostomy to break up the stone
   4. *Extracorporeal shock wave lithotripsy*: use of shock waves while the client's flank is under water
   5. *Pyelolithotomy*: direct visualization of the renal pelvis via a large flank incision and removal of the stone
   6. *Nephrolithotomy*: direct visualization of the kidney via a large flank incision and removal of the stone
   7. *Pyeloureterolithotomy*: direct visualization of the ureter via a large flank or lower abdominal incision and removal of the stone

- The nurse provides preoperative care

   1. Provides routine preoperative care
   2. Provides individualized instructions dependent on the procedure to be performed.

- Postoperative care is dependent on which procedure is performed and the type of drainage tubes, such as nephrostomy tubes, ureteral stents, or Penrose drains.
- The nurse provides postoperative care

   1. Provides routine postoperative care
   2. Monitors surgical drains and catheters (ureteral, urethral, and/or nephrostomy) for excess bleeding and drainage
   3. Monitors hourly urinary output from each catheter for adequate amounts and the presence of hematuria
   4. Inspects the dressing(s) for bleeding and/or urine and changes the dressings as ordered

NDx: POTENTIAL FOR INFECTION

- The nurse

   1. Administers broad-spectrum antibiotics, such as aminoglycosides and cephalosporins, as ordered
   2. Ensures adequate caloric intake representing a balance of the four food groups
   3. Encourages 2 to 3 L of fluid intake per day

NDx: POTENTIAL FOR INJURY

- The nurse
    1. Administers drugs, as ordered, to prevent hypercalciuria, such as thiazide diuretics, orthophosphate, and sodium cellulose phosphate
    2. Administers drugs, as ordered, to prevent hyperoxaluria, such as allopurinol (Zyloprim) and/or vitamin B_6 (pyrodoxine)
    3. Administers drugs, as ordered, for hyperuricuria, such as allopurinol
    4. Administers antibiotics, as ordered, such as penicillins, and acetohydrosamic acid for struvite stones
    5. Administers medication, as ordered, to alkalinize the urine, such as 50% sodium citrate
    6. Provides diet modifications dependent on stone type, in consultation with the dietitian
    7. Limits calcium intake for calcium stones
    8. Limits dark green foods such as spinach because oxalate increases as calcium decreases
    9. Reduces purine intake such as boned fish and organ meats for clients with uric acid stones
    10. Encourages ambulation to promote calculi passage
    11. Provides and encourages a liberal fluid intake
    12. Strains urine in filter paper to collect passed stone fragments

Discharge Planning

- The nurse teaches
    1. Medication information for antibiotics or pH-altering drugs, including purpose, method, duration of administration, and desired effects and side effects
    2. How to test urine pH daily
    3. Importance of balancing regular exercise with rest
    4. Diet instructions depending on stone type
- The nurse
    1. Encourages continued adequate fluid intake, including the rationale, to prevent dehydration and promoting urine flow
    2. Provides postoperative care instructions, including to keep the incision dry, shower instead of bathing, and monitor the incision for redness, swelling, and drainage
    3. Teaches the client to report symptoms of recurrent infection, such as fever, chills, and general malaise

U

4. Emphasizes the importance of follow-up visits with the physician(s)

For more information on urolithiasis, see *Medical-Surgical Nursing: A Nursing Process Approach*, **pp. 1857–1863.**

Urothelial Cancer

OVERVIEW

- Urothelial cancers are malignancies of the urothelium, which is the lining of transitional cells in the renal pelvis, ureters, urinary bladder, and urethra.
- Most tumors occur in the urinary bladder; consequently *bladder cancer* is a general term used to describe urothelial cancer.
- The urothelium is described initially in terms of cellular dysplasia.
- The *first stages* have nonspecific cellular alteration.
- In the *second stage* of cell growth, there are superficial low- or high-grade, flat or papillary lesions.
- The *third stage* refers to local invasion of the tissues.
- *Stage 4* represents metastasis into the lymphatics or vasculature.
- Effects of tumors include local inflammation, ischemia, hemorrhage, and urinary obstruction.

COLLABORATIVE MANAGEMENT
Assessment
- The nurse records the client's
  1. Sex, age, and race
  2. Active and /or passive exposure to cigarette smoke

3. Occupation to determine exposure to harmful environmental agents

- The nurse assesses for
  1. Abdominal tenderness or discomfort
  2. Bladder distention
  3. Abdominal asymmetry
  4. Changes in color, frequency, or amount of urine
  5. Painless hematuria
  6. Dysuria
  7. Frequency
  8. Urgency

Planning and Implementation

NDx: POTENTIAL FOR INJURY
Nonsurgical Management

- The chemotherapy agents used in the treatment of urothelial cancer include thiotepa (Tespa), cisplatin (Platinol), doxorubicin (Adriamycin), and mitomycin (mitomycin C).
- Radiation therapy may be done in combination with chemotherapy.

Surgical Management

- *Cystectomy*, or surgical removal of the bladder with urinary diversion to remove the cancerous bladder, is performed.
- Surgical techniques include
  1. *Partial cystectomy*, in which a portion of the urinary bladder is removed
  2. *Radical cystectomy*, in which there is extensive surgical removal of the bladder and dissection of adjacent muscle and tissue, with placement of a permanent urinary diversion
  3. *Cutaneous ureterostomy*, in which one ureter is brought to the skin surface and an ostomy pouch is worn
  4. *Ureteroureterostomy*, where one ureter is surgically joined to the other, a single cutaneous stoma is formed, and an ostomy pouch is worn
  5. *Bilateral cutaneous*, or *double-barreled ureterostomy*, a variation of ureteroureterostomy, with the ureters lying side by side on the skin surface and an ostomy pouch is worn
  6. *Ileal conduit* (ureteroileal urinary conduit, ileal bladder, ileal loop, Bricker's procedure, or ureterileostomy), in which a portion of the ileum is isolated from the ileum of the small intestine; one end is closed and both ureters are surgically

U

inserted into the isolated portion of the ileum; the open end of the ileum is brought to the skin surface, and an ostomy pouch is worn

7. *Colon conduit*, constructed similarly to the ileal conduit but a portion of the sigmoid colon is used

8. *Utererosigmoidostomy*, the diversion of the ureters into the sigmoid whereby urine empties into the rectum and there is no control of urinary flow

9. *Ureteroileosigmoidostomy*, in which the ureters are diverted into an isolated portion of the ileum and anastamosed to the sigmoid whereby urine exits by the rectum

10. *Continent internal ileal reservoir* (Kock pouch), in which a portion of the ileum is isolated, creating a pouch; the ureters are implanted into the pouch's side and a special nipple valve connects the pouch to the exterior skin, preventing reflux of urine into the renal pelvis from the points of ureteral entry into the pouch

- The nurse provides preoperative care
  1. Provides routine preoperative care
  2. Provides educational counseling about the urinary diversion and postoperative care requirements
  3. Assists in the selection of the stoma site (with the enterostomal therapist)

- Postoperative care depends on the type and extent of the surgical procedure; the nurse
  1. Maintains drainage tubes, including a Foley catheter and Penrose drains
  2. Assesses for abdominal distention
  3. Assesses the urinary stoma for edema
  4. Monitors urinary flow
  5. Assesses for skin excoriation
  6. Monitors for electrolyte imbalances
  7. Provides routine postoperative care

Discharge Planning

- The nurse
  1. Provides dietary instructions, including the avoidance of gas-forming foods if urinary diversion is into the gastrointestinal tract
  2. Teaches care of the external pouch, including application, skin care, pouch care, methods of adhesion, and drainage mechanisms
  3. Instructs the client on catheterization techniques following Kock pouch procedure

4. Teaches the client to replace electrolytes and monitor for long-term losses
5. Provides educational and psychologic counseling on the impact of urinary diversions on self-image and self-esteem

For more information on urothelial cancer, see *Medical-Surgical Nursing: A Nursing Process Approach,* **pp. 1868–1876.**

Uterine Displacement

• Uterine displacement is a variation in normal uterine placement resulting from congenital or acquired weakness of pelvic support structures.

• The most common variation is posterior displacement of the uterus, or retroversion, where the uterus is tilted posteriorly and the cervix rotates anteriorly.

• Other variations include retroflexion, anteversion, and anteflexion.

• Uterine displacement may result in prolapse of the uterus into the vagina.

• Physical findings include
  1. No symptoms
  2. History of backaches
  3. Secondary amenorrhea
  4. Infertility
  5. Dyspareunia (painful intercourse)
  6. Pelvic pressure or heaviness

• Interventions are based on the severity of symptoms and include
  1. Knee-chest positioning

633

2. Insertion of a vaginal pessary (a device placed in the vagina to hold the uterus in the correct position)

For more information on uterine displacement, see *Medical-Surgical Nursing: A Nursing Process Approach*, **pp. 1703–1705**.

Uterine Leiomyoma

OVERVIEW

- Uterine leiomyomas, also called myomas and fibroids (fibroid tumors), are the most frequently occurring benign pelvic tumors.
- Myomas develop from the uterine myometrium and are attached to it by a pedicle or stalk.
- Myomas are classified according to their position in the layers of the uterus and anatomic position.
- The most common types are
  1. Intramural (contained in the uterine wall within the myometrium)
  2. Submucosal (protrude into the cavity of the uterus)
  3. Subserosal (may grow laterally and extend into the broad ligament)

COLLABORATIVE MANAGEMENT

Assessment

- The nurse records the client's history of abnormal bleeding.
- The nurse assesses for
  1. Complaints of a feeling of pelvic pressure
  2. Constipation
  3. Urinary frequency or retention

4. Increased abdominal size
5. Dyspareunia (painful intercourse)
6. Infertility
7. Abdominal pain occurring with torsion of the fibroid or pedicle
8. Uterine enlargement on abdominal, vaginal, and/ or rectal examination

Planning and Implementation

NDx: FEAR AND ANXIETY

Nonsurgical Management

• The client who is asymptomatic or who desires childbearing is observed and examined for changes in the size of the leiomyoma every 3 to 6 months.

• If the woman is postmenopausal, the fibroids usually shrink.

Surgical Management

• Surgical treatment is dependent on whether future childbearing is desired, the age of the woman, the size of the fibroid, and associated symptoms.

• A *myomectomy* (removal of the leiomyomas with preservation of the uterus) is done to preserve childbearing capabilities.

• *Hysterectomy* is the usual surgical management in the older woman who has multiple symptomatic leiomyomas.

• A *total* hysterectomy involves the removal of the uterus, by either a vaginal or abdominal approach.

• A *subtotal* hysterectomy, removal of the uterus except the cervix, is rarely performed.

• *Panhysterectomy*, or total abdominal hysterectomy (TAH), includes the removal of the uterus, ovaries, and fallopian tubes.

• A *radical* hysterectomy involves removal of the uterus, lymph nodes, the upper third of the vagina, and the surrounding tissues.

• Preoperative care includes routine measures and a complete psychological evaluation.

• The nurse
  1. Explores the client's feelings about the loss of the uterus, including childbearing, self-image and femininity, or sexual functioning
  2. Identifies the support system.
  3. Discusses the client's fear of rejection from her sexual partner.

• Postoperative care for the client undergoing abdominal hysterectomy is similar to that of any other client having abdominal surgery.

U

- The nurse provides postoperative care for a client with a vaginal hysterectomy
  1. Assesses for vaginal bleeding
  2. Provides perineal care
     a. Sitz baths
     b. Heat lamps
     c. Ice packs

Discharge Planning

- The client/family education required is dependent on the specific treatment.
- The nurse instructs the postoperative abdominal or vaginal hysterectomy client
  1. To avoid or limit stair climbing for 1 month
  2. To avoid tub baths and sitting for long periods
  3. To avoid strenuous activity or lifting anything weighing more than 10 to 20 lb
  4. To expect certain physical changes, including cessation of menses, inability to become pregnant, weakness and fatigue in the convalescence period, and absence of menopausal symptoms unless the ovaries are removed
  5. To participate in moderate exercise such as walking
  6. To consume foods that aid in healing, such as foods high in protein, iron, and vitamin C
  7. To avoid sexual intercourse for 3 to 6 weeks
  8. To observe for signs of complications, including infection
  9. To expect emotional reactions/changes
  10. To keep follow-up visits with the physician(s)

For more information on uterine leiomyoma, see *Medical-Surgical Nursing: A Nursing Process Approach*, **pp. 1709–1714.**

Uterine Prolapse

- Uterine prolapse is more serious than uterine displacement.
- Three stages are described, according to the degree of descent of the uterus.
  1. *Grade I*: The uterus bulges into the vagina, but the cervix does not protrude through the entrance to the vagina.
  2. *Grade II*: The uterus bulges further into the vagina, and the cervix protrudes through the entrance to the vagina.
  3. *Grade III*: The body of the uterus and cervix protrude through the vaginal entrance; the vagina is turned inside out.
- Uterine prolapse is caused by congenital defects, persistent high intra-abdominal pressure related to heavy physical labor or exertion, or any cause that weakens pelvic support.
- Physical findings include
  1. Client's report of "something in the vagina"
  2. Dyspareunia
  3. Backache
  4. Feeling of heaviness or pressure in the pelvis
  5. Bowel and/or bladder problems (e.g., incontinence)
  6. Protrusion of the cervix during pelvic examination
- Interventions are based on the degree of prolapse
  1. Insertion of a pessary
  2. Surgical vaginal hysterectomy

U

For more information on uterine prolapse, see *Medical-Surgical Nursing: A Nursing Process Approach*, **pp. 1705–1706.**

Uveitis

- Uveitis is a general term for inflammatory diseases of the uveal tract of the eye.
- *Anterior uveitis*
    1. Includes iritis, an inflammation of the iris; iridocyclitis, an inflammation of both the iris and ciliary body; and cyclitis
    2. Is manifested by moderate periorbital aching, tearing, blurred vision, and photophobia; small, irregularly shaped, nonreactive pupil; purplish discoloration of the cornea; and hypopyon, an accumulation of purulent material in the anterior chamber.
- *Posterior uveitis*
    1. Includes retinitis, an inflammation of the retina, and chorioretinitis, an inflammation of both the retina and choroid
    2. Is manifested by slow, insidious onset of symptoms, including visual impairment; small, irregularly shaped, nonreactive pupil; and vitreous opacities that are seen as black dots against the background of the fundus.
- Treatment is symptomatic
    1. Atropine eyedrops (which cause blurred vision) to put the ciliary body to rest
    2. Steroid drops to decrease inflammation
    3. Timolol (Timoptic) if intraocular pressure is increased
    4. Treating the underlying systemic disease
    5. Warm compresses
    6. Darkened room, wearing sunglasses

For more information on uveitis, see *Medical-Surgical Nursing: A Nursing Process Approach,* **pp. 1052–1053.**

Vaginal Cancer

OVERVIEW

• Primary vaginal cancer, a rare disease, usually occurs as an extension of cervical, endometrial, or vulvar cancers.

• Most vaginal cancers are squamous cell carcinomas that develop in the upper one-third of the vagina.

• Adenocarcinomas are associated with intrauterine exposure to diethylstilbesterol as a result of maternal ingestion during pregnancy.

• The spread of vaginal cancer depends on the tumor location; upper vaginal lesions spread in the same manner as cervical cancer, whereas lower lesions spread similarly to vulvar cancer.

• Early metastasis occurs.

• Predisposing factors associated with development of vaginal cancer include

1. Repeated pregnancies
2. Sexually transmitted diseases such as herpes virus and papilloma virus infection
3. Age (most occur after age 50)

• Both nonsurgical and surgical interventions may be used to treat women with vaginal cancer.

• Noninvasive malignancy and early-stage vaginal cancers may be treated with a variety of measures.

COLLABORATIVE MANAGEMENT

Nonsurgical Management

• Laser therapy is performed after iodine staining of the vagina to identify the areas for laser.

• Local application of 5-fluorouracil cream to the vagina daily for 1 week is another treatment.

• Internal radiation therapy (IRT) is used alone for treatment of cancer limited to the vaginal wall.

• External radiation therapy, combined with IRT, is used for treatment of cancer that extends beyond the vaginal wall.

• Complications of radiation therapy include vaginal stenosis and adhesions and vaginal drainage.

• The nurse

1. Teaches the client to use a vaginal dilator
2. Assesses for sexual dysfunction

• Chemotherapy is used for recurrent disease, although there is no effective therapy.

Surgical Management

- Local wide excision is performed for localized lesions.
- Partial or total vaginectomy (removal of part or all of the vagina) is performed for invasive disease.
- The nurse
  1. Informs the client that vaginectomy affects sexual function
  2. Counsels the client on alternative sexual activities
- Radical hysterectomy or pelvic exenteration may also be performed depending on the extent of the cancer.

For more information on vaginal cancer, see *Medical-Surgical Nursing: A Nursing Process Approach*, **pp. 1730–1731.**

Vaginal Fistula

- Trauma is the primary cause of vaginal fistula, an abnormal opening between two adjacent areas.
- Other causes include complications from surgery, obstetric complications, spread of malignancy, or radiation therapy.
- Types of vaginal fistula include
  1. Urethrovaginal (urethra)
  2. Vesicovaginal (bladder)
  3. Rectovaginal (rectum)
- Symptoms depend on the location of the fistula and include
  1. Urine, flatus, or feces leaking into the vagina
  2. Irritation or excoriation of the vulva and vaginal tissues

3. Unpleasant odor (fecal or urine) in the vagina
4. Complaints of feeling wet or dribbling in the vagina

- Management is dependent on the location of the fistula.
- Treatment measures are focused on perineal hygiene
  1. Sitz baths
  2. Perineal cleaning with mild unscented soap and water
  3. Low-pressure douching
  4. Sanitary napkins or undergarments, such as Depends
  5. Applying deodorizing powders
  6. Use of heat lamps
  7. Applying vitamin A and D ointment
- Surgery is not performed if infection or inflammation is present.
- Postoperative care after fistula repair is aimed at preventing infection and avoiding stress on the repaired area.

For more information on vaginal fistula, see *Medical-Surgical Nursing: A Nursing Process Approach*, **p. 1707.**

Vaginitis, Atrophic

- Atrophic vaginitis occurs in postmenopausal women as a result of a lack of endogenous estrogen production.
- Physical findings include
  1. Pale, thin, dry mucosa
  2. Itching
  3. No odor

4. Scant white or pink discharge
5. Dyspareunia, postcoital bleeding

• Treatment is with a topical conjugated estrogen cream.

For more information on atrophic vaginitis, see *Medical-Surgical Nursing: A Nursing Process Approach*, **pp. 1700–1701.**

Vaginitis, *Candida Albicans*

• *Candida albicans*, also known as candidiasis, moniliasis, and yeast infection, is the most common form of vaginitis.

• Symptoms appear in women during their reproductive years, usually developing in the premenstrual period.

• Change in vaginal pH encourages growth of *C. albicans*, a gram-positive fungus, and recurrences are frequent.

• Predisposing factors include pregnancy, diabetes, oral contraceptives, frequent douching, antibiotic therapy, and poor hygiene.

• It is not considered a sexually transmitted disease.

• Physical findings include
  1. Odorless, white or yellow, cheesy discharge
  2. Patches on vaginal walls and cervix
  3. Inflamed vaginal walls and cervix

• Treatment includes miconazole nitrate (Monistat), clotrimazole (Gyne-Lotrimin), or nystatin

(Mycostatin) vaginal creams or suppositories for 7 days.

For more information on *Candida albicans* vaginitis, see *Medical-Surgical Nursing: A Nursing Process Approach*, **pp. 1699–1700.**

Vaginitis, *Gardnerella Vaginalis*

- *Gardnerella* is a common form of vaginitis and one of the most contagious and most common sexually transmitted diseases.
- The infection is benign and does not invade the vaginal mucosa.
- Physical findings include
  1. Gray-white discharge
  2. Fishy odor
  3. Itching
  4. Normal vaginal mucosa
  5. 10% to 40% asymptomatic
- Treatment includes oral metronidazol (Flagyl), ampicillin, or tetracycline.

For more information on *Gardnerella vaginalis* vaginitis, see *Medical-Surgical Nursing: A Nursing Process Approach*, **pp. 1700–1701.**

Vaginitis, Simple

- Vaginitis is an inflammation of the lower genital tract.

- Vaginitis develops when there is a disturbance of hormone balance and bacterial interaction in the vagina, caused by changes in normal flora, alkaline pH, insertion of foreign objects such as tampons or condoms, chemical irritants such as douches or sprays, and medications, especially antibiotics.

- Client history includes
  1. Onset of symptoms
  2. Characteristics and color of discharge
  3. Odor of discharge
  4. Associated symptoms such as itching and dysuria
  5. Type of contraceptive used
  6. Recent antibiotic use
  7. Sexual activity
  8. History of previous vaginal infection
  9. Hygiene practices such as douching and tampon use

- Physical examination includes
  1. Abdominal palpation for tenderness and pain
  2. External genitalia inspected for erythema, edema, excoriation, odor, and discharge
  3. Vaginal examination to note the source of the discharge and/or inflammation

- Interventions include special hygiene practices
  1. Perineal cleaning from front to back after urination and defecation
  2. Wearing cotton underwear
  3. Avoiding strong douches and feminine hygiene sprays
  4. Avoiding tight-fitting pants

- Client education focuses on preventive measures and information on infection transmission.

For more information on simple vaginitis, see *Medical-Surgical Nursing: A Nursing Process Approach*, **p. 1699.**

Vaginitis, *Trichomonas Vaginalis*

- *Trichomonas vaginalis* is a parasitic protozoan transmitted by sexual activity.
- *T. vaginalis* frequently occurs in women aged 16 to 35 years.
- Symptoms appear during or immediately after menstruation.
- Predisposing factors include a nonacidic vaginal pH, pregnancy, illness, diets, and gastrointestinal disturbances.
- Physical findings include
  1. Green, yellow, or white, frothy, foul-smelling discharge
  2. Vaginal itching
  3. Strawberry spot on the cervix
- Treatment is oral metronidazol (Flagyl).

For more information on *Trichomonas vaginalis* vaginitis, see *Medical-Surgical Nursing: A Nursing Process Approach*, **pp. 1699–1700.**

Varicocele

- A varicocele is a cluster of dilated veins posterior to and above the testis.
- A varicocele is diagnosed by scrotal palpation; the scrotum feels "wormlike."

V

- Most varicoceles are unilateral and on the left side of the scrotum, but they also occur bilaterally.

- Varicoceles can cause infertility by altered spermatogenesis due to increased scrotal temperature from venous stasis.

- Surgical removal (varicocelectomy) is performed via an inguinal incision in which the spermatic veins are ligated in the cord or through an incision adjacent to the superior iliac spine in which the spermatic veins are ligated in the retroperitoneal space.

- Postoperative instructions include
  1. Placing a rolled towel under the scrotum while in bed
  2. Applying ice, if necessary, to decrease swelling
  3. Using a scrotal support while ambulating
  4. Notifying the physician for increasing discomfort at the incision or in the scrotum

For more information on varicocele, see *Medical-Surgical Nursing: A Nursing Process Approach*, **p. 1766.**

Varicose Veins

- Varicose veins are distended, protruding veins that appear darkened or tortuous.

- The vein walls weaken and dilate; venous pressure increases, and the valves become incompetent.

- Incompetent valves enhance vessel dilation, and veins become tortuous and distended.

- Varicose veins occur primarily in clients requiring prolonged standing; they also occur in pregnant women and in clients with systemic problems, such as heart disease, obesity, and a family history of varicose veins.

- Clinical manifestations include
  1. Pain after standing

2. Fullness in the legs
3. Distended, protruding veins
- Conservative treatment measures include
  1. Wearing elastic stockings
  2. Elevating the extremities as often as possible
- Surgical intervention entails *ligation* (tying) and *stripping* (removal) of the affected veins under general anesthesia.
- Postoperatively the nurse
  1. Assesses the groin and entire leg through the elastic (Ace) bandage dressing
  2. Instructs the client to keep the legs elevated and to perform range-of-motion exercises
  3. Discharges the client to the home, as ordered, by the first postoperative day and instructs the client to
     a. Continue wearing elastic stockings
     b. Exercise by walking
     c. Limit sitting for long intervals, and when sitting keep the legs elevated
     d. Avoid standing in one place
- Sclerotherapy as a management modality involves injection of sclerosing agent into the varicosed vein. This procedure may be done as the primary treatment or after surgical ligation and stripping.

For more information on varicose veins, see *Medical-Surgical Nursing: A Nursing Process Approach*, **pp. 2227–2228.**

Vulvar Cancer

OVERVIEW

- Vulvar cancer is slow growing, stays localized for a long period, and metastasizes late.
- Most vulvar cancers are squamous cell carcinomas and develop in the absence of premalignant changes in the epithelium.

- The first change is usually vulvar atypia or mild dysplasia.

- The cancer spreads directly to the urethra, the vagina, and/or the anus and through the lymphatic system to the inguinal, femoral, and deep iliac pelvic nodes.

COLLABORATIVE MANAGEMENT

- The nurse records the client's
    1. Age
    2. Family history of cervical cancer or diabetes
    3. Obesity
    4. Possible sexually transmitted diseases
- The nurse assesses for
    1. Irritation or itching in the perineal area
    2. Bleeding (a late sign)
    3. Multifocal lesions on the labia
- Management depends on the extent of the spread.
- Laser therapy is done for premalignant vulvar lesions.
- Chemotherapy, in the form of a topical application of 5-fluorouracil, is used for carcinoma in situ.
- External radiation therapy follows surgery for deep pelvic node involvement.
- Surgical interventions include
    1. Local wide *excision* of the lesion
    2. *Simple vulvectomy*, the removal of the vulva, the labia majora, the labia minora, and possibly the clitoris (used less frequently)
    3. *Skinning vulvectomy*, the removal of the superficial skin of the vulva, without removal of the clitoris, and replacement of the skin with a split-thickness skin graft
    4. *Modified radical* or *radical vulvectomy*, for invasive cancer, involving the removal of the entire vulva—skin, labia, clitoris, subcutaneous tissues, and possibly inguinal and femoral node dissection
- The nurse performs specific preoperative procedures
    1. Shaves the abdomen and perineum
    2. Administers a douche
    3. Administers an enema
    4. Inserts an indwelling urinary catheter
- For postoperative nursing care, see Cystocele.
- Client/family education is focused on
    1. Relief of postoperative discomfort, including medications

2. Diet instructions, including vitamin C, iron, and protein
3. Changes in body image and sexual function

For more information on vulvar cancer, see *Medical-Surgical Nursing: A Nursing Process Approach*, **pp. 1728–1730.**

Vulvitis

- Vulvitis is an inflammatory condition of the vulva associated with pruritis (itching) and a burning sensation.
- The vulvar skin is sensitive to hormonal, metabolic, and allergic influences; symptoms can be caused by systemic conditions, by direct contact with an irritant, or by extension of infections from the vagina.
- The most common skin disease affecting the vulva is contact dermatitis caused by irritants such as feminine hygiene sprays, fabric dyes, soaps and detergents, and allergens.
- Primary infections affecting the vulva include herpes genitalis and condyloma acuminatum (venereal warts).
- Secondary infections are caused by organisms responsible for vaginitis, including candidiasis.
- Common parasitic infections include pediculosis pubis (crab lice) and scabies (itch mites).
- Other causes include atrophic vaginitis, vulvar kraurosis (a postmenopausal disorder causing dryness and atrophy), vulvar leukoplakia (postmenopausal atrophy and thickening of vulvar tissue), cancer, and urinary incontinence.
- Physical findings include
  1. Itching

2. Burning sensation
3. Erythema, edema, and superficial skin ulcerations
4. White and thickened vulvar tissue
5. Dry and scaly skin

- Treatment depends on the cause and includes
  1. Antibiotics
  2. Removal of irritants or allergens
  3. Treatment for pediculosis and scabies
  4. Interventions to relieve itching, such as sitz baths, Burow's compresses, and application of topical steroids

- Client education focuses on preventive measures.

For more information on vulvitis, see *Medical-Surgical Nursing: A Nursing Process Approach*, **pp. 1701–1702.**

Wart, Common

- Warts, or verrucae, are small tumors caused by infection of the keratinocytes with the papillomavirus.

- Warts occur singly or in groups.

- *Common* warts are raised, flesh-colored papules with a rough, hyperkeratotic surface, commonly occurring on the hands and fingers.

- *Flat* warts appear as elevated reddish-brown or flesh-colored papules with flat tops and minimal scale.

- *Plantar* warts are painful warts occurring on the bottom of the foot and are usually covered with thick callus.

- *Venereal* warts (condylomata acuminata) are sexually transmitted neoplasms involving the external genitalia, rectum, urethra, vagina, and cervix; they have a soft, cauliflower appearance.

- Wart treatment is aimed at destroying keratinocytes containing the virus and includes
    1. Cryosurgery (preferred)
    2. Surgical excision
    3. Electrodesiccation and curettage
    4. Topical caustic agents

For more information on warts, see *Medical-Surgical Nursing: A Nursing Process Approach*, **pp. 1207–1208.**

Wart, Venereal

- *Condylomata acuminata*, also known as genital warts, is caused by the papillomavirus.
- Genital warts are sexually transmitted and often are seen with other sexually transmitted diseases.
- Warts are exacerbated in pregnant women and the elderly.
- Sites commonly affected include the urinary meatus, vulva, labia majora, vagina, cervix, penis, scrotum, anus, and perianal areas.
- The incubation period is usually 1 to 3 months.
- Venereal warts are initially single, small papillary growths that grow into cauliflower-like masses.
- They are strongly associated with genital dysplasia and carcinoma.
- Treatment interventions include
    1. Wart removal
        a. Cryotherapy with liquid nitrogen or a cryoprobe
        b. Carbon dioxide laser
        c. Podophyllum resin application
        d. Electrocautery
        e. Surgical removal

W

   2. Symptom treatment
   3. Treatment of sexual partner
- Client education includes
   1. Use of condoms
   2. Mode of transmission and incubation period
   3. Recurrence is likely
   4. Annual Pap smears for females

For more information on venereal warts, see *Medical-Surgical Nursing: A Nursing Process Approach*, **pp. 1782–1783.**

Appendix A
Nursing Interventions for Physiologic Changes Related to Aging

TABLE A.1 Interventions for Changes of Aging That Become Surgical Risk Factors

Change	Interventions	Rationales
CARDIOVASCULAR SYSTEM		
Decreased cardiac output. Increased diastolic blood pressure. Decreased peripheral circulation.	1. Determine normal activity levels and when client tires. 2. Monitor vital signs. 3. Teach leg exercises and turning in bed.	1. To prevent fatigue. 2. To establish baseline data and to detect deviations. 3. To promote circulation.
RESPIRATORY SYSTEM		
Reduced vital capacity. Loss of lung elasticity. Decreased oxygenation of blood.	1. Teach coughing and deep breathing. 2. Monitor respirations.	1. To prevent respiratory complications. 2. To establish baseline data.

RENAL SYSTEM

Decreased blood flow to kidneys.
Reduced ability to excrete waste products.

1. Monitor intake and output.

2. Monitor electrolyte status.

1. To detect dehydration, fluid overload, and decreased renal function.

2. To detect imbalances.

NEUROLOGIC SYSTEM

Sensory deficits.
Slower reaction time.

1. Orient client to surroundings.
2. Allow extra time for client teaching.

1, 2. Client's orientation and presence of sensory deficits call for individualized preoperative teaching plan.

MUSCULOSKELETAL SYSTEM

Increased incidence of deformities related to osteoporosis or arthritis.

1. Assess level of mobility.
2. Teach turning, positioning.
3. Encourage ambulation.

1–3. To prevent complications of immobility.

TABLE A.2 Interventions for Changes in the Musculoskeletal System Related to Aging

Change	Interventions	Rationales
BONE		
Decreased density Prominent bony structure	Teach safety tips to prevent falls. Prevent pressure on bony prominences.	Porous bones are more likely to fracture. There is less soft tissue to prevent skin breakdown.
VERTEBRAL COLUMN		
Kyphotic posture; widened gait, shift in the center of gravity	Teach proper body mechanics; instruct the client to sit in supportive chairs with arms.	Correction of posture problems prevents further deformity; the client should have support for bony structures.
SYNOVIAL JOINT		
Cartilage degeneration Decreased ROM	Provide moist heat, such as shower. Assess the client's ability to perform ADLs and mobility.	Moist heat increases blood flow to the area. The client may need assistance with self-care skills.
MUSCLE		
Atrophy, decreased strength Slowed movement	Teach exercises. Do not rush the individual; be patient.	Exercises increase muscle strength. The client may become frustrated if hurried.

TABLE A.3 Interventions for Changes in the Nervous System Related to Aging

Change	Interventions	Rationales
Recent memory loss	1. Reinforce teaching by repetition and written teaching aids.	1. Visual and auditory reinforcement enhances recall of information.
Decreased touch sensation	1. Remind the client to look where his or her feet are placed when walking.	1. The client is prone to falling if the feet are not placed correctly.
	2. Instruct the client to wear shoes that provide good support when ambulating.	2. Proper footwear helps prevent slipping and falls.
	3. If the client is unable, change the client's position frequently (every hour) while in bed or chair.	3. Moving the client frequently helps to prevent pressure sore formation.
Change in perception of pain	1. Ask the client to describe the nature and specific characteristics of pain.	1. Elderly clients often believe that their pain is related to the aging process, although pain is not typically an age-related change.
	2. Monitor additional assessment variables to detect possible health problems.	2. Behavior changes, such as increased confusion, are often more indicative of major health problems (like myocardial infarction) than complaints of pain.

Table continued on following page

657

APP

INDEX

TABLE A.3   Interventions for Changes in the Nervous System Related to Aging *continued*

Change	Interventions	Rationales
Change in sleep patterns	1. Ascertain individual sleep patterns and preferences. 2. Adjust the client's daily schedule to sleep pattern and preference as much as possible, e.g., evening versus morning bath.	1. Assessment of the client's usual sleep patterns provides a baseline for comparison in determining sleep changes. 2. The client needs to maintain his or her routine for sleep to the extent possible as a change can lead to disorientation and increased confusion.
Altered balance or coordination	1. Instruct the client to move slowly when changing positions. 2. If needed, advise the client to hold on to handrails when ambulating. 3. Assess the need for an ambulatory aid, such as a cane.	1. Slow movement helps to prevent falls. 2, 3. A handrail or ambulatory aid may assist balance and share weight bearing for the client to help prevent falls.

TABLE A.4 Interventions for Changes in the Integumentary System Related to Aging

Change	Interventions	Rationales
Epidermis		
Decreased thickness in epidermal layer	Handle the client gently when moving or providing care.	Skin is very fragile and prone to tearing.
Decreased epidermal mitotic activity	Assess wound healing and use proper technique for wound care.	Wounds usually heal slowly and are subsequently prone to infection.
Decreased epidermal mitotic homeostasis	Assess the skin for changes, especially changes in pigmentation or the occurrence of lesions.	Skin is susceptible to hyperplasias, such as hyperkeratoses and skin cancers (especially in sun-exposed areas).
Increased epidermal permeability	Use mild soap (like Ivory) and lotion on the skin.	Harsh soap and other topical application can cause skin irritation, especially rashes.
Flattening of the dermal-epidermal junction	Move the client in bed or to a chair by picking the client up rather than pulling the client across the linen.	The skin is susceptible to shearing forces, resulting in blisters, purpura, skin tears, and pressure-related skin problems.
Dermis		
Decreased dermal blood flow	Apply lotion often to lubricate the skin.	The skin is susceptible to dryness, leading to cracks and sores.
Degeneration of elastic fibers	Assess body image changes and what the changes mean to the client.	The decreased tone and elasticity of the skin cause wrinkles and sagging, which may result in altered body image.
Abnormal nerve endings	Teach the client to use a thermometer to test the temperature of bath water or dish water.	Decreased sensory perception can prevent the client from accurately assessing temperature; burns may result.

Table continued on following page

659

APP

INDEX

TABLE A.4 Interventions for Changes in the Integumentary System Related to Aging *continued*

Change	Interventions	Rationales
Subcutaneous layer		
Redistribution of adipose tissue	Assess body image changes and what the changes mean to the client.	"Bags," cellulite, and a double chin may cause altered body image.
Thinning of subcutaneous fat layer	Keep the client warm.	The client has an increased susceptibility to hypothermia.
Hair		
Decreased number of hair follicles and rate of growth/decreased number of active melanocytes in follicle	Assess body image changes and what the changes mean to the client.	Hair thinning and graying may cause altered body image.
Nails		
Decreased rate of growth and blood flow	Assess for fungal infection.	Nails are prone to recurrent fungal infections.
Glands		
Decreased eccrine and apocrine (sweat) gland activity	Apply lotion often to lubricate skin; assess skin warmth.	Skin is susceptible to dryness and decreased cooling.

TABLE A.5 Interventions for Changes in the Digestive System Related to Aging

Change	Interventions	Rationales
STOMACH		
Atrophy of gastric mucosa is characterized by a decrease in the ratio of gastrin-secreting cells to somatostatin-secreting cells. This change leads to decreased hydrochloric acid (hypochlorhydria). Decreased hydrochloric acid leads to decreased absorption of iron and vitamin B_{12} and to proliferation of bacteria. Atrophic gastritis occurs secondary to bacterial overgrowth.	1. Encourage frequent feedings of bland foods high in vitamins and iron. 2. Assess for epigastric pain.	1. To prevent gastritis and to ensure adequate intake of vitamins and iron. 2. To detect gastritis.
LARGE INTESTINE		
Peristalsis decreases, and nerve impulses are dulled. Decreased sensation to defecate can result in postponement of bowel movement, which leads to constipation and impaction.	1. Encourage high-fiber diet and 1500 mL of fluids daily (if not contraindicated). 2. Encourage as much activity as tolerated.	1, 2. To increase sensation to defecate.

Table continued on following page

APP

INDEX

661

TABLE A.5 Interventions for Changes in the Digestive System Related to Aging *continued*

Change	Interventions	Rationales
PANCREAS		
Distention and dilation of pancreatic ducts change. Calcification of pancreatic vessels occurs with a decrease in lipase production.	1. Encourage small, frequent feedings. 2. Assess for diarrhea.	1. To prevent steatorrhea. 2. To detect steatorrhea.
Decreased lipase results in decreased fat absorption and digestion. Steatorrhea, or excess fat in the feces, occurs because of decreased fat digestion.		
LIVER		
A decrease in the number and size of hepatic cells leads to decreased liver weight and mass. This change and an increase in fibrous tissue lead to decreased protein synthesis and changes in liver enzymes. Enzyme activity and cholesterol synthesis are diminished.	1. Assess all clients for adverse effects of all drugs, even those administered in normal doses.	1. To detect toxicity.
Decreased enzyme activity depresses drug metabolism, which leads to accumulation of drugs, possibly to toxic levels.		

TABLE A.6 Interventions for Changes in the Endocrine System Related to Aging

Change	Interventions	Rationales
POSTERIOR PITUITARY		
Increased secretion of antidiuretic hormone	1. Assess for dilute urine and polyuria. 2. Encourage fluid intake.	1, 2. To prevent complications, especially dehydration.
GONADS		
Decreased ovarian function	1. Teach the client signs and symptoms of estrogen. 2. Promote exercise and calcium intake.	1. To improve the client's ability to cope with changes. 2. To slow bone loss and prevent complications related to osteoporosis.
PANCREAS		
Decreased glucose tolerance	1. Identify clients at risk: overweight, excess of fat in the diet, or little physical exercise. 2. Teach the client signs and symptoms of hyperglycemia.	1. To avoid complications. 2. To improve the client's recognition of hyperglycemia, which can occur after meals.
THYROID		
Decreased peripheral metabolism	1. Assess for signs of hypothyroidism, especially constipation, lethargy, dry skin, or mental deterioration.	1. To distinguish signs of hypothyroidism, which often resemble clinical features of aging.

TABLE A.7 Interventions for Changes in the Urinary System Related to Aging

Change	Interventions	Rationales
Bladder capacity decreases	1. Encourage the client to use the toilet, bedpan, or urinal at least q 2 h. 2. Respond as soon as possible to the client's indication of the need to void.	1, 2. To prevent episodes of urinary incontinence.
Tendency to retain urine develops	1. Observe the client for signs and symptoms of urinary tract infection, such as confusion (or increased confusion) and urinary frequency (dysuria is *not* a common finding in the elderly).	1. To detect infection and underlying urinary retention.
Nocturia increases	1. Ensure adequate nighttime lighting. 2. Ensure the availability of a toilet, bedpan, or urinal.	1. To prevent injury. 2. To prevent episodes of urinary incontinence.
Urinary sphincter weakens	1. Respond as soon as possible to the client's indication of the need to void. 2. Provide thorough perineal care after each voiding.	1. To prevent episodes of urinary incontinence. 2. To prevent skin irritation.

TABLE A.8 Interventions for Changes in the Respiratory System Related to Aging

Change	Interventions*	Rationales
CHEST WALL		
Anteroposterior diameter increases. Slope changes. Progressive kyphoscoliosis occurs. Decreased mobility occurs. Osteoporosis is possible.	1. Discuss normal changes of aging. 2. Discuss the need for increased rest periods during exercise.	1. Clients may be anxious because they must work harder to breathe. 2. Older clients have less tolerance for exercise.
ALVEOLI		
Alveolar membranes thicken. Diffusion capacity decreases. Elastic recoil decreases. Dilation of bronchioles and alveolar ducts occurs. Ability to cough decreases.	3. Encourage vigorous pulmonary toilet (i.e., turn, cough, and deep breathe), especially if the client is confined to bed or has had surgery.	3. There is increased potential for mechanical or infectious respiratory complications in these situations.

Table continued on following page

665

TABLE A.8 Interventions for Changes in the Respiratory System Related to Aging *continued*

Change	Interventions*	Rationales
LUNGS		
Residual volume increases.	4. Include inspection, palpation, percussion, and auscultation in lung assessments.	4. All four techniques are needed to detect normal age-related changes.
Decreased capacity results in less efficient oxygen and carbon dioxide exchange.	5. Assess the client's respiration for abnormal breathing patterns.	5. Periodic breathing patterns can occur (e.g., Cheyne-Stokes).
Elasticity decreases.	6. Encourage frequent oral hygiene.	6. Oral hygiene aids in removal of secretions.
PHARYNX AND LARYNX		
Muscles atrophy.	7. Have face-to-face conversations with the client when possible.	7. Voices of clients may be soft and difficult to understand.
Vocal cords become slack.		
Laryngeal muscles lose elasticity and cartilage.		
PULMONARY ARTERY		
Increased vascular resistance to blood flow through pulmonary vascular system occurs.	8. Assess the client's level of consciousness.	8. Clients can become confused during acute respiratory conditions.
Risk of hypoxia increases.		

*Interventions 1–6 apply to all structures; 7 and 8 are specific for those structures.

TABLE A.9 Interventions for Changes in the Cardiovascular System Related to Aging

Change	Interventions	Rationales
CARDIAC VALVES		
Thicken and stiffen owing to lipid accumulation, degeneration of collagen, and valve fibrosis.	1. Assess heart sounds for murmurs.	1. Systolic ejection murmurs are common in the elderly owing to valve thickening and stiffness.
CONDUCTION SYSTEM		
Decrease in number of pacemaker cells and increase in fibrous tissue and fat in the SA node. Few muscle fibers in the atrial myocardium and bundle of His.	1. Assess ECG and heart rhythm for dysrhythmias or heart rate less than 60 beats/min.	1. SA node may lose its inherent rhythm.
LEFT VENTRICLE		
Increases in size. Becomes stiff and less distensible. Longer ejection phase and delay in early diastolic filling to compensate for stiff ventricle, allowing the heart to more effectively "empty."	1. Assess ECG for longer PR and QT intervals. 2. Assess for activity intolerance. 3. Assess heart rate at rest and with activity.	1. Conduction time increases. 2. Ventricular changes result in decreased stroke volume, ejection fraction, and cardiac output; the heart is less able to meet increased oxygen demands. 3. Maximal heart rate with exercise is decreased.

Table continued on following page

667

APP

INDEX

TABLE A.9 Interventions for Changes in the Cardiovascular System Related to Aging *continued*

Change	Interventions	Rationales
BLOOD FLOW IN CORONARY VESSELS		
Distribution changes, with more blood flowing to venous vessels and sinusoids and less flowing to coronary arteries.	1. Assess for activity intolerance.	1. The heart is less able to meet increased oxygen demands.
AORTA AND LARGE ARTERIES		
Thicken and become stiffer and less distensible. Systolic blood pressure increases to compensate for stiff arteries. Systemic vascular resistance increases as a result of less distensible arteries, so the left ventricle pumps against greater resistance, contributing to left ventricular hypertrophy.	1. Assess blood pressure. 2. Assess for activity intolerance and shortness of breath.	1. Hypertension may occur, which must be treated to avoid target organ damage. 2. Left ventricular hypertrophy decreases cardiac output and may lead to CHF.
BARORECEPTORS		
Becomes less sensitive.	1. Assess blood pressure with the client lying and sitting or standing. 2. Assess for dizziness when the client changes from a lying to a sitting or standing position. 3. Teach clients to change positions slowly.	1–3. Orthostatic (postural) changes occur owing to ineffective baroreceptors. Changes may include a drop in blood pressure of 10 mmHg or more, dizziness, or fainting.

Appendix B
Guidelines for Common
Client Problems

TABLE B.1 Guidelines for Positioning Burn Victim

Affected Body Part	Position of Function	Interventions
Head and neck	Hyperextension	Place a towel roll under client's neck or shoulder under spine
Posterior neck	Flexion	Have client turn head side to side
Chest	Shoulder	Place client supine No pillows Place folded towel under spine between scapula
Lateral trunk	Flexion to uninvolved side	Place client on back with arm on affected side over head
Anterior shoulder	Abduction and external rotation	Maintain upper arm at 90 degree abduction from lateral aspect of trunk
Posterior shoulder	Slight flexion and internal rotation	Keep arm slightly behind midline
Elbow	Extension and supination	Keep joint in extended position

670

TABLE B.2   The Client Using a Continuous Passive Motion (CPM) Machine

Interventions	Rationales
1. Ensure that the machine is well padded with sheepskin or other similar material.	1. The metal of the machine can damage skin and underlying tissues.
2. Check the cycle and range-of-motion settings at least once per shift (every 8 h).	2. The settings should be specified by the physician. The client or staff may change the settings unintentionally.
3. Ensure that the joint being moved is properly positioned on the machine.	3. If the extremity is not properly positioned, nerve or soft-tissue damage can occur.
4. If the client is confused, place controls to the machine out of the client's reach.	4. A confused client may change the settings.
5. Assess the client's response to the CPM machine.	5. The machine may increase the client's pain or cause other concerns.
6. Turn off the machine while the client is having a meal in bed.	6. Motion and noise from the machine can prevent the client from eating.
7. When the machine is not in use, do not store it on the floor.	7. The machine may become soiled or damaged.

671

TABLE B.3 The Client Who Has Undergone Myelography

Interventions	Rationales

1. Check the client's neurologic status immediately after the client returns to the room and every 1–2 h for the first 24 h (or according to institutional policy). If a change from pretest status is present, notify the physician immediately.
   a. Vital signs.
   b. Ability to move all extremities.
   c. Loss of sensation in extremities.
   d. Complaint of severe pain in back or extremities.
	1. The contrast medium can temporarily or permanently injure the spinal cord, spinal nerves, or brain. The nurse compares pretest and posttest findings.

2. Check the needle puncture site for bleeding or other drainage when assessing neurologic status. If present, notify the physician immediately.	2. The spinal needle can cause local tissue trauma. If the site does not close, CSF can leak from the subarachnoid space, causing a CSF deficit and possibly severe headache.

3. Observe for adverse effects of contrast medium.
   a. Headache.
   b. Nausea or vomiting.
   c. Neurologic changes, such as disorientation or seizure.
	3. These adverse effects can be uncomfortable or life-threatening and must be treated.

4. Maintain proper client positioning.
   a. The client remains flat in bed for 8–12 h after iophendylate administration (may turn from side to side).
   b. The client sits at a 15- to 45-degree angle for 8–16 h, followed by 8 h flat in bed, after administration of metrizamide or other water-based medium.
5. Give prescribed pain medication as needed.
6. Check the client's ability to void. If the client has not voided within 8 h after the test, notify the physician.
7. Do not give CNS depressants or stimulants or phenothiazines for 24 h after the test. Observe for episodes of seizure.
8. Force oral fluids and maintain IV fluid administration if needed. Offer at least 8 oz/h.
9. Explain interventions to the client.

4. Positioning depends on the type of dye used.
   a. Clients who received iophendylate have a CSF deficit of 6–15 mL from the procedure. If placed upright, the client can leak additional CSF, contributing to a severe headache.
   b. Clients who receive a water-based medium are at risk for its ascension into the brain tissue, causing neurologic damage.
5. Clients often have mild to moderate discomfort at the needle site. They may also have a headache.
6. The spinal needle can traumatize sacral nerves, which innervate the bladder.
7. These drugs lower a person's seizure threshold, increasing the risk of seizure activity.
8. Increasing fluid intake promotes CSF production, prevents dehydration from vomiting, and promotes excretion of water-based contrast medial.
9. Providing the client with information often promotes compliance and allays anxiety.

TABLE B.4 The Client with a Cast

Interventions	Rationales
1. Monitor neurovascular status of casted extremity every 1–2 h for the first 24 h and every 4 h thereafter.	1. Neurovascular status indicates tissue perfusion.
a. Perform circulation check	a, b. Adequate tissue perfusion prevents tissue necrosis and compartment syndrome.
b. Ask client if cast feels too tight.	
c. Have cast cutter available.	c. If the cast restricts circulation, it must be cut to relieve pressure.
2. Maintain integrity of cast.	2. A disrupted cast can cause complications in healing.
a. Turn client every 1–2 h.	a. Repositioning allows a plaster cast to dry and prevents skin breakdown.
b. Use palms of hands when handling wet cast.	b. Use of palms prevents indentations of the cast, which can cause pressure ulcers.
c. Do not turn client by holding on to abductor bar, e.g., hip spica.	c. The bar can bend or break.
d. Do not cover a wet cast or place it on a plastic-coated pillow.	d. Coverings and plastic prevent drying of a cast.
e. Protect other parts from irritation from the rough surface of cast made from synthetics.	e. The rough surface can injure skin and soft tissue.
f. Keep set plaster cast dry during bathing by covering it completely with plastic (also, tuck plastic into ends to prevent water seepage under the cast).	f. Wetting a plaster cast can change its shape.

g. Immerse synthetic cast in water during bathing, if permitted.
h. Clean soiled plaster cast with mild detergent and damp cloth as necessary.
i. Inspect cast when performing circulation checks for crumbling and cracking.
3. Maintain skin integrity.
   a. Examine skin around cast edges for redness and irritation.
   b. Trim edges of cast to prevent roughness
   c. Petal edge with 1- to 2-in adhesive strips if stockinet edging is not used.
   d. Do not use lotion or powder on skin around cast.
   e. Teach client not to place foreign objects beneath cast (e.g., wire hanger to scratch under cast).
   f. Smell cast for foul odor and palpate for hot areas every shift.
   g. Inspect cast for increase in drainage every shift.

g. Most synthetic casts do not change shape when wet.
h. Extreme soiling can cause skin infection.
i. A disruption in cast integrity can reduce its effectiveness in immobilization.
3. Healthy skin prevents infection, irritation, and other complications.
   a. Skin breakdown can lead to infection.
   b. Rough edges can cause skin breakdown.
   c. Protecting cast edges prevents skin irritation.
   d. These substances provide media for bacterial growth.
   e. Sharp objects can cause skin breakdown under the cast.
   f. Foul odor and hot areas may indicate infected skin beneath the cast.
   g. Increased drainage may indicate bleeding or purulent exudate from an infected area under cast.

TABLE B.5 The Client Receiving Nasogastric Tube Feeding

Interventions	Rationales
1. Check tube for placement in stomach every 8–12 h by injecting 30 mL of air into the tube while listening over the stomach area with stethoscope (should hear a "swooshing" sound).	1. Prevents feeding from entering lungs.
2. Flush tube every 4 h with 30–50 mL of water (may not be necessary if a continuous feed is used). Flush well when medications are given.	2. Maintains patency of the tube.
3. Secure the tube to the nose with tape so that the tube does not cause pressure on the nares; change the tape every 1–2 d.	3. Prevents tube dislodgement; prevents pressure necrosis of the nares.
4. Provide feeding at hourly rate prescribed by the physician or dietitian.	4. Provides adequate calories and other nutrients to meet the client's daily requirements. (Water is given as a bolus to maintain adequate fluid and electrolyte balance.)
5. Keep the head of bed elevated.	5. Helps to prevent aspiration of the feeding solution into the lungs.
6. Check for residual in the stomach every 4 h or according to hospital policy or physician's orders.	6. Prevents overdistention of the stomach, which can cause nausea and vomiting.
7. Monitor the client's weight and serum albumin and serum electrolyte values.	7. Determines if the client's daily nutritional needs are being met.

TABLE B.6 The Client with a Nasointestinal Tube

Interventions	Rationales
1. Before inserting a Cantor or Harris tube, fill the balloon bag's upper portion with mercury and aspirate all air from the bag.	1. Tubes vary with regard to filling with mercury before or after insertion.
2. Follow institutional policy and physician's orders for tube insertion.	2. Policies vary.
3. After the tube is inserted into the esophagus, place the client on his or her right side.	3. This position facilitates advancement of the tube through the pylorus.
4. If ordered, advance the tube 2–4 in at a time, and change the client's position.	4. Slow advancement decreases the possibility of kinks.
5. Do not secure the tube firmly until it has reached its desired position.	5. This inhibits advancement of the tube.
6. As the tube is being advanced, allow drainage to occur by gravity and monitor the drainage. If it stops, obtain physician's order to inject 10 cc of air. Do not irrigate with fluid.	6. The absence of drainage may indicate clogging of the tube.
7. Confirm tube placement on x-ray films.	7. Abdominal x-ray films are the only way to ensure that the tube has reached the small intestine.
8. If using Miller-Abbott tube, fill the balloon lumen with mercury when the tube reaches the stomach.	8. This procedure facilitates passage of the tube through the pylorus into the small intestine.
9. Clamp the balloon lumen and label it as mercury lumen.	9. Labeling prevents accidental mercury withdrawal through suction.
10. If ordered, attach the suction lumen to intermittent low suction when the tube reaches the specified destination.	10. Suction facilitates decompression, after the tube is in the proper position.
11. Keep client NPO and provide scrupulous mouth care every 2 h and prn.	11. Loss of GI contents can lead to dehydration.
12. When withdrawing the tube, remove the mercury from the balloon first, and pull the tube back 6 in/h.	12. Withdrawal should be done slowly to avoid separation of the balloon in the intestine.

TABLE B.7 The Client with a T Tube

Interventions	Rationales
1. Assess the amount, color, consistency, and odor of drainage at least q 4 h, then q 8 h. In the initial postoperative periods, expect bloody drainage, which changes to green-brown bile. Bile output will be 400 mL/d with a gradual decrease in amount. Report bile drainage amounts in excess of 1000 mL/d.	1. Close observation of bile flow is necessary to ensure patency of the bile duct and proper T tube placement. A decrease in bile flow in the early postoperative period may indicate obstruction or bile leakage into the peritoneal cavity. Excessive output may lead to a decrease in volume status with electrolyte imbalances.
2. Collect and administer excess bile output to the client by the nasogastric tube or give synthetic bile salts, such as dehydrocholic acid (Decholin).	2. Bile or bile salt replacement therapy is done to reduce excessive losses and prevent electrolyte imbalance.
3. Report sudden increases in bile output after a normally decreasing output pattern is established (9–10 d postoperatively).	3. Sudden increase may indicate ductal obstruction below the T tube site.
4. Assess for foul odor and purulent drainage, which indicate infection or extensive inflammation. Report changes in drainage to the physician.	4. Infection may require additional medical management with antibiotics.
5. Inspect the skin around the T tube insertion site for signs of inflammation, including redness, swelling, and erythema, and observe for frank bile leakage. Keep the dressing dry. (Utilize the hospital's procedure and provide drain care and dressing change per protocol. Site is usually cleaned and dressing changed daily.)	5. Bile drainage is irritating and excoriating to the skin. Bile leakage may indicate dislodgment of the T tube.

678

6. Keep the drainage system below the level of the gallbladder. Maintain the client in semi-Fowler's position.
7. *Never* irrigate, aspirate, or clamp a T tube without a physician's order.
8. Assess the drainage system for pulling, kinking, or tangling of tubing, especially when the client is positioned toward the right side. Assist the client with early turning and ambulation.
9. When ordered by the physician, raise the drainage bag to the level of the abdomen (usually on the fourth or fifth postoperative day). Then, assess for feelings of fullness, nausea, or pain.
10. Clamp the T tube for 1–2 h per physician's orders before and after meals. Assess the client's response for tolerance of food.
11. Observe stools for return of brown color 7–10 d postoperatively.

6. This position allows for free-flowing bile drainage.
7. These precautions prevent disruption of the suture line by bile backflow.
8. This allows for free-flowing bile drainage and prevents tube dislodgment.
9. This helps to check for patency of the common bile duct.
10. Clamping helps to check for digestion of foods.
11. As ductal edema subsides after surgical manipulation, the amount of bile is decreased and routed via the normal channel to the duodenum. The bile drainage decreases in the T tube drainage system and is channeled directly to the duodenum, where it is utilized for digestion of fats and fat-soluble vitamins.

TABLE B.8 The Client with a Tracheostomy

During this procedure, the nurse must ensure that the tracheostomy tube is secured at all times to prevent dislodgment. This procedure can be done with two people; one person changes the ties while the other person secures the tube. If the one-person technique is used, the old tracheostomy ties must remain intact until the new ties have been secured.

Interventions	Rationales

1. Assemble the following equipment:
  a. Equipment for suctioning.
  b. Scissors.
  c. Sterile water.
  d. Sterile gloves.
  e. Tracheostomy kit, which includes
    ■ Containers for sterile water and peroxide.
    ■ Sterile precut tracheostomy dressing.
    ■ Tracheostomy ties.
    ■ Pipe cleaners.
    ■ Tracheostomy brush.
    ■ Cotton-tipped swabs.
    ■ Forceps.
    ■ 4 × 4 in gauze pads.
	1. Having all materials and equipment initially together prevents the nurse from leaving the sterile field unattended during the procedure.

2. Wash hands.	2. Proper hand washing prevents contamination of the tracheostomy site.
3. Explain the procedure to the client and assist the client to a comfortable position that facilitates easy access to the tracheostomy.	3. A thorough explanation before the procedure may alleviate the client's anxiety.

4. Suction the tracheostomy tube.

5. Remove old dressings and excess secretions.

6. Open the tracheostomy kit and pour a solution of one-half strength hydrogen peroxide and sterile water in equal amounts into one bowl; pour sterile water into the other bowl.

7. Put on sterile gloves.

8. Remove the inner cannula and clean it.
   a. Immerse the inner cannula in the hydrogen peroxide solution.
   b. Use the tracheostomy brush and pipe cleaners to clean secretions from the inside inner cannula.
   c. Rinse the inner cannula in the bowl of sterile water; pat it dry.
   d. Reinsert the inner cannula into the outer cannula; ensure that the locking mechanism is engaged; reconnect the ventilator or oxygen source.
   e. If the client is using a ventilator, replace the inner cannula with an extra one or an adapter so that the client continues to use the ventilator while tracheostomy care is accomplished.

9. Clean the stoma site and then the tracheostomy plate with half-strength hydrogen peroxide solution followed by sterile water and then dry them; ensure that none of the solution enters the stoma.

4. The inner cannula is easier to clean if excess secretions are removed prior to the cleaning procedure.

5. Old secretions provide a medium for bacterial growth, which could result in an infection of the stoma.

6. Solutions are poured prior to donning gloves to prevent glove contamination.

7. A tracheostomy is a surgical opening into the skin that provides an entry for pathogens; sterile gloves prevent contamination of the stoma.

8, 9. Secretions adhere to the inner cannula, stoma site, and outer cannula, which can become a medium for bacterial growth.

Table continued on following page

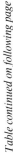

TABLE B.8 The Client with a Tracheostomy *continued*

Interventions	Rationales

10. Change tracheostomy ties if they are soiled.
  a. Velcro ties can be used according to the manufacturer's directions.
  b. Use tracheostomy ties from the tracheostomy kit.
    ■ Cut a hole ⅜ in from one end of each tape.
    ■ Pass a short length of tape with the hole through one end of the cannula's flange loops.
    ■ Take the other end of the tie and thread it all the way through the hole and pull firmly. Repeat on the opposite side.
    ■ Bring the ties around the side of the neck and tie them in a square knot.
    ■ Tie in a square knot (not a bow) that allows one finger to be placed between the tape and the neck. The knot must be in a visible place on either side of the neck. The position of the knot is rotated to the other side with each tie change to prevent skin breakdown and pressure.
11. Place a new tracheostomy dressing if desired. Do not use cut gauze pads.
	10. Tracheostomy ties are often soiled with old secretions.
	
	11. Gauze pads that are cut by the nurse may have loose fragments that can fall into the stoma; precut manufacturer pads should be used instead.

TABLE B.9 The Client Triggering a Ventilator Alarm

Cause	Interventions
HIGH-PRESSURE ALARM	
Sounds when peak inspiratory pressure (PIP) reaches the set alarm limit (usually 10–20 mmHg above the client's baseline PIP).	
There is an increased amount of secretion in airways.	Apply suction as needed.
The client coughs, gags, or bites on oral endotracheal tube (ETT).	Insert oral airway to prevent biting on ETT.
The client is anxious or fights the ventilator.	Provide emotional support to decrease anxiety. Explain all procedures to the client. Provide sedation or paralyzing agent per the physician's order. Auscultate breath sounds.
Airway size decreases related to wheezing or bronchospasm.	Consult with the physician for management of bronchospasm. Auscultate breath sounds.
Pneumothorax occurs.	Consult with the physician regarding a new onset of decreased breath sounds or unequal chest excursion, which may be due to a pneumothorax.
The artificial airway is displaced; the ETT may have slipped into the right mainstem bronchus.	Assess the chest for unequal and equal breath sounds and chest excursion. Obtain a chest x-ray film as ordered to evaluate the position of the ETT. After the proper position is verified, tape the tube securely in place. Assess the system, moving from the artificial airway toward the ventilator.
Obstruction in tubing occurs because the client is lying on the tubing or there is water or a kink in the tubing.	Empty water from the ventilator tubing and remove any kinks.

Table continued on following page

683

TABLE B.9   The Client Triggering a Ventilator Alarm continued

Cause	Interventions
There is increased PIP associated with deliverance of a sigh.	Adjust the pressure alarm.
Decreased compliance of the lung is noted; a trend of gradually increasing PIP is noted over several hours or a day.	Evaluate the reasons for the decreased compliance of lungs. Increased PIP occurs in ARDS.
LOW EXHALED VOLUME ALARM	
Sounds when there is a leak in the ventilator circuit or in the artificial airway of the client.	
A leak in the ventilator circuit prevents breath from being delivered.	Assess all connections and all ventilator tubing for disconnection.
The client stops spontaneous breathing in the SIMV or CPAP mode.	Evaluate the client's tolerance of the mode.
A cuff leak occurs in the ETT tracheostomy tube.	Evaluate the client for a cuff leak. A cuff leak is suspected when the client is able to talk (air escapes from the mouth) or when the pilot balloon on the artificial airway is flat. Keep exhalation part horizontal.
The exhalation valve on Bear I or II is wet.	Unsnap and check the membrane for dampness. If the sensor is wet, gently dab dry and resnap.

Note: PIP, peak inspiratory pressure; ETT, endotracheal tube; ARDS, adult respiratory distress syndrome; CPAP, continuous positive airway pressure; SIMV, synchronized intermittent mandatory ventilation.

Appendix C
Isolation Precautions

TABLE C.1 Category-Specific Isolation Precautions

	Private Room*	Masks	Gowns	Gloves
Strict isolation (for varicella-zoster (chicken pox); pharyngeal diphtheria; shingles (zoster), localized in an immunocompromised client or disseminated)	Always	Always	Always	Always
Contact isolation (for acute respiratory tract infection in infants and young children; disseminated herpes simplex; methicillin-resistant *Staphylococcus aureus*; pediculosis; scabies)	Always	For close contact	If soiling with infective material is likely	If contact with infective material is likely
Respiratory isolation (for measles; meningococcal meningitis, pneumonia, or meningococcemia; mumps; pertussis)	Always	For close contact	No	No

Acid-fast bacteria isolation (for tuberculosis [primary pulmonary or pharyngeal])	Always	If client is coughing	Only to prevent gross contamination	No
Enteric precautions (for enteroviral infection, including infectious gastroenteritis meningitis; [e.g., giardiasis, salmonellosis, shigellosis]; hepatitis A, *Clostridium difficile* enterocolitis)	Only if the client's hygiene is poor	No	If soiling with infective material is likely	If contact with infective material is likely
Drainage and secretion precautions (for minor or limited abscess, wound, burn, or skin infection; conjunctivitis)	No	No	If soiling with infective material is likely	If contact with infective material is likely
Blood and body fluid precautions (for AIDS; hepatitis B: non-A, non-B hepatitis; malaria)	Only if the client's hygiene is poor	If contact with blood or body fluids is likely	If contact with splashes of blood or body fluids is likely	If contact with blood or body fluids is likely

*In most instances when a private room is required, clients infected with the same organism may share a room.

687

TABLE C.2 Blood and Body Fluid Precautions

These precautions are to be used with all clients to protect health care providers from blood-borne communicable diseases.

Gloves should be worn for contact with blood and body fluids, nonintact skin, and mucous membranes of all clients; for handling surfaces or items that are soiled with blood and body fluids; and for performing venipuncture and other vascular access procedures. Gloves should be changed after each client contact.

Masks or protective goggles should be worn during procedures that are likely to cause splashes of blood or body fluids.

Gowns or aprons should be worn during procedures that are likely to result in splashes of blood or body fluids.

Hand washing should be done immediately on contact with blood or other body fluids. One should wash hands as soon as gloves are removed.

Needles and sharp instruments should be placed in puncture-resistant containers for disposal to prevent injuries from needles or other sharp items. Needles should not be recapped, bent, or removed from the syringe.

Mouth-to-mouth resuscitation should be performed using mouthpieces or other ventilation devices.

Based on Centers for Disease Control. (1987). Recommendations for prevention of HIV transmission in health-care settings. *Morbidity and Mortality Weekly Report, 36*(2S), 3–17.

Appendix D
Quick Reference to High-Flow Oxygen Delivery Systems

TABLE D.1 Comparison of High-Flow Oxygen Delivery Systems

System	FIO₂ Delivered	Interventions	Rationales
Venturi's mask	24%–100% FIO_2 with flow rates of 4–10 L/min; provides high humidity.	1. Perform constant surveillance to ensure accurate flow rate for specific FIO_2. 2. Keep the orifice for the Venturi adapter open and uncovered. 3. Provide a mask that fits snugly and tubing that is free of kinks. 4. Assess the client for dry mucous membranes. 5. Change to a nasal cannula during mealtimes.	1. An accurate flow rate ensures FIO_2 delivery. 2. If the Venturi orifice is covered, the adapter does not function and oxygen delivery varies. 3. FIO_2 is altered if kinking occurs or if the mask fits poorly. 4. Humidity or aerosol can be added to the system to prevent the drying effect of oxygen. 5. Oxygen is a drug that needs to be given continuously.
Aerosol mask, face tent, tracheostomy collar	24%–100% FIO_2 with flow rates of at least 10 L/min; provides high humidity.	1. Assess that aerosol mist escapes from the vents of the delivery system during inspiration and expiration.	1. Humidification should be delivered to the client.

Device	Nursing Interventions	Rationale
	2. Empty condensation from the tubing.	2. Emptying prevents the client from being lavaged with water and promotes an adequate flow rate.
	3. Keep the aerosol water container full.	3. Adequate humidification is ensured.
T piece	24%–100% FIO_2 with flow rates of at least 10 L/min; provides high humidity.	1. Empty condensation from the tubing.	1. Condensation interferes with flow rate and may drain into the tracheostomy if not emptied.
	2. Keep the exhalation port open and uncovered.	2. If the port is occluded, the client can suffocate.
	3. Position the T piece so that it does not pull on the tracheostomy or endotracheal tube.	3. The weight of the T piece pulls on the tracheostomy and causes pain or erosion of skin at the insertion site.
	4. Make sure the humidifier creates enough mist. A mist should be seen during inspiration and expiration.	4. An adequate flow rate is needed to meet the inspiratory effort of the client. If not, FIO_2 is decreased.

INDEX

694

698

APP

INDEX

705

APP

INDEX

APP

INDEX

713

717

APP

INDEX

FAST (fluoroallergosorbent test), chemonucleosis and, 50
Fat embolism syndrome, 228
Fatigue, in leukemia, 381
  in rheumatoid arthritis, 573
Fatigue fracture, 223
Fatty liver, 219
FBD (cystic disease; dysplasia; fibrocystic breast disease), 219–220
Fear. *See also* Anxiety.
  in brain tumors, 69–70
  in cervical cancer, 120–122
  in dysfunctional uterine bleeding, 195
  in endometrial cancer, 202–204
  in uterine leiomyoma, 635–636
Feeding. *See also* Altered nutrition; Diet; Nutrition.
  by nasogastric tube. *See* Nasogastric (NG) tube, feeding by.
  enteral, in pancreatic carcinoma, 469
  parenteral. *See* Total parenteral nutrition
    (hyperalimentation; TPN).
Femoral fractures, 232–233
Femoral hernia, 288
Femoropopliteal bypass, in peripheral vascular disease,
    arterial, 494
Femorotibial bypass, in peripheral vascular disease, arterial,
    494
Fenoterol (Berotec), in respiratory acidosis, 564
Fibrinolysin, in peripheral vascular disease, 498
Fibroadenoma, breast, 74
Fibrocystic breast disease (cystic disease; dysplasia; FBD),
    219–220
Fibroid. *See* Uterine leiomyoma (fibroid; myoma).
Fibroma, ovarian, 453
Fibrosarcoma, 61
Fibular fractures, 233
Filter, umbrella, in pulmonary contusion, 535
Filtering procedures, in glaucoma, 249
Finger replacement, in degenerative joint disease, 171
First-degree burn, 81
Fissure, anal, 26–27
  primary and secondary, 26
Fistula, anal, 27
  gastrojejunocolic, in peptic ulcer disease, 486
  in Crohn's disease, 158–159
  vaginal. *See* Vaginal fistula.
Fistulizing sclerectomy, in glaucoma, 249
Fixation, external, in fractures, 227
Flaccid bladder, 547
Flagyl (metronidazole), in brain abscess, 64
Flail chest, 220–221
Flap (closed) amputation, 21
Flat warts, 650
Fleet (sodium phosphate) enema, in anorexia nervosa, 37
Flexoject. *See* Orphenadrine (Banflex; Flexoject; Myolin;
    Norflex).
Florinef (fludrocortisone), in adrenal hypofunction, 12
Floxuridine (FUDR), in pancreatic carcinoma, 468
Flu (influenza), 359–360
Fludrocortisone (Florinef), in adrenal hypofunction, 12

APP

INDEX

731

APP

INDEX

736

APP

INDEX

Platelet transfusions, in autoimmune thrmobocytopenic purpura, 47
Platinol. *See* Cisplatin (Platinol).
PLE (pacinar emphysema; panlobar emphysema), 135
PMS (premenstrual syndrome), 519–520
Pneumoconiosis, 433, 434
Pneumocystic carinii pneumonia, in acquired immunodeficiency syndrome, 8
Pneumonectomy, thoracotomy with, in lung cancer, 388
Pneumonia, 505–507, 575
  community-acquired, 505
  hospital-acquired, 505
  Pneumocystic carinii, in acquired immunodeficiency syndrome, 8
Pneumonitis, toxic, 434
Pneumothorax, 507–508
  tension, 609–610
Poisoning, food, 221–222
Poliomyelitis (polio), 508
  postpolio syndrome (PPS) and, 519
Polycystic kidney disease (PKD), 509–511
Polycystic ovary (Stein-Leventhal) syndrome, 452
Polydipsia (excessive thirst), in diabetes mellitus, 181
Polymyxin B, bacitracin with (Polysporin), in burn injury, 88
Polymyxin B, in myasthenia gravis, 420
Polyneuritis, idiopathic, acute. *See* GB; Guillain-Barré syndrome (acute idiopathic polyneuritis; infectious polyneuritis; Landry's paralysis).
Polyneuritis/polyneuropathy, 511–512
Polyneuritis/polyneuropathy, glove and stocking polyneuropathy and, 511
Polyp(s), cervical, 123
  gastrointestinal, 512–513
    pedunculated, 512
  laryngeal, 375–376
  nasal, 425
Polypectomy, gastrointestinal polyps and, 513
  nasal polyps and, 425
Polyphagia (excessive eating), in diabetes mellitus, 181
Polysporin (Bacitracin with polymyxin B sulfate), in burn injury, 88
Polyuria (frequent and excessive amount of urination), in diabetes mellitus, 181
Portal (alcohol-induced; Laennec's; nutritionsl) cirrhosis, 139
Portal systemic encephalopathy, in cirrhosis, 141
Portal-systemic shunting procedures, in cirrhosis, 143
Portocaval shunt, in cirrhosis, 143
Port-wine stain, 279
Positioning, burn injury and, 670t
  in back pain, 49
Positive end-expiratory pressure, in flail chest, 221
  in pulmonary contusion, 534
Postanesthesia care unit (PACU; recovery room), 514
Postasium-sparing diuretics, in chronic renal failure, 556
Postcholecystectomy syndrome, in cholelithiasis, 133
Postmenopausal bleeding, 513–514
Postmenopausal (type I) osteoporosis, 441

APP

INDEX

APP

INDEX

Rifamycin (rifampin), in meningitis, 403
Right ventricular (RV) failure, 275–276
RIND (reversible ischemic neurologic deficit), 114
Ringworm (tinea corporis), 596
Rinne's test, hearing loss and, 272, 273
    in otosclerosis, 448
Risk factors, surgical, age-related changes as, nursing
        interventions for, 654t–655t
Rival. See Diazepam (E-Pam; Neo-Calme; Rival; Valium).
Robaxin. See Methocarbamol (Delaxin; Robaxin; Skelaxin).
Rods, Luque, in scoliosis, 578
Role performance, altered. See Altered role performance.
Rolling (paraesophageal) hernia, 289–290
ROM (range-of-motion) exercises. See Exercise(s), range-of-
        motion (ROM).
Rubber band ligation, in hemorrhoids, 282
Running traction, 226
Rupture, of patellar tendon, 370
RV (right ventricular) failure, 275–276

Sacular aneurysm, 30
Salem sump, in intestinal obstruction, 362
Salicylates. See also Aspirin.
    in lupus erythematosus, 391
    in rheumatoid arthritis, 571–572
Salivary hypersecretion, reflex (waterbrash), 243
Salpingo-oophorectomy, bilateral, in endometrial cancer, 203
        in ovarian cancer, 450
        in ovarian cyst, 452
    unilateral, in epithelial ovarian tumor, 454
Sarcoidosis, pulmonary, 536
Sarcoma, chondrosarcoma as, 61
    Ewing's, 61
    fibrosarcoma as, 61
    osteogenic (osteosarcoma), 61
Scabicides, in scabies, 577
Scabies, 577
Scapular fractures, 232
Scleral buckling procedure, in retinal hole/tear/detachment,
        569
Sclerectomy, fistulizing, in glaucoma, 249
Scleroderma, systemic (progressive systemic sclerosis; PSS),
        527–528
Sclerosis, otosclerosis and, 447–449
Sclerotherapy, in cancer, 100
    in cirrhosis, 143
    in hemorrhoids, 282
    in varicose veins, 647
Scoliosis, 577–578
Screws, fractures and, 226
Scrub nurse, 364
Seasonal allergies (allergic rhinitis; hay fever; perennial allergic
        rhinitis), 14
Second-degree burn, 81
Secretions, drainage and secretion precautions and, 355, 687t
Sedatives, preoperative, 525
Segmental resection, thoracotomy with, in lung cancer, 388

758